Breast reconstruction following mastectomy

Breast reconstruction following mastectomy

NICHOLAS G. GEORGIADE, M.D., F.A.C.S.

Professor and Chairman,
Division of Plastic, Reconstructive, and Maxillofacial Surgery,
Duke University School of Medicine,
Durham, North Carolina

with 379 illustrations

The C. V. Mosby Company

ST. LOUIS • TORONTO • LONDON   1979

Printed in the United States of America

The C. V. Mosby Company
11830 Westline Industrial Drive, St. Louis, Missouri 63141

Library of Congress Cataloging in Publication Data

Georgiade, Nicholas G   1918-
  Breast reconstruction following mastectomy.

  Bibliography: p.
  Includes index.
    1. Mammaplasty. 2. Mastectomy—Complications
and sequelae. 3. Mastectomy—Psychological aspects.
I. Title. [DNLM: 1. Mastectomy. 2. Surgery,
Plastic.   WP910 G352b]
RD539.8.G46   618.1′9   79-15679
ISBN 0-8016-1807-X

GW/CB/B   9 8 7 6 5 4 3 2 1   01/A/088

Contributors

Edward Clifford, Ph.D.

Professor of Medical Psychology,
Department of Psychiatry and
Division of Plastic Surgery,
Duke University School of Medicine,
Durham, North Carolina

Gregory S. Georgiade, M.D.

Associate in Plastic Surgery, Division of Plastic,
Reconstructive, and Maxillofacial Surgery,
Duke University School of Medicine,
Durham, North Carolina

**Nicholas G. Georgiade, M.D.,
F.A.C.S.**

Professor and Chairman,
Division of Plastic, Reconstructive,
and Maxillofacial Surgery,
Duke University School of Medicine,
Durham, North Carolina

Gregg H. D. Kesterson, M.S.

Research Associate,
Endocrine Oncology Laboratory,
Department of Medicine & Pathology,
Duke University School of Medicine,
Durham, North Carolina

Kenneth S. McCarty, Jr., M.D., Ph.D.

Director, Endocrine Oncology Laboratory;
Assistant Professor, Division of Endocrinology,
Department of Medicine;
Assistant Professor, Department of Pathology,
Duke University School of Medicine,
Durham, North Carolina

Robert McLelland, M.D.

Associate Professor of Radiology;
Chief, Mammography Section;
Director—Breast Cancer Detection
Demonstration Project,
Duke University School of Medicine,
Durham, North Carolina

Ronald Riefkohl, M.D.

Assistant Professor,
Division of Plastic, Reconstructive,
and Maxillofacial Surgery,
Duke University School of Medicine,
Durham, North Carolina

H. F. Seigler, M.D., F.A.C.S.

Professor of Surgery,
Associate Professor, Immunology,
Duke University School of Medicine,
Durham, North Carolina

Donald Serafin, M.D., F.A.C.S.

Associate Professor,
Division of Plastic, Reconstructive,
and Maxillofacial Surgery,
Duke University Medical Center,
Durham, North Carolina

Foreword

One of the most impressive of the recent advances in surgery has been the progress in the field of breast reconstruction following mastectomy. It is fortunate that in this text a widely acknowledged leader and innovative contributor in this expanding area has undertaken the editorship of an unusually thorough and important work. Moreover, he is himself substantially involved in many portions of this outstanding book.

It is a great tribute to women that in the recent past a tremendous interest has been kindled in the concept of reconstruction of the breast following mastectomy in a manner designed to emphasize both beauty and sensuous pleasure. It is no longer feasible to hold the view that the majority of women accept external mammary prostheses as the answer to removal of an organ long recognized to have both anatomic and psychologic importance. During the past decade, Nicholas Georgiade has made impressive contributions to many aspects of the problems associated with these patients. The in-depth understanding that he and his colleagues have accumulated about this complex subject is remarkable, including the relationships to the various histopathologic processes, the timing of the procedure, the prevention of complications, and the continuous stream of original and innovative ideas that they have contributed to the field. They have garnered a very large series of patients with breast reconstruction following mastectomy with an almost negligible incidence of complications and with superb cosmetic results.

In this monograph the editor has selected outstanding authorities in each of the areas involved, including the psychologic effects of mastectomy, surgical-anatomic aspects, the role of mammography, and the importance of accurate characterization of the histopathologic lesion. The exacting surgical techniques, many of which have been pioneered by the editor, greatly increase the importance of this text to the operating surgeon. Of particular significance are the careful descriptions provided of management of the nipple-areolar complex as well as the updated use of microsurgical composite tissue transplantation in mammary reconstruction.

There can no longer be any doubt that the field of reconstructive surgery of the breast following mastectomy has fully arrived, and this collection is the most thorough and scientific work in this increasingly important field.

David C. Sabiston, Jr., M.D.

James B. Duke Professor of Surgery and Chairman,
Department of Surgery, Duke University Medical Center,
Durham, North Carolina

Preface

Since the introduction of the radical mastectomy by Halsted in 1890, emphasis has been on the surgical ablation of the carcinomatous breast and associated regional lymph nodes. In recent years surgical extirpation has been augmented by radiation or chemotherapy in an attempt to improve survival rates. After therapy an extreme deficiency of healthy, well-vascularized skin is frequently evident at the mastectomy site.

The modified radical mastectomy introduced in 1948 by Patey has largely supplanted the radical mastectomy as the primary surgical mode of therapy when controlled clinical series revealed no adverse effect on patient survival. Surgical treatment thus has become less ablative, facilitating reconstructive attempts.

von Langenbeck in 1875 and Kocher in 1880 introduced the composite resection for the surgical treatment of malignancies of the head and neck. Although a biologically different epithelial neoplasm was involved, regional lymphadenectomy combined with primary extirpation proved to be of definite value in improving survival statistics, as in breast carcinoma. A significant functional and cosmetic loss ensued, making further reconstruction necessary. In the face of a local primary recurrence following such extensive surgery, survival rates were abysmally low, approximately 15%. With the recognition and appreciation of these statistics, reconstruction, which previously had been postponed to an indefinite date, was undertaken early. If survival is not adversely affected, *why not* reconstruct these surgically mutilated patients?

During recent years an increased patient awareness of the possibility for breast reconstruction has been generated in nonprofessional periodicals and commercial media, reflecting new surgical techniques and changing scientific attitudes. Carcinoma of the breast was also recognized as being a systemic disease and not a local one, occurring bilaterally with alarming frequency.

The functional loss was not as disabling as that resulting from major surgical ablation in the head and neck but was equally devastating emotionally to the patient. Concepts such as "self-image" and "femininity" were examined and their clinical significance in the mastectomy patient was finally appreciated.

Physician awareness also increased, with emphasis being no longer solely on cure from this elusive, mutilating disease but on the restoration of breast contour and form as well. *Why not* carry out reconstruction following radical mastectomy, particularly if survival is not adversely affected?

As reconstructive efforts at the mastectomy site increased, greater attention was directed to the contralateral breast. Subcutaneous mastectomy specimens revealed a significant increased incidence of premalignant disease as well as a 6% to 7% incidence of occult carcinoma. The bilaterality of certain types of breast malignancy as well as the multifocal nature of others was graphically demonstrated. Plastic and reconstructive surgeons became not only concerned with the ablated breast but also acutely aware of the malignant potential of the opposite breast. Reconstruction was no longer a single surgical exercise but a philosophy of surgical management of an elusive disease entity requiring careful planning and assimilation of recent scientific thought.

Concepts such as these could not evolve without a critical appraisal of results following mastectomy and particularly without improvement in surgical techniques of tissue transfer to deficient recipient sites.

The evolution of modern techniques of reconstruction has also been significantly molded by the following advancements: (1) the use of early chest flaps by Tansini as described in d'Este in 1912; (2) the use of abdominal flaps in the 1920s and 1930s; (3) the use of dermis as described by Loewe in 1913 (now utilized as supporting dermal grafts under mastectomy scars); and (4) the constant improvement of synthetic materials for breast mound reconstruction. Recent contributions in microsurgery and an increased appreciation of the usefulness of musculocutaneous flaps have facilitated the reconstructive efforts following mastectomy.

Because scientific thought and surgical technique are constantly changing, this text attempts to correlate the current views of pathologists, psychologists, and endocrinologists as well as oncologic and reconstructive surgeons.

The timing and indications for reconstruction following mastectomy are critically evaluated with regard to eventual prognosis. New techniques of breast mound reconstruction as well as methods of nipple-areolar reconstruction are described and illustrated in detail.

Many problems remain as yet unsolved. The incidence and description of both premalignant and malignant disease of the contralateral breast require further clarification. Breast carcinoma has only recently been evaluated as a systemic rather than a local disease and treatment redirected appropriately. Considerable investigation still needs to be done. Finally any enthusiasm for new surgical techniques to reconstruct the breast should not detract from the supreme challenge of eliminating the mutilation and death of many women from this dread disease.

The accumulation of these ideas on reconstruction of the breast was simplified and aided by many people. I especially wish to thank my associates, Drs.

Donald Serafin, Connell Shearin, and Ronald Riefkohl, and our residents, Drs. Richard Morris, Richard Gregory, Gregory Georgiade, Alexander Stradoudakis, Carl Quillen, Kenna Given, Philip Polack, and David Smith, who have added much to the care of these patients.

I would also like to thank the many fine surgeons here at Duke and those in this country and abroad who referred their premastectomy and postmastectomy patients to us as well as those who were kind enough to share their patients with us, giving us the opportunity to serve them better.

The seemingly endless attention to detail in carefully and accurately completing this text is the work of Mrs. Ruth Jones, our Associate, and Mrs. Faye Beasley, our Executive Secretary.

Nicholas G. Georgiade

Contents

1 Psychological effects of the mastectomy experience, 1
Edward Clifford

2 The reconstruction experience: the search for restitution, 22
Edward Clifford

3 Surgical anatomy of the breast, 35
Donald Serafin

4 Mammography in the diagnosis of breast cancer, 54
Robert McLelland

5 Clinical significance of histopathologic lesions observed in subcutaneous mastectomy specimens, 67
Kenneth S. McCarty, Jr.
Gregg H. D. Kesterson
Nicholas G. Georgiade

6 Surgical management of fibrocystic disease of the breast, 86
Nicholas G. Georgiade
Ronald Riefkohl

7 Surgical treatment of cancer of the breast (extirpation) and how it relates to reconstruction; team relationship: adjuvant therapy and its relation to surgery, 124
H. F. Seigler
Nicholas G. Georgiade

8 Reconstruction of the breast: rationale, prognosis, and timing, 131
Donald Serafin

9 Clinical significance of histopathologic lesions observed in the contralateral breast in patients with breast carcinoma, 152

Kenneth S. McCarty, Jr.
Gregg H. D. Kesterson
Nicholas G. Georgiade

10 Reconstruction of the breast mound after mastectomy, 164

Nicholas G. Georgiade
Ronald Riefkohl
Gregory S. Georgiade

11 Latissimus dorsi musculocutaneous flap, 191

Ronald Riefkohl
Nicholas G. Georgiade

12 Microsurgical composite tissue transplantation: reconstruction of the breast, 215

Donald Serafin

13 Management of the nipple-areolar complex in reconstruction, 239

Nicholas G. Georgiade

Breast reconstruction following mastectomy

CHAPTER 1

Psychological effects of the mastectomy experience

Edward Clifford

Mention of mastectomy brings forth a number of reactions, most of which are negative in character. Mastectomy has been labeled an "emotional" operation, and women who have experienced the procedure have been called "birds with broken wings" or "shattered vases which cannot be mended."[3,55] Rhetoric aside, the time has come to examine the current state of knowledge about mastectomy. A number of concepts will be examined, and the evidence supporting these concepts will be presented. It is the purpose of this chapter to review the available literature and to present a framework with which the psychologic aspects of mastectomy can be presented most effectively.

Most of the reports about mastectomy stem from clinical practice with patients with breast cancer. For the most part, rigorous research is lacking; for example, control groups are infrequently used. Unsupported or poorly supported statements are frequently made and repeated until they become accepted because they have gone unchallenged. Conclusions appear and seem to reflect consensual clinical judgments. One finds individual experiences with mastectomy,[14] reports of surgeons with patients,[39] conceptions of femininity,[43] and sporadic attempts to organize the literature. This chapter systematizes the literature so that complex issues associated with mastectomy can be examined.

Conceptually the literature can be divided into two sections, each of which will be discussed. The cultural context in which breast cancer and the subsequent mastectomy occurs is explored for relevant variables first. Following this, psychosocial factors associated with mastectomy during the presurgical, hospitalization, and postsurgical periods will be presented. The postsurgical period will include an examination of the short- and long-term effects of the mastectomy experience.

CULTURAL CONTEXT

All behavior, including reactions to breast cancer and mastectomy, takes place within a cultural context. The culture provides a framework of prevailing values and attitudes toward illness and dying, about appropriate sex roles and concepts of femininity and masculinity, and for the development of feelings of self-esteem

1

and self-worth. The experience of having breast cancer and of having a breast amputated needs to be examined within these social contexts. Two themes have been selected for examination because of their relevance to the experience of mastectomy. The first is concerned with attitudes toward cancer, the reason for mastectomy; the second is concerned with the concept of femininity, which is commonly believed to be assaulted in breast removal.

Attitudinal framework

"I fear pain; I fear dying slowly: I fear losing control; and oddly, I fear hospitals."[26]

In our society cancer is rarely mentioned within a positive context; the word itself produces fear. Holland[29] enumerates several fears commonly associated with cancer. In the context of fears of death, pain, and mutilation, the person faces an uncertain future. Fears may also center about possible loss of work, separation from family, becoming dependent on others for care and financial support, and becoming isolated or alienated from family and friends.

Cancer is perceived as a death sentence; many patients are aware that health professionals rarely talk of cures, whereas prognoses are generally put in terms of 5- to 10-year survival rates. In addition to its lethal nature, there are other shared anxieties about cancer. The disease process is insidious in the sense that it occurs silently; it is invasive and destructive and capable of spreading. This disease process is perceived to be beyond the control of the person and frequently beyond the control of the attending physician.[10]

Associated with cancer is the spectre of a lingering and painful death. Whereas there is a belief in the ability of medicine to modify or halt the inexorable course of the disease, there are anxiety-arousing reactions to the aggressive treatment of cancer (ablative surgery, radiotherapy, and chemotherapy). In the face of anxiety patients undergo their treatments with a degree of uncertainty about the outcome, not knowing whether or not the cancer has been eradicated, contained, or metastasized. In addition to not being able to control the disease process, full cooperation with a physician cannot guarantee that the course of treatment will be successful.[10]

In our society there is also the expectancy that medicine can and will be able, in the long run, to conquer disease processes. In the case of breast cancer, emphasis is placed on early detection so that the physician can have a fighting chance of success. Thus each potential patient must deal with pessimistic portrayals of cancer as a fatal disease process as well as optimistic hopes about the progress in medicine and the ability of the physician to treat the illness successfully.

Beliefs about cancer and mastectomy. The Gallup Organization surveyed a national sample of 1000 women above the age of 18 years for the American Cancer Society.[1] Unaffected women tended to overestimate the incidence of breast cancer; only 8% were able to approximate that 50 in 1000 women would develop breast cancer during their lifetime. Kushner[36] cites a slightly higher incidence rate of 6%. A large proportion of the women surveyed (61%), however, expressed optimism about survival after the diagnosis of breast cancer had been made. This accompanied a belief, which was widespread (74%), that a great deal of medical progress had been made over the past two decades in early diagnosis and cure.

The survey concluded that questions about the cause of cancer revealed extensive confusion and ignorance on the part of the women interviewed. Forty per cent of the women were not aware of the increased risk of cancer with age. In addition 62% believed breast cancer to be caused by injury or a blow to the breast. As further evidence of confusion, the report cites the finding that one fourth of these women believed that breast-feeding decreased the chance of getting cancer whereas 43% of them believed that the use of birth control pills increased the chance of getting cancer of the breast. To bolster its point of view, the report stated that no hard scientific evidence existed to support these beliefs. Kushner,[36] however, after interviewing scientists in breast cancer research, points out that not one of them believed that oral contraceptives were safe insofar as breast cancer is concerned.

The survey suggested that women seemed to lack awareness about the extent to which breast cancer is treated with extensive surgery. In general the women were familiar with the terms *simple mastectomy* (79%), *radical mastectomy* (66%), and *lumpectomy* (62%), although some confusion existed about the precise meanings of these terms. For example, the word *radical* implied the use of extreme measures. This confusion may account for the women believing that early detection of breast cancer would lessen the need for radical procedures.[1] Sutherland's patients equated dangerous and destructive surgery with radical surgery, leading him to suggest that the term *definitive surgery* would be less traumatic and better understood.[54]

The American Cancer Society survey indicated that women feared mastectomy for two reasons: the fear of cancer was of primary concern, followed closely by uneasiness about the impairment of womanhood. When asked what their first thoughts after mastectomy would be, their responses paralleled the concerns already mentioned. They would want to know whether or not the procedure had been successful in eliminating the cancer. They also expressed concerns about the type of emotional adjustments they would have to make to the loss of the breast.

Predetection behaviors. It has been estimated that of all cases of breast cancer, 95% of symptoms are initially discovered by the women themselves.[44] Although women may discover the problem, it appears that it is rarely found through a process of regular self-examination. A high proportion of the women (77%) sampled in a Gallup poll[1] were aware of breast self-examination; however, only 30% practiced it and not necessarily on a regular monthly basis. Fear and anxiety appeared to contribute to the low levels of breast self-examination. Forty-six percent of the women in the sample indicated that such self-examination would cause them to have needless worries, and 47% of the women not practicing breast self-examination explained their behavior with avoidance responses. These women mentioned not being able to take the time for the examination and did not mention specific fears.

Delay or lagtime. Since most women find the suspicious breast symptom by themselves, it seems reasonable to direct attention to their subsequent behaviors. Certainly there is much emphasis on reporting to a physician promptly, and most women do. Not all women are prompt, however, and the interval between symptom discovery and having it evaluated by a physician has been labeled "delay." The definition of delay is arbitrary; for example, Buls, Jones, Bennett, and Chan[6] define delay as a period of 1 month or more between self-detection and physician evaluation, whereas Cameron and Hinton[8] extend the period to 3 months or more. No information is given as to why specific periods are selected. Worden and Weisman[62] question the use of the term *delay*. They point out, for example, that within a 3-month period most women have seen a physician. Further, they emphasize the arbitrary nature of selecting a 3-month cutoff period because there is no consistent evidence that beyond this time limit the woman's health is endangered significantly. They propose using the term *lagtime,* which in their opinion is less value-laden and blame-placing.

Several investigators have examined the relationships between lagtime and demographic variables such as age of the woman, educational level, and parity. When women with greater and shorter lagtimes were compared, obtained differences could not be attributed to age.[8,22,58] Relationships to educational level have been found—lagtime increases with less education.[8,58] Finally, women with fewer children tended to have shorter lagtimes.[58,62]

Reasons for lengthening the period between discovery and evaluation have also been sought in numerous areas. For example, the lagtime period is not correlated with breast size[6] or with the presence of pain.[8] In one study, however, the absence of pain was found to contribute to increased lagtime.[58] The extent of previous life crises is not related to lagtime,[22] although difficulties with one's husband[7,62] and problems revolving about domestic matters[7,8] are related to increased lagtime.

The woman's subconscious awareness that a malignancy is present appears to affect lagtime. Lagtimes were obtained from women interviewed immediately prior to biopsy. Subsequently these lagtimes were contrasted for those whose biopsies revealed malignancy and those with a benign growth. Women with malignancies had greater lagtimes than women whose growths were benign.[8,22] In a similar retrospective approach, the lagtimes of women with breast cancer were compared to the lagtimes of women with other types of cancer. Either there was no difference in lagtime when the groups of women were compared[15,62] or the lagtime for women with breast cancer was less.[45]

Two psychologic explanations—anxiety and denial—are frequently invoked to explain increased lagtime. Whereas most investigators stress that a variety of fears—usually of cancer and of breast loss—increase lagtime,[6] Magarey and Todd[40] indicate that anxiety can decrease as well as increase lagtime, perhaps explaining the results of Cameron and Hinton[8] that anxiety played no role in lagtime in their study. Denial and avoidance responses have also been noted to be factors in lagtime.[7,22,40,62] These responses are difficult to classify, and the classification is usually dependent on the orientation of the investigator. For example, if women do not use the word cancer in describing symptomatology, this can be interpreted as disinclination or denial or avoidance. Similarly, if a woman professes ignorance, the lack of information can be attributed to a denial process, since such information appears to be available readily.

A number of intrapersonal explanations have been put forth to account for increased lagtime. Holland[30] suggests that the period between discovery and evaluation is stressful and that reasons for increased lagtime can be found in the woman's characteristic pattern of coping with stress. Schon[52] believes that these reactions are related to failure in coping, which is further related to a fear of emotional disorganization if the suspected diagnosis is confirmed. Lagtime has been related to feelings of introversion,[8] to feelings of powerlessness, and to a history of isolation in childhood.[62] Contrary to these negative personality characteristics, Fisher[15] finds women with greater lagtimes to be more autonomous, more independent, and to possess a clearer sense of personal identity. Women with greater lagtimes are relatively unconcerned with body vulnerability and exhibit a false sense of body security.

Clearly a variety of factors contribute to increased lagtime. Some of the factors are demographic—it is not too surprising to find that better educated women tend to involve the health care system sooner. Also, it is not too surprising to find that situational factors contribute to greater lagtime—concerns about the relationship with one's husband or concern about pressing familial matters may take precedence. The presence of anxiety is not unexpected, but, as Chesser and Anderson[9] point out, the anxiety is at a moderate level and allows the women to cooperate in their treatment. Anxiety, as well, may be the motivating force that impels women to seek informed evaluations.

Predisposing characteristics. Enlow, Krant, Rezzonico, and Schain[12] suggest that women who develop breast cancer place blame on themselves and attribute the development of the cancer to their own sins and their guilt for things they did or did not do. A number of investigators also turn to the examination of psychologic culpability. Giovacchini and Muslin[17] report interesting changes in behavior in psychoanalysis of a patient who developed breast cancer during treatment. Prior to the detection of the cancer the patient went through a period of ego regression. She was able to regain her psychic equilibrium after biopsy and surgical treatment. The authors concluded that invasive diseases are traumatic to psychologic aspects of ego equilibrium. Goldfarb, Drieson, and Cole,[18] following the psychodynamic tradition, describe several psychologic themes differentiating breast cancer patients from noncancer patients. Their breast cancer patients, prior to detection, exhibited feelings of despair, hopelessness, and helplessness and were unable to express hostility. These women suffered from maternal domination, demonstrated immature sexual adjustments, and were incapable of accepting the loss of a significant object in their lives.

Two relatively recent studies examined personality differences between women who were biopsied and found to have breast cancer and those who were biopsied and found to have benign tumors. Greer and Morris[23] examined 160 women (ninety-one benign, sixty-nine malignant) with an extensive battery of psychologic tests on the day prior to biopsy. The investigators concluded that breast cancer patients demonstrated persistently throughout adult life a pattern of behavior characterized by an abnormal release of emotions. These women tended to extreme suppression of anger and other feelings. No significant relationships were obtained for extraversion scores, feelings of hostility or the directionality of the hostility, neuroticism, or the use of denial as a means of coping with stress. In addition no differences were found between the two groups of women in their marital relationships, interpersonal relationships, leisure activities, work activities, or verbal intelligence. In a similar fashion Schonfield[53] examined 112 Israeli women the day before biopsy with a large number of psychologic tests. Twenty-seven of these women were found to have malignancies. There was no evidence that women who developed malignancies suffered losses of significant others in the years preceding the development of their tumors to any greater extent than women whose diagnoses were benign. For the most part, differences between these two groups of women were nondetectable.

Breasts and femininity

There are implicit and explicit assumptions about the nature of femininity and the relationship of breasts (or rather the loss of them) to femininity. Most prevalent is the emphasis on the cultural setting that stresses, or overemphasizes, the role of breasts in a figure- and clothes-conscious society. There is also emphasis on a sense of femininity arising internally that relates the importance of breasts to the meanings ascribed to them by individual women. Finally there is an implicit assumption that femininity can be defined by a subtractive process, that is, the woman becomes less feminine with loss or injury of a significant body part or function, particularly if it is sexually relevant.

Cultural considerations. For the most part, males and females are immediately recognizable and discriminated. Among other characteristics (for example, movement, hair), the presence of breasts is a persistent identifying characteristic of women. This discrimination can even be found in early cave drawings, probably drawn by males, in which breasts are emphasized.[24] If femininity is solely defined by easily identified physical characteristics, the genitalia and the breasts are exclusively female physical attributes. Loss of a body part does not change gender; thus the person's sexual identification would not change accordingly.

Behavioral definitions of femininity are more difficult to state with any degree of preciseness, let alone universal agreement. Any such definition is bound by the culture, the subculture, and the historical era in which the definition is promulgated. Further, behavioral roles, particularly as society changes, are not necessarily exclusive to male or female gender. For the most part, society relies on currently expected behaviors or culturally relevant standards or norms. Thus femininity can be defined in terms of the roles that women usually play, or are expected to play, in our society. Roles that are uniquely feminine are those of wife and mother.

Breasts and motherhood are functionally and symbolically related. The functional relationship between the breast and the feeding of infants is obvious. Since this relationship exists, Anstice[3] is able to take the position that the breast assumes an emotional meaning for everyone, beginning in infancy. Since motherhood is also associated with nurturance, comfort, and love, the breast acquires a symbolic value and is associated with this asset of femininity.[24]

Femininity is defined in terms of sexual behavior as well. Within sexuality the breast is seen as being of crucial importance. The size and shape of the breasts are related to sexual attractiveness and to acceptability as a woman to those who base their identification on them.[52] Schain[50] points out that, from early adolescence on, the emergence and the condition of her breasts become a significant aspect of a woman's identity. Each woman eventually interprets what her breasts mean to her as a sexual being, that is, the degree of stimulation and satisfaction she receives from being viewed and caressed.[56] Breasts are sexually stimulating to the male, and seeing them may be a more potent sexual stimulus than viewing the genitalia.[5] If male sexual behavior is breast dependent, women whose breasts are deemed inadequate lose, or fail to achieve, value as an object of male sexual desires.[43] Meyers[43] states that these women lose value in the sexual marketplace.

Women may come to accept for themselves the values placed on breast size and shape encountered in high fashion,[44] where attention is focused on the accentuation of the breast or on the hiding of real or imagined breast imperfections. In addition women in our society are generally aware of their body contours and dimensions, and breast-waist-hip measurements take on the characteristic of a vital statistic[55] that is compared to standards for an ideal feminine figure. For some women, particularly if the size and shape of the breasts and other body dimensions are of value to them, satisfaction can be achieved through varying degrees of exhibitionism, as exemplified by the use of scanty bathing suits and low-cut dresses.[54]

Internal sense of femininity. Do breasts define femininity? Certainly, as Schain[50] points out, their mere presence or absence can affect a woman's well-being; yet to assess femininity requires one to know the woman's feelings about her breasts, the sensations and pleasures she derives from them, and the personal meanings she ascribes to them. Worden and Weisman[63] take the position that concepts of femininity are vague and may range from narcissistic attention and devotion to physical appearance to amorphous ruminations about a sense of inner worth.

For the individual woman, concepts of femininity are dependent on her sexual identity, which has evolved and been influenced by relationships with parents and by experiences during development.[51] Green[21] perceives the development of femininity as a diffuse internalization process influenced by others who relate to a woman's needs for approval and acceptance. Concepts of femininity can vary from woman to woman, and they are affected by her personal history, including familial factors, interpersonal experiences, personality patterns, age, and the culture or subculture in which she lives.

Subtractive process. The loss or damage of a sexually significant body part is viewed as creating a spoiled or discounted identity. Whereas gender does not change with breast removal, women are perceived to be, or may perceive them-selves to be, less feminine. If, in a woman's self-image, breasts are emphasized, the loss of a breast may destroy or disrupt her body image[16] and compromise or diminish her self-esteem.[56] For women who view their breasts as another body appendage having no special significance, losing a breast does not require a reevaluation of the self or bring femininity into question.[60]

The characterization of mastectomy as mutilative[55] carries with it the notion that femininity has been assaulted as well. Wabrek and Wabrek[56] perceive the loss of a breast to be an insult and suggest that it is nonsensical to believe that a marriage, even a good one, can easily survive the trauma. They suggest that both the woman and her husband need to adapt to a new status and deal with their own feelings. Green,[21] on the other hand, is of the opinion that the assault on the woman's body does not universally result in the woman perceiving herself to be less feminine. Feelings of injured or compromised femininity would only arise in those women for whom breasts signify a feminine identity.

There is a threat to the expression of sexuality, both in terms of stimulation and responsiveness, with the loss of a sexually significant body part. In this sense, the woman becomes less feminine and difficulties in sexual relationships are expected to emerge following mastectomy.[34] Labby[37] states that a period of sexual deprivation can take place following mastectomy, which results in the loss of an important means of tension reduction for the woman. He states, categorically, that the removal of a breast endangers femininity more than the removal of any genital organ or organs. Green[21] found feelings expressed by mastectomized women to be similar to those described for emasculated males.

MASTECTOMY EXPERIENCE

Each woman comes to the mastectomy experience with her unique set of personality characteristics, internalized and externalized attitudes toward her sex and her sexual functioning, feelings about her worth as a person, a history of satisfactory and/or unsatisfactory interpersonal relationships, and a cultural and societal heritage influencing her judgments, attitudes, and behaviors as well as various other unknown concerns. For purposes of convenience, the beginning of the mastectomy experience is taken as the woman's encounter with the health care system where the diagnosis will be confirmed. The experiences continue with surgery and the ensuing hospitalization period. Postsurgical experiences consist of the woman's return to home, family, and community. Whereas a number of women have written articulately and movingly about their individual experiences,[26,49] Kushner,[36] as a science reporter and as a woman who recently experienced mastectomy, interviewed clinicians and scientists throughout the world to produce a comprehensive review for the lay public. Emphasis in this chapter, however, will be on direct clinical and research evidence.

Presurgical experiences

Owen[44] estimates that 95% of the women discover the suspicious symptom themselves. Most of them seek evaluations from their physicians within a 30-day period. For the most part, the ultimate decision about whether a malignancy is present or not is dependent on biopsy. Schain,[50] citing an unpublished study by Schneidman, points out that a one-stage rather than a two-stage biopsy procedure is prevalent. In the Schneidman study, for example, 88% of the women had a one-stage biopsy involving a biopsy combined with surgery in one procedure, should the pathologist report a malignancy present. In this situation the woman is certain of the diagnosis only after the surgery has been performed. The two-stage biopsy involves the biopsy, followed at a later time by the surgery. In this case the woman is aware of the diagnosis before the surgery.

Psychologically there may be different effects of the two procedures. The one-stage procedure can be psychologically ambiguous, since the diagnosis is uncertain and there is room for confused communication. For example, the woman may believe the symptom to be benign only to find that she has had a mastectomy. On the other hand, the lack of delay between diagnosis and surgery may prevent a further period of anxiety from occurring. The two-stage procedure allows the woman and the physician to deal with the situation with certainty. Once the diagnosis is confirmed, it becomes possible, even in the face of anxiety, to discuss the surgery and its aftermath. For some women this procedure may enhance their feelings that they have a measure of control over their lives and that they can influence decisions concerning themselves.[50] Since most of the presurgical experiences reported involve the use of the one-stage biopsy, the following discussion will reflect this state of affairs.

Stress and communication. A number of investigators take the point of view that the period immediately prior to biopsy is stressful.[7] It is its perception and interpretation that is unique to the individual woman.[33] When stress is present, information processing is reduced, giving rise to the observed discrepancy between a woman's recollection of what she was told about the most likely diagnosis and the actual communication.[9] Stress, in this case, affects the communication received from the physician.

The physician, if only to communicate more effectively, should be aware of the woman's stress. Unfortunately, although women may be emitting signals, their stress is not always perceived. For example, women attending a breast clinic exhibited nonverbal signs of distress that tended to be ignored by the physician.[38] The verbal cues of being upset are also rarely picked up by either surgeons or nurses.[41]

Women may be hesitant to reveal their feelings to the physician. In a large-scale, prospective study of 450 women, Maguire[41] found that there was a reluctance on the part of the women to reveal their concerns directly. When asked about how they were feeling, for example, most of them responded in terms of physical health, rather than in terms of the issues of most concern to them at the moment. Perhaps this reluctance to communicate is related to the common complaint that the information received is inadequate or to the feeling that they will not be heard or understood.

Whereas Owen[44] takes the point of view that surgeons are very informative, she remains a relatively lonely voice. Clark[10] states that the physician's inclination is to concentrate on the presenting medical problem rather than on the person who is the patient. Quint[47] finds that her mastectomy patients were given generalities rather than specifics about breast cancer and surgery. She asserts further that physicians and nurses make it difficult for patients to ask direct questions. This is exemplified in the statement by a surgeon who stated that the woman should be told about the diagnosis and surgery without going into details, while stressing the probability of a complete and permanent cure.[39]

Psychologic reactions. Depression and anxiety are the most frequently mentioned feeling states; Maguire[42] found that 40% of the women in his prospective study were anxious or depressed on admission to the hospital. Further, he found that as the time for hospitalization approached there was an increase in reported irritability and sleeplessness. Chesser and Anderson[9] also noted these behavioral characteristics and found that the greater the tendency to display this behavior prior to hospitalization, the greater the depression or anxiety after surgery. Anxiety, however, may not be a completely negative characteristic, since it may enable the woman to marshal her strengths to cope with the situation. The anxiety may be tempered with hopeful optimism, may be openly expressed, and is healthy in terms of what needs to be faced.[16] Finally, the anxiety may allow the woman to participate in the necessary care regimens. However, not all anxiety serves an energizing function; when the anxiety is too intense or overwhelming, its presence can interfere with treatment and recovery.

For some women this initial experience has an unreal quality[7] accompanied by a multiplicity of fears ranging from those associated with the anesthetic and surgery to familial concerns.[19] The initial period, for some, is one of disbelief followed by anger and depression, which then give way to attempts to deal with reality,[29] in which the majority of women are able to cope with the situation.[33] Katz and his colleagues[33] propose three criteria for assessing the capacity of a woman to cope with forthcoming biopsy and mastectomy. These include (1) the degree of emotional or affective distress, (2) the extent to which ordinary functioning has been disrupted, and (3) the degree to which her defensive reserve has been impaired. Whereas there were momentary breakdowns of behavior during the interviews prior to biopsy (crying, agitation, feelings of tenseness), these did not affect the ability of the women to cope effectively with the presurgical experience.[33]

In a parallel study Katz and his colleagues[32] examined the women's ego defenses in response to stress during the presurgical period, finding that a moderate amount of distress facilitated more realistic and effective handling of the threat. They found that women whose defense mechanism included a stoic-fatalistic approach, who were dependent on the use of prayer and faith as a means of coping, or who tended to use denial in association with rationalization exhibited fewer psychologic concerns and less physiologic disruptions than women not using these defensive approaches. Further, women who tended to use either projection or displacement as a means of coping exhibited a greater degree of defensive failure. In the main the defenses of these women were operating with great success. However, Katz and his collaborators go on to say that the effective defense selected was not necessarily one that was healthy or reality oriented.

Postsurgical hospitalization experiences

Quint would define mastectomy as a critical experience for the woman that functions as a turning point in her life. This crisis precipitates a reevaluation of the self and a revision of personal identity.[46] It starts the realization with an immediate confrontation of the loss of the breast,[61] which is usually established by self-examination after surgery or by asking the first available person to tell her if she had her breast removed,[40] because, as in the preoperative phase, patients are frequently allowed to assume the initiative in seeking information.

Cyclical reactions. Whereas depression is frequently mentioned as a reaction to mastectomy,[12] at least two investigators[20,30] posit an identifiable pattern of responding. According to Grandstaff,[20] the pattern begins with denial, which is expressed in feelings of disbelief or shock. These feelings give way to anger and frustration because of feelings of powerlessness or hopelessness. In turn anger gives way to depression, frequently accompanied by weeping. In time these reactions give way to acceptance. Before final acceptance, some would interpose a period of mourning and grieving for the lost breast and state that only after this process has taken place is the woman able to accept the loss of the breast.[12,35,51]

Depression, however, appears to be far from universal. Maguire,[41] for example, found depressive and anxiety responses in slightly more than one third of his sample of women. Worden and Weisman[63] take the point of view that the association of depression with mastectomy is, in a sense, fallacious, since only 20% of their sample exhibited postmastectomy depression along with other aspects of the depressive cycle. They do point out, however, that the number of women experiencing mastectomy is large and that 20% represents a sizable number of women who are so affected.

Distress reactions. There is little doubt that a significant number of women experience some kind of emotional distress subsequent to mastectomy, as many as 56% in the Maguire[42] study. Of these women who experienced emotional distress, 10% of them had severe reactions including panic, uncontrolled weeping, and depression. They also exhibited impairments of concentration, sleep, appetite, and the ability to converse with others.

Despite feelings of distress, women may believe that they must meet the world with a brave front most of the time[20] and keep up a veneer of cheerfulness.[3] Perhaps this occurs because of a pressure on the woman to adjust quietly and easily to the surgery.[56] The woman may have to face her illness alone because talking about it is discouraged by many people.[47]

Some women display a remarkable lack of concern, whereas others are relieved apparently because the uncertainty has been resolved.[42] Women who knew the diagnosis prior to surgery may find the mastectomy reassuring, since it has been demonstrated that the cancer was operable rather than inoperable.[30] Questions do arise about the success of the operation,[56] and once assured of the results the women may then be able to turn their attention to a new *status quo*.

Reactions to viewing self. Sooner or later the woman looks at the results of the surgery, the first viewing most frequently taking place in the hospital. Some would consider the decision to view or not to view as a crisis point.[20] Others stress the shock-like state induced by viewing the self for the first time that gives rise to feelings of mutilation and repulsion.[13] For Quint[46] the shock lies not in the absence of a breast, but in the horrible scar. Many believe that the absence of a breast in conjunction with the scars of ablative surgery force a confrontation resulting in reconceptualizations of the self and the body image.[60] No universality of reaction can be expected, for, as Schain[50] notes, reactions to viewing the self after mastectomy are highly varied, ranging from disgust, fear, and anger to guilt, indifference, and resignation.

Self-concept and body image concerns. There is a fairly common assumption that the self-esteem of women is compromised when a breast is lost,[21] threatened,[30] disturbed,[16] depreciated,[41] or diminished.[63] However, in a careful study comparing forty women with breast cancer and fifty women with other types of cancer, Worden and Weisman[63] found that loss of self-esteem was not a dominant pattern. Loss of self-esteem, accompanied by depression, occurred with equal frequency in both samples of women. Approximately 20% of the women demonstrated lowered self-esteem scores on psychologic tests.

Historically body image refers to a number of body attitudes and rarely is conceptualized as a single variable. For purposes of discussion, the body image variable will be viewed as a single composite attitude about the body, its appearance, and its functioning. Reactions to viewing one's body, as we have seen, may result in feelings of mutilation and loss. As the self-concept becomes depreciated, the image of one's body goes through a similar loss of esteem. If a woman defines herself in body image concepts or if a professional identity depends on the use of the body, breast loss can become traumatic. The change in body contour, Woods[60] asserts, requires the woman to adapt to a new image.

The woman may also come to believe that the body has proved its vulnerability and remove the trust she once placed in her body.[56] The period of hospitalization may involve psychologic wound healing within the context of the physical healing process following surgery. Despite the rapidity of the physical change and the rapidity with which the confrontation takes place, a period of time may be required for the integration of a new image or the modification of the old one.

Not all women react with overt body image concerns. Whether one calls it denial or a defense against breast loss, some women deemphasize the importance of the lost breast, saying, in effect, that the breast was not large enough to see in the first place.[50] The extent of body image concerns in women undergoing mastectomy was also investigated by Worden and Weisman,[63] who found that 80% to 90% of their sample of women with breast cancer and other types of cancer reported no significant symptoms related to impaired body image. Nevertheless, this type of concern occurs with sufficient frequency to require attention.

Fears and concerns. Within the hospital environment, before the woman loses the status of being a patient, she has an opportunity to contemplate the future. Schain[50] states that many concerns are not admitted to the self at this time. Immediate pressures cause many of the psychologic problems to be tucked away. Involved as a patient, the woman may be concerned more immediately with problems of physical comfort, the quality of the hospital food, controlling visitors to the room, and aspects of patient-staff relationships.

The most omnipresent fear concerns cancer and its control or eradication and the implications for life.[4] These women have fears about suffering pain, being bedridden, and becoming a burden on their families.[41] Whether or not the marital relationship is a good one, women may be concerned about a possible loss of love from the husband because he may no longer find her attractive.[41] She may imagine a loss of sexual feelings on her own part.[56] She may also be concerned about her children and how they will react to her cancer, her hospitalization, and her surgery.[20] If these fearful ruminations take place during periods of depression or lowered self-esteem, the future can look bleak indeed. The existence of these fears and concerns may be related to an attempt to deal with the stress, during which the worst is anticipated and in which the woman may be attempting to marshal her psychologic forces to cope with the pressures of returning home. It has been previously noted that, for the most part, women are able to cope effectively.[63]

Postsurgical experiences

Psychologic reactions to mastectomy seem to endure over lengthy periods of time. It is of prime importance to learn what happens to these women during convalescence and recovery.

Reactions of husbands. Although the role of husbands is being introduced in this section, they have had important functions throughout the mastectomy experience. Expecting the husband to be a source of support may or may not be realistic if information about the husband-wife relationship is lacking. Hobbs,[28] among others, stresses the fact that the marital relationship postsurgically is a function of the quality of that relationship before the mastectomy. If the marital relationship is essentially indifferent or poor, the needed support, even as reflected in physical care, may be given only as a token.[54] Sutherland[54] believes that a good preoperative relationship will usually be continued, whereas Wabrek and Wabrek[56] assert strongly that it is nonsensical to believe that a good marriage easily survives the trauma of the mastectomy experience.

Husbands are viewed both as sources of support for their wives and as denying or withholding support.[7] Whereas there is considerable emphasis on the negative aspect of the husband's behavior in some studies, Maguire[41] finds that most couples were brought together despite the strain placed on the marriage.

Anstice[2] states that, before support can be given, the husband needs information and guidance, particularly about his wife's feelings. Supposedly, in this case, the counselor knows more about the wife's feelings than does the husband. The position could be taken, however, that at least some husbands and wives communicate fully without external teaching.

The basic support the wife appears to need is to be reassured that she is of value as a human being[30] and that the change in contour does not matter.[13] Valuing his wife, along with increasing his sensitivity to her needs and feelings, seems to be the most effective way for the husband to demonstrate support.

The husband also has needs, internal feelings, fears, and concerns. He must deal with his own uncertainties and his own conflicting emotions.[4] The events surrounding the mastectomy may instigate feelings of helplessness and powerlessness.[20] He may become unsure of himself and of how to react and unsure of his wife's needs and of whether or not he will be able to meet them.[4] Certainly he is concerned with the outcome and has fears for his wife's survival.[20] The emotional state of husbands has been neglected; Wabrek and Wabrek[56] assert that husbands need opportunities to voice feelings, concern, and fears.

When the wife permits the husband to view the results of surgery for the first time, his reactions may be observed carefully by her. The husband may want to relate to his wife in an appropriate fashion, but he may be afraid that he will not be able to accomplish it.[20] If the husband reacts negatively or if his reaction is perceived negatively, his wife may withdraw and experience feelings of rejection.[20] In viewing the operative site, his own sensibilities may be violated,[34] particularly if he has strong fears of disfigurement.[60]

Sexual behavior can be affected. Fear of hurting his wife may inhibit the husband from touching the scar.[34] Conversely she may be afraid of being hurt; this can be used as an excuse to sleep in separate beds,[28] to avoid the resumption of sexual intercourse,[52] or to avoid sexual contact completely. In part these reactions can lead to a cycle of sexual dysfunction.[56] Because of his own anxiety the husband can reinforce his wife's withdrawal by withdrawing, exacerbating her feelings of rejection.[52] Finally the husband has to deal with his own sexuality and the meanings he ascribes to the breast. He may perceive the absent breast as a threat to his sexual satisfaction[52] or as a threat to his own masculinity.[60]

Short-term effects

The woman returns home with feelings of weakness, and it is usually anticipated that she will require approximately 12 weeks after surgery to regain her strength.[50] This period of decreased physical vitality, particularly if it is accompanied with feelings of being physically and sexually hurt,[2] can lead to protracted invalidism.[54] The immediate convalescent period can be one of exhaustion accompanied by frequent crying and irritability.[46] In addition there may be problems of wound healing that have further emotional consequences.[47] There are frequent concerns about death and cancer recurrence,[47] stimulated in some cases by return visits to the surgeon and by therapeutic regimens. These concerns and other concerns about the future continue during the year and reach a peak approximately 7 months after the mastectomy.[59] Maguire[42] has noted that feelings of despair, mixed with feelings of bitterness and resentment, are prominent. These feelings are frequently accompanied by endless questioning about why cancer had to be present. Obvious emotional stress is present, reaching a peak 2 to 3 months postoperatively.[63]

Depressive reactions are common—as many as 83% of the women report experiencing it.[42] This occurs during convalescence and continues throughout the year.[3] The intensity of the depression varies, and approximately 30% experience marked to moderate depression 3 to 4 months after the mastectomy.[42] Depressive reactions may be heightened with anticipatory grief over possible death, a phenomenon more pronounced within the first few months, and with an inability to discuss these feelings with the husband or anyone else.[20]

For some women crying spells are uncontrollable and inexplicable and they may be given antidepressants and/or tranquilizers. For example, most of Green's mastectomy patients had been given tranquilizers for several months after surgery.[21] The women may have to deal with other inexplicable sensations; phantom breast sensations, for example, occur in 23% to 36% of women sampled.[31,48,57] Combined with sleeplessness and frightening dreams, these sensations can cause women to question whether or not they are experiencing a nervous breakdown.[25]

Social and interpersonal problems. One of the decisions the woman has to make revolves about the sharing of the mastectomy experience with others, that is, who is to be told what.[30] Establishing communication about the mastectomy may prove difficult, particularly where there is a tendency toward social isolation and a wish to withdraw from people.[3] If the woman experiences body image disturbances and her self-esteem is compromised, she may not be able to function adequately with others.[16]

The reactions of other people to her become significant, and she may get mixed messages from them.[7] Some friends and acquaintances offer kindness, understanding, and practical help. Others may be afraid or worry about intruding on her. Still others change the nature of the relationship so that it is characterized by avoidance, and they become more and more distant.[14]

Some women have little difficulty in resuming their former social activities,[42] although there is a general tendency for leisure and social activities to diminish during the first year after the mastectomy.[38] A small proportion of women (12%) found interpersonal relationships worsening during the 4-month period after mastectomy. The impoverishment of social relationships, combined with withdrawal reactions, may give rise to the feelings of loneliness and isolation noted by Labby[37] and to the sense of conversational isolation commented on by Woods.[61]

Self-respect and a sense of self-esteem are maintained through the conduct of valued life activities.[61] Winick and Robbins[59] queried 863 patients who attended their postmastectomy program and found that 84% reported the resumption of normal activities within 4 months. Seventy-four percent of the working women returned to work within 3 months. This finding contrasts with Maguire's study, in which only 10% returned to full-time work. Maguire[42] also reported that when women returned to work they experienced difficulty in coping with the job. Perhaps the more positive results reported by Winick and Robbins can be attributed to their postmastectomy program.

Sexual and marital problems. In the presence of lowered self-esteem and increased self-consciousness, the sexual life of the woman may become a difficult area of adjustment for her and sexual activity may not be enjoyed.[34] Maguire[41] found that sexual relations were commonly affected; some women completely lost interest, whereas others exhibited a marked lessening in desire and enjoyment. Reduced sexual activity may increase the woman's anxiety about her capacity to function sexually, whereas, at the same time, lack of activity may be experienced as sexual deprivation, lessening chances of tension reduction. Conversely, particularly if the woman questions her femininity, there may be increased emphasis on sexual activity and extreme emphasis on achieving frequent and/or multiple orgasms. This latter behavior may have the effect of inducing a sexual dysfunction cycle, further disrupting the marriage.[56]

Maguire[41] found that sexual and marital problems were more likely to occur in younger women. The older women, aged 60 years and above, seemed to adapt fairly readily. The quality of the marital and sexual relationship was dependent on the relative importance of sex to the woman and her perceptions of her husband. Subsequently Maguire[42] stated that the woman's reaction depended on how emotionally invested the woman was in her breast. Some women went to great lengths to avoid being seen by their husbands while dressing or bathing. Others would create excuses to avoid intercourse. Some women insisted on wearing a prosthesis during sexual intercourse.[34] Others rejected revealing bed clothes and adopted styles designed to conceal.[52] The marriage is in danger for these women not only because of the sexual problems but also because the problems indicate communication difficulties and a basic lack of trust in oneself or in one's partner.

Prosthetic and clothing problems. Each woman must decide about the extent of camouflage needed.[46] Although a prosthesis may be desired, its use may have to be delayed if there are problems of wound healing. Getting a well-designed prosthesis is frequently a problem and a source of embarrassment and worry.[2] Proper fit, cost, and availability are also concerns,[50] with many women finding counseling about the prosthesis inadequate.[42]

For some women, daily dressing and undressing create an emotional upheaval and attention is focused on the choice of clothes to be used to hide the defect.[52] The thought of having to buy new clothes may induce feelings akin to panic.[42] There is a change in clothing life-style, and women encounter difficulties in obtaining a proper fit.[4] Not all problems of concealment and proper fit are related to the absence of a breast, per se; the presence of lymphedema and the attendant arm swelling also have effects.[4] In a follow-up study of eighty-six postmastectomy women, Roberts, Furnival, and Forrest[48] noticed the presence of lymphedema in 46% of the women whose mastectomies included axillary clearance.

The choice of clothing style and the search for an adequate prosthesis are related to self-consciousness about appearance and the embarrassment that is experienced, aside from issues of personal comfort.[2] Patients may become concerned about whether acquaintances or strangers can detect the mastectomy.[7] Shopping for lingerie may induce frustration, anxiety, and anger,[50] particularly if help is needed from a saleswoman.

Long-term effects

A few studies have attempted to assess the long-term effects of mastectomy. Maguire[42] found that, at the end of a year, depression is still a considerable problem, although anxiety is much less. Forty-two percent of the women sampled had moderate to marked impairment of social and work activities, whereas 25% experienced difficulties in sexual and interpersonal relationships. Maguire also found that 25% of these women took hypnotics, antidepressants, or tranquilizers regularly. Curiously the prescription of medication appeared to have little relationship to the woman's mood state, for many women who were especially depressed received no medication.

In a retrospective study of 100 postmastectomy women, Buls, Jones, Bennett, and Chan[6] found that the anxiety and embarrassment present in one third of the sample did not diminish with time. Frank embarrassment in social situations continued to be quite common. Social habits were altered in one third of the sample, and these were expressed mainly in the style of dress and the avoidance of recreational activities such as swimming.

Healy[27] followed 271 postmastectomy women prospectively. Slightly fewer than 40% of the women developed lymphedema, and for a significant group of women the lymphedema was limiting. Women were self-conscious about the enlarged arm and reported that they had difficulty in fitting clothes. The fear of cancer recurrence was still present.

In a well-controlled study, Craig, Constock, and Geiser[11] obtained from the cancer registry the names of 134 women who had breast cancer. These women were matched to population and neighborhood samples of women. These investigators found the quality of survival of the women who had breast cancer remarkably similar to that of the other groups of women. There was no evidence of increased psychosocial disability associated with mastectomy. There was no difference in either present or future orientation for the three groups of women. The women had identical patterns in recreational activities, and the great majority rated themselves as happy. The authors compared their results favorably with previous studies indicating that 83% of women with mastectomies resumed their preoperative responsibilities within 2 years and that a similar proportion of women were exercising these responsibilities 5 years later.

CONCLUSIONS

Unfortunately much of the data reported are obtained from poorly conceived and poorly conducted studies. In many of them, even the semblance of experimental design is lacking. Statements are made that are probably more representative of the author's viewpoint than of the women concerned. This area of inquiry is too important and too fraught with social significance to allow the present state of affairs to continue much longer.

It is quite clear that reactions to the mastectomy experience are highly varied rather than universal. It is also quite clear that the majority of women who experience mastectomy are able to cope quite well. Despite the presence of anxiety, depression, and uncertainty, the women appear to be able to draw on an inner reserve to meet adversity and not become completely overwhelmed by it. In addition to inner resources, most women are able to rely on their husbands for additional support and strength.

Whereas most women cope effectively with the mastectomy experience over the long range, a significant proportion of them tend to be overwhelmed initially and for a period of time following the mastectomy. In the face of impoverished inner resources, external sources of support may help them compensate for experienced inadequacy. The kind of support needed can begin with the recognition of the woman's feelings and progress to the investment of trust in her surgeon, the people taking care of her, and the significant people in her environment. Trust is gained and maintained by responsivenss and by careful listening as information is being shared.

REFERENCES

1. American Cancer Society: Women's attitudes regarding breast cancer, Occup. Health Nurs. **22:**20-23, February 1974.
2. Anstice, E.: Coping after mastectomy, Nurs. Times **66:**882-883, 1970.
3. Anstice, E.: The emotional operation, Nurs. Times **66:**837-838, 1970.
4. Asken, M. J.: Psychoemotional aspects of mastectomy: a review of recent literature, Am. J. Psychiatry **132:**56-59, 1975.
5. Baker, J. L., Kolin, I., and Bartlett, E.: Psychosexual dynamics of patients undergoing mammary augmentation, Plast. Reconstr. Surg. **53:**652-659, 1974.
6. Buls, J. G., Jones, I. H., Bennett, A. C., and Chan, D. P.: Women's attitudes to mastectomy for breast cancer, Med. J. Aust. **2:**336-338, 1976.
7. Butler, A.: Breast cancer, Can. Nurse **72**(6):17-22, 1976.
8. Cameron, A., and Hinton, J.: Delay in seeking treatment for mammary tumors, Cancer **21:**1121-1126, 1968.
9. Chesser, E. G., and Anderson, J. L.: Psychological considerations in cancer of the breast, Proc. R. Soc. Med. **68:**793-795, 1975.
10. Clark, R. L.: Psychologic reactions of patients and health professionals to cancer. In Cullen, J. W., Fox, B. H., and Isom, R. N., editors: Cancer: the behavioral dimensions, New York, 1976, Raven Press.
11. Craig, T. J., Constock, G. W., and Geiser, P. B.: The quality of survival in breast cancer: a case-control comparison, Cancer **33:**1451-1457, 1974.
12. Enlow, A. J., Krant, J. J., Rezzonico, J. M., and Schain, W. S.: Rehabilitation and programming rehabilitation: panel discussion. In Vaeth, J. M., editor: Breast cancer, Basel, 1976, S. Karger.
13. Ervin, C. V.: Psychologic adjustment to mastectomy, Med. Aspects Hum. Sexuality **7**(2):42-65, 1973.
14. Evans, J.: Mastectomy—the patient's point of view, Nurs. Mirror Midwives J. **140** (14):62, 1975.
15. Fisher, S.: Motivation for patient delay, Arch. Gen. Psychiatry **16:**676-678, 1967.
16. Friel, F. B., Nicolay, G. C., and Frank, M. D.: Adverse emotional reactions to disfigurative surgery: detection and management, Conn. Med. **31:**227-881, 1967.
17. Giovacchini, P. L., and Muslin, H.: Ego equilibrium and cancer of the breast, Psychosom. Med. **27:**524-532, 1965.
18. Goldfarb, C., Drieson, J., and Cole, D.: Psychophysiologic aspects of malignancy, Am. J. Psychiatry **123:**1545-1552, 1967.
19. Goldsmith, H. S., and Alday, E. S.: Role of the surgeon in the rehabilitation of the breast cancer patient, Cancer **28:**1672-1675, 1971.
20. Grandstaff, H. W.: The impact of breast cancer on the family. In Vaeth, J. M., editor: Breast cancer, Basel, 1976, S. Karger.
21. Green, R. L., Jr.: The emotional aspects of hysterectomy, South. Med. J. **66:**442-444, 1973.
22. Greer, S.: Psychological aspects: delay in the treatment of breast cancer, Proc. R. Soc. Med. **67:**470-473, 1974.
23. Greer, S., and Morris, T.: Psychological attributes of women who develop breast cancer: a controlled study, J. Psychosom. Res. **19:**147-153, 1975.
24. Grossman, A. R.: Psychological and psychosexual aspects of augmentation mammaplasty, Clin. Plast. Surg. **3:**167-170, 1976.
25. Harrell, H. C.: To lose a breast, Am. J. Nurs. **72:**676-677, 1972.
26. Harris, J.: I have cancer, Nurs. Mirror **138**(11):1-2, 1974.
27. Healy, J. E., Jr.: Role of rehabilitation medicine in the care of the patient with breast cancer, Cancer **28:**1666-1671, 1971.

28. Hobbs, P.: Community aspects of breast cancer, Nurs. Mirror **140**(14):52-54, 1975.
29. Holland, J. C. B.: Coping with cancer: a challenge to the behavioral sciences. In Cullen, J. W., Fox, B. H., and Isom, R. N., editors: Cancer: the behavioral dimensions, New York, 1976, Raven Press.
30. Holland, J. C. B.: The clinical course of breast cancer: a psychological perspective. In Vaeth, J. M., editor: Breast cancer, Basel, 1976, S. Karger.
31. Jarvis, J. H.: Post-mastectomy breast phantoms, J. Nerv. Ment. Dis. **144:**266-272, 1967.
32. Katz, J. L., Weiner, H., Gallagher, T. F., and Hellman, L.: Stress, distress and ego defenses: psychoendocrine response to impending breast tumor biopsy, Arch. Gen. Psychiatry **23:**131-142, 1976.
33. Katz, J. L., and associates: Psychoendocrine aspects of cancer of the breast, Psychosom. Med. **32:**1-18, 1970.
34. Kent, S.: Coping with sexual identity crises after mastectomy, Geriatrics **30**(10):145-146, 1975.
35. Klein, R.: A crisis to grow in, Cancer **28:**1660-1665, 1971.
36. Kushner, R.: Breast cancer: a personal history and investigative report, New York, 1975, Harcourt Brace Jovanovich, Inc.
37. Labby, D. H.: Sexual concomitants of disease and illness, Postgrad. Med. **58:**103-111, 1975.
38. Lee, E. C. G., and Maguire, G. P.: Proceedings: emotional distress in patients attending a breast clinic, Br. J. Surg. **62:**162, 1975.
39. Leis, H. P., Jr.: Surgical approach to breast cancer, N.Y. State J. Med. **73:**1992-1996, 1973.
40. Magarey, J., and Todd, P. B.: Breast loss and delay in breast cancer: behavioral science in surgical research, Aust. N.Z. J. Surg. **46:**391-393, 1976.
41. Maguire, P.: The psychological and social consequences of breast cancer, Nurs. Mirror Midwives J. **140**(14):54-57, 1975.
42. Maguire, P.: The psychological and social sequelae of mastectomy. In Howells, J. G., editor: Modern perspectives in the psychiatric aspects of surgery, New York, 1976, Brunner/Mazel, Inc.
43. Meyers, T. J.: The psychologic effects of gynecologic surgery, Pacific Med. Surg. **73:** 429-432, 1965.
44. Owen, M. L.: Special care for the patient who has a breast biopsy or mastectomy, Nurs. Clin. North Am. **7:**373-382, 1972.
45. Polivy, J.: Psychological effects of mastectomy on a woman's feminine self-concept, J. Nerv. Ment. Dis. **164:**77-87, 1977.
46. Quint, J. C.: The impact of mastectomy, Am. J. Nurs. **63**(11):88-92, 1963.
47. Quint, J. C.: Institutionalized practices of information control, Psychiatry **28:**119-132, 1965.
48. Roberts, M. M., Furnival, I. G., and Forrest, A. P.: The morbidity of mastectomy, Br. J. Surg. **59:**301-321, 1972.
49. Rollin, B.: First you cry, New York, 1977, The New American Library Inc.
50. Schain, W.: Psychological impact of the diagnosis of breast cancer on the patient. In Vaeth, J. M., editor: Breast cancer, Basel, 1976, S. Karger.
51. Schoenberg, B., and Carr, A. C.: Loss of external organs: limb amputation, mastectomy and disfiguration. In Schoenberg, B., Carr, A. C., Peretz, D., and Kutscher, A. H., editors: Loss and grief: psychological management in medical practice, New York, 1970, Columbia University Press.
52. Schon, M.: The meaning of death and sex to cancer patients, J. Sex Res. **4:**288-302, 1968.

53. Schonfield, J.: Psychological and life experience differences between Israeli women with benign and cancerous breast lesions, J. Psychosom. Res. **19:**229-234, 1975.
54. Sutherland, A. M.: Psychological observations in cancer patients, Int. Psychiatry Clin. **4:**75-92, 1967.
55. Torrie, A.: Mastectomy—"the emotional operation," Nurs. Mirror **132**(22):34-35, 1971.
56. Wabrek, A. J., and Wabrek, C. J.: Mastectomy: sexual implications, Primary Care **3:** 803-810, 1976.
57. Weinstein, S., Vetter, R. J., and Sersen, E. A.: Phantoms following breast surgery, Neuropsychologia **8:**185-197, 1970.
58. Williams, E. M., Baum, M., and Hughes, L. E.: Delay in presentation of women with breast diseases, Clin. Oncology **2:**327-331, 1976.
59. Winick, L., and Robbins, G. F.: Physical and psychologic readjustment after mastectomy: an evaluation of Memorial Hospital's PMRG program, Cancer **39:**478-486, 1977.
60. Woods, N. F.: Influences on sexual adaptation to mastectomy, J. Obstet. Gynecol. Neonatal Nurs. **4**(3):33-37, 1975.
61. Woods, N. F.: Psychologic aspects of breast cancer: review of the literature, J. Obstet. Gynecol. Neonatal Nurs. **4**(5):15-22, 1975.
62. Worden, J. W., and Weisman, A. D.: Psychosocial components of lagtime in cancer diagnosis, J. Psychosom. Res. **19:**69-79, 1975.
63. Worden, J. W., and Weisman, A. D.: The fallacy in postmastectomy depression, Am. J. Med. Sci. **273:**169-175, 1977.

CHAPTER 2

The reconstruction experience: the search for restitution

Edward Clifford

Publications about breast reconstruction following mastectomy are usually speculative and concerned with the advisability of the procedure or its probable results. Factual information is not readily available.

Despite this dearth of information, considerable concern is expressed about the psychologic effects of enduring a mastectomy experience. Whereas it appears that a majority of women are able to cope quite well despite the presence of some anxiety, depression, and uncertainty, some women experiencing mastectomy appear to be overwhelmed by the experience. We do not know, in any systematic fashion, what impels the search for restitution. It is not known whether or not it is the woman with impoverished inner resources or the stronger, more assertive woman who seeks breast reconstruction.

In order to examine the motivations and reactions of women who undergo breast reconstruction, unstructured and open-ended psychologic interviews were conducted with sixty-five women who were in the process of having their breasts reconstructed.[1] These women were asked to share their experiences and feelings about breast cancer, mastectomy, and reconstruction. In addition background information was obtained. The results of these clinical interviews will be presented in the context of information obtained from the literature about mastectomy and reconstruction.

WOMEN EXPERIENCING RECONSTRUCTION

Only women who were in some phase of breast reconstruction following mastectomy were involved in this study. All had had breast cancer and had experienced mastectomy. Four had had breast reconstruction in conjunction with mastectomy. Women were involved in the study in serial order as they arrived at Duke University Medical Center for an examination or for admission. They were asked to volunteer their participation; no woman refused to do so. Many expressed an eagerness to talk about what they had experienced.

The women ranged in age from 30 to 71 years, with the average age being 45.77 years. Two, however, exceeded 60 years of age; most were between 40 and 49 years of age. All but eight had at least finished high school; schooling averaged 12.74 years. Twenty-five percent classified themselves as full-time house-wives, whereas 75% were employed. Employed women tended to work full time rather than part time.

Eighty percent of the women were married. Of the rest, four were widowed, four were either divorced or separated, four were in the process of becoming divorced or separated, and one was contemplating divorce. The current marriage was the second one for 17% of the women. Two had been divorced twice and another had been divorced three times. The average length of the current marriage was 21.45 years, with the marriage length ranging from 6 months to 45 years. The typical woman had two children; only six of the married women had no children.

RECALLED REACTIONS TO MASTECTOMY

Reactions to the mastectomy were solicited because these reactions could be related to the search for restitution. Conceivably the desire for breast reconstruction may be related to adverse psychologic reactions to the mastectomy. Similarly the search for restitution may signify a basic characterological defect implying that the woman has not adapted well to her breast loss and that she cannot or will not accept the breast loss.[5]

Much of the information obtained is retrospective, for a considerable amount of time had elapsed in most cases (an average of 5.41 years) since the mastectomy had taken place. The interval between the mastectomy and these clinical interviews ranged widely; four patients were examined within 2 weeks, whereas three patients had experienced mastectomy approximately 25 years ago and one woman had this experience 31 years ago. Because the recall of information is retrospective, it is possible that the information obtained reflects current feelings about the experience rather than being an accurate portrayal of what actually occurred. The passage of time may have dulled some reactions, or persistent concerns over this long a time span could represent an adaptive failure.

Concerns about cancer

A sizable group of women (32%) said that they accepted their cancer matter-of-factly, voicing the feeling that they were now minimally concerned about it, 5.88 years, on the average, after their mastectomies. No single reaction to having had cancer involved more than 25% of the women. Fifteen (23%) still expressed a fear of suffering, thirteen (20%) were still concerned with the threat of death, and nine (14%) were afraid of cancer recurrence. An occasional woman was worried about the quality of life that had been adversely affected by having cancer, whereas a few women experienced difficulty in communicating about and obtaining information about their cancers.

In this sample at least, the clinical evidence does not support Asken's[2] contention that concerns about cancer are the most omnipresent fear experienced by these women. Whereas the fears of suffering pain, being bedridden, or being a burden on the family, which were reported by Maguire[10] are present, most women in this study do not emphasize such reactions. It is possible that these effects are moderated for these women with the knowledge that their breasts are going to be reconstructed. They have been reassured as well that the recurrence of cancer is not a significant problem, otherwise reconstructions would not be attempted.

Husband's reactions

Previous studies have not attempted to differentiate perceptions of differing roles of husbands in the mastectomy experience. Conceivably husbands can react to cancer as a disease process in a different manner than they would to breast amputation. This study attempted to examine women's perceptions of their husbands' reactions to cancer as a separate question from their husbands' reactions to the mastectomy itself.

Whereas the supportiveness of fourteen (22%) of the husbands could not be determined, most husbands (53.5%) were perceived as being supportive; only sixteen (24.5%) were not. When husbands were viewed positively, their wives saw them as offering reassurance, expressing positive concerns, and being available when needed. Nonsupportive husbands were viewed as being noncommunicative, more concerned with their own fears than with the wife's anxieties, and unable to offer the emotional support the wife felt she needed.

Defensive or coping strategies

During the course of the interview, as the women were recalling their experiences with cancer, it became apparent that they employed a number of differing coping strategies. No single defense mechanism was used by a majority of the women. Seventeen (26%) tended to deny, avoid, or suppress any mention of the fact that they had cancer. It is possible that the interviewer failed to earn fully the trust of some of these women, resulting in their not sharing their feelings with him rather than using a denial mechanism.

The use of prayer or religious faith was used as a coping mechanism by 20% of the women, and an equal proportion stated that their faith and trust in the physician enabled them to deal effectively with having cancer. Twelve (18%) related some defensive breakdown reflected in emotional turmoil as a reaction to having cancer. Two of these women attempted suicide; an additional three women had been in psychiatric treatment.

In many cases women combined coping strategies; the general tendency was to use more than one mechanism. Suppression or denial, however, tended to occur alone. The results reported here are congruent with those reported by Katz, Weiner, Gallagher, and Hellman[8] in that multiple rather than single defense mechanisms are involved. The results are congruent with theirs as well in the emphasis placed by the woman on the use of prayer and faith as a means of coping.

Breast loss

The women in this sample varied widely in the interval between mastectomy and seeking breast reconstruction. Since an average of 5.41 years had passed, many of these women had the opportunity to accommodate to the loss of the breast.

Apparently the passage of time had not dulled some of the feelings about the mastectomy. Despite the length of time that had elapsed since breast loss, 77% of the women could attach a date to the surgical procedure. Thirty women (46%) gave spontaneously the month and year of the mastectomy, whereas twenty (31%) recalled the anniversary by mentioning the month, day, and year spontaneously. A few women gave approximate dates, for example, about 6 years ago.

Whereas the date of the surgery could be recalled with precision, the impression was obtained that many could not describe accurately the surgery. Women were confused about terminology, particularly where the word *radical* was used; they tended to interpret the term as meaning something drastic rather than relating it to the extensiveness of the surgical procedure. This finding is in keeping with the results of the survey undertaken for the American Cancer Society in which some confusion existed about the precise meanings of surgical terms associated with mastectomy.[1] Perhaps Sutherland's[13] suggestion that the term *definitive surgery* would cause less confusion has merit.

Expressed concerns about breast loss. A few women (9%) stated that they had no concerns about breast loss. It is of considerable interest to note that all four women experiencing simultaneous mastectomy and reconstruction were in this group. For the other women, concerns were multiple, for example, a woman could express dissatisfaction with body contour *and* with herself as a person. The predominant response (55%) centered about negative reactions to body contour, that is, feeling unbalanced or lopsided. Thirty-two percent of the women expressed feelings of self-consciousness, particularly in a social context such as when they were buying clothing or wearing a bathing suit or in situations in which they might have to disrobe in front of other women. An equal number of women believed that their self-concept as individuals and as women had been affected. Concepts of femininity were not necessarily related to concerns about sexuality; most frequently an inner sense of femininity seemed to be involved. These women stressed their own views of femininity rather than the views of others about their femaleness predominated. Along with heightened self-consciousness, 17% of the women experienced strong negative feelings when they viewed themselves in the mirror or while bathing.

Ten women continued to experience depressive-like or angry feelings. Two of these women were currently psychiatric outpatients. For the most part, women in this sample did not receive psychiatric or psychologic assistance. At some time in their postmastectomy experience, an additional six women, excluding the two currently in treatment, experienced some contact with a mental health professional. It is not clear, however, whether these women would have needed some form of assistance independently of the mastectomy.

Anxiety about husbands did not appear to be a predominant factor. This may be because of the fact that most husbands were viewed as providing support and being available when needed at the initial phases of the mastectomy experience. Only 8% of the women expressed concerns about their spouse's reaction to the mastectomy. Perhaps husband support allowed the wife to concentrate more on her own reactions. From these interviews it becomes apparent that these women are primarily involved with feelings about themselves as persons rather than with their acceptability to others.

Husband's reactions to mastectomy. For the most part husbands were perceived as being supportive (63%), some (28%) were seen as not being supportive at all, and perceived support could not be determined in the remainder (9%). Where the husband was characterized as being supportive, his wife saw him as giving assurance and as being accepting. One husband was characterized as being verbally supportive, although he was unable to look at or touch his wife at the mastectomy site. According to their wives, 17% of the men were unable to offer any verbal support at all, and an additional 11% refused to look at or touch their wife in the area of the mastectomy. An occasional woman, anticipating her husband's reluctance, would not expose herself in order to spare him.

Quality of marriage. It has been noted that four women were in the process of becoming divorced or separating from their husbands subsequent to mastectomy and that an additional woman was contemplating divorce. Divorce and separation, however, are not the only criteria for estimating the quality of the marriage.

Although not specifically asked about the marriage, 63% of the remaining fifty-two married women spontaneously characterized the quality of their marriages. Fifteen (29%) had positive feelings about their marriages or believed that the marriage was improving since the surgery. A slightly greater proportion (35%) stated that their marriages were poor and/or deteriorating. Impoverished marriage, however, was not related necessarily directly to the mastectomy, for many women indicated that the marriage was poor or failing before breast loss. Within the impoverished married group, four women reported that they were having extramarital affairs. An additional four women stated that their husbands were having such affairs.

There is an interesting discrepancy between the assessment of the marriage and the perception of husband support. Apparently husbands were able to provide some support even in the face of a marriage that was poor or unhappy. Perhaps the husbands were able to marshal support in the face of a crisis but were unable to do so in a continuing, long-term relationship with their wives. These women, however, differentiate between the quality of the support received and the quality of the marriage.

Sexual behavior. In part the quality of the marriage is related to satisfactions obtained in sexual behavior. Of the women who were not divorced or in the process of being divorced or separated, 77% expressed their feelings about their sexual experiences. Sixty-two percent of these women believed that no change took place in sexual behavior following the mastectomy. Of this group, twenty-one women indicated that their sex life was good, whereas eleven stated that it was as poor before as after the mastectomy. Eight women indicated that a change in sexual behavior had taken place. Relationships had improved for two and had become poorer for six women.

The women did not, nor were they asked to reveal, specific details about their sexual practices. Five women mentioned dissatisfaction with the husband's behavior. In these cases the husband seemed to have a low sex drive or he refused to look at his wife during sexual intercourse. More frequently it was the woman's sexual behavior that was involved. Fourteen women gave some details about themselves. One positive change was reported; one woman felt less inhibited in her sexual expression since the mastectomy. The remaining women were all adversely affected. Four reported a decrease in sex drive; nine refused to have the husband see or touch her in the area of the absent breast. Of the latter women, two insisted on remaining covered during intercourse.

The type of support received by the woman, the quality of her marriage, and the satisfaction she receives from her sexual experiences are interrelated. The picture that emerges demonstrates the difficulties encountered by many marriage partners; the effect of the mastectomy on the marriage is much more difficult to articulate. Apparently these women see themselves as coping with problematic marriages at the same time that they must deal with what is happening to them as a result of the mastectomy. Whereas a good marriage does not negate the impact of the mastectomy on the woman, the quality of her relationship with her husband can serve as a base from which she may be able to cope better with the mastectomy. The poor marriage, on the other hand, with its attendant lack of emotional support, may exacerbate feelings of self-doubt and adversely affect the woman's capacity to cope effectively with the mastectomy experience.

SEARCH FOR RESTITUTION

There were several aspects of breast reconstruction that these women were asked to share with the interviewer. Since motivating factors were of primary interest, women were asked to state how they had come to learn about breast reconstruction; they were also asked to state what their expectations were. Following this, the women were asked about their reactions to what had been accomplished for them with breast reconstruction. Finally they were asked specifically to share any negative experiences they had with breast reconstruction.

An initial phase of the search for restitution for these women began with their learning about the availability of breast reconstruction. In contrast to the mastectomy experience in which there was extensive contact with the health-care system, most patients seeking reconstruction seek the surgery by themselves. Frequently, in this sample, patients learned about breast reconstruction through newspaper publicity, from friends or relatives, or from former patients. Twenty-five percent of these women were stimulated to seek surgery because of newspaper reports, and an additional 17% were told about the availability of the surgery by friends, relatives, or former patients. Twenty-eight percent of the sample were informed about the availability of breast construction by their physicians, and an additional 6% were experiencing simultaneous mastectomy and reconstruction.

These findings are congruent with those reported for women seeking breast augmentations. Perhaps because augmentation and reconstruction are elective procedures, women typically do not learn about the availability of them from their physicians; friends and former patients seem to be most active in referring new patients.[3]

Expectations of reconstructive breast surgery

Some physicians believe that the search for breast reconstruction signifies a basic characterological defect in the woman seeking the procedure, whereas for others breast reconstruction is the only realistic way to deal with the problem of disfigurement. The former point of view is exemplified by Goldsmith and Alday,[5] who assert that the pressure for reconstruction comes from women who have difficulty in accepting breast loss. They imply that the desire for this procedure is indicative of a lack of adaptation on the woman's part; she is unable to accept and adapt to her postmastectomy status. In contrast Asken[2] believes that reconstruction is the only solution to the continuing problem of disfigurement, whereas Kent[9] states that reconstruction is the most dramatic type of help a physician can offer. Further, breast reconstruction can be expected to produce positive emotional responses in those who experience it.[4]

Little attention has been paid to the process by which the woman decides to seek breast reconstruction. Possibly anxieties about surgery and her recovery from cancer may be exacerbated when further breast surgery is contemplated.[11] The woman may be met with arguments about being accepted the way she is, implying that reconstruction is needless. If this is the case, such arguments may intensify further any self-doubts she may be experiencing at the time. In a retrospective study of 270 women seeking augmentation mammaplasties, Baker, Kolin, and Bartlett[3] found that 84% of the women responding to their questionnaires indicated that personal need was the primary motivation. The strength of the desire is attested to by their finding that 58% of the women queried stated that opposition from the husband or other family members would not deter them from seeking augmentation.

Each woman has to face her own expectancies as well, and these may not be voiced or discussed. Schain[11] believes that it is crucial for the woman to discuss her fantasies and motivations for reconstruction. This, however, may be accomplished best with psychologic assistance in helping her examine her perceptions in the context of what surgery realistically can offer. For Schain a *risk-reward ratio* is involved in which the woman must balance the gains expected against potential unacceptable outcomes.

In this sample of women very few had difficulty in stating what they hoped to accomplish by having their breasts reconstructed; only two women were unable to provide some rationalization for having the reconstruction. The stated motivations were classified according to thematic content. These illustrative comments and the number of women involved are listed in Table 2-1.

It is quite evident that the primary motivation is restitution, mentioned by

Table 2-1. Expectations of reconstructive breast surgery—thematic content

Categorization	Illustrative comments	Number of women	Per-centage
Restoration	To be whole again; to be a woman again; to look like I used to; to be like myself; to feel more natural; to be normal again	45	69
Relief of clothing or prosthetic problems	To get rid of uncomfortable prosthesis; to get rid of clothing problems; want to wear swimming suits; to be able to wear a natural bra; so that I can dress nice; want to look well in clothes; to look good in night-gowns; more convenient than prosthesis	32	49
Becoming less self-conscious or embarrassed	To lose self-consciousness; to feel less con-spicuous; people will stop staring; ashamed for people to see me; to feel more comfortable; would not have to hide in the bathroom to change clothes; to feel more like a woman	27	42
Improving appearance	To complete the aesthetic picture; to improve contour; to improve looks; to look more natural; to have breasts the same size; won't have to look at a flat chest anymore; I like bosoms and I like to let them show	26	40
Improving feelings	To feel better, make me more relaxed; better internal feelings; to feel happier; to get rid of depression; to feel better mentally; to feel better about myself; help me keep my sanity	10	15
Improving marital relationships	Husband will have better outlook; gift to husband, I like to reveal my bosom to him; to save the marriage; to improve sex; to become more sexually attractive; hoping husband and sex life would change	10	15
Changing life-style	Hope to marry again; have a new life; start a new life	3	5
No expectations	I don't know; I can't tell you	2	3

69% of the women. A sizable proportion of these women are still concerned about appearance as well as with realistic problems associated with clothing selection and the discomfort of prosthetic devices.

Although the average interval between mastectomy and reconstruction was slightly more than 5 years, these women remained self-conscious about their appearance and aware of discomfort. In the absence of a control group, it is difficult to determine whether such reactions are realistic or are indicative of an underlying chronic agitation. Certainly one need not accept an appearance marred by a deformity when corrective procedures are available. The drive for restitution exists in sufficient strength to be one of the primary motivations for this sample of women.

Relatively few women chose to seek restitution because it would improve their marriage or the quality of their sex life. This finding is related, in all probability, to the corollary finding that most of the marital and sexual problems existed before the mastectomy. For some women, however, breast reconstruction was associated with hoped-for improvements in the marriage or in their life-style.

Clearly these women are seeking restitution; they wish to be returned to their former state. The data support Gifford's[4] contention that women seek reconstruction because they desire realistic breasts that can be incorporated into their body concepts. The data would also agree with others that along with restitution women seek to enhance their self-esteem, become less self-conscious about appearance, become less dependent on prostheses, return to former clothing preferences, make their marriages a bit more secure, and increase their enjoyment of sex.[3,4,6,7]

Finally there is little evidence that adaptive failure has taken place. Several women needed psychiatric assistance. They might have done so anyway or with any stress in their lives. However, relatively few women appeared to search for restitution because of an inner turmoil. On the contrary these women seemed to be demanding normality by rejecting what appeared to them to be a remedial physical defect.

Timing of reconstruction

The timing of the reconstruction may be significant. Snyderman and Guthrie[12] believe that reconstructive surgery should be planned before the mastectomy is performed. They assert that knowing that reconstruction is planned serves to reduce the negative consequences of the surgery. Asken[2] is of the opinion that offering women the option of breast reconstruction before the mastectomy has psychologic value, if only to provide a source of comfort. No data are reported in the literature about the effects of simultaneous versus delayed reconstruction. There were four women in this sample who experienced simultaneous mastectomy and reconstruction. None of these women displayed any of the negative psychologic effects seen in some of the others. However, the data are insufficient to allow generalizations.

Reactions to reconstruction

The women in this sample were in various phases of the reconstruction experience. Several women were interviewed before the first reconstructive surgery, whereas several others were interviewed very shortly after a surgical procedure, which possibly contaminates reactions. In addition several women had not completed all of the reconstructive procedures, so that their responses could not reflect their feelings about the end product. As a result a total of forty-one women served as a subsample from whom information was obtained about reactions to reconstruction.

For a large proportion of these women (76%), restitution has resulted in the expression of positive feelings. This finding is congruent with that of Gifford.[4]

Table 2-2. Reactions to reconstructive breast surgery—thematic content*

Categorization	Illustrative comments	Number of women	Percentage†
Positive feelings	Wonderful; great; enthusiastic; happy; pleased; like a kid on Christmas morning; feel better; prevented me from committing suicide; feel normal	31	76
Appearance	Looks better now; size of breasts are O.K.; size of breasts improved; smaller size is an improvement	23	56
Satisfaction with results	Glad I had it done, procedure is simpler than I thought; in the long run it is a lot better; I would recommend this to other women; I have to adjust to being smaller, but that is no problem; surgeon is next in importance to Jesus Christ	11	27
Marriage	Husband is delighted; husband is pleased; sex life is better; sex life is more relaxed	11	27
Self-consciousness	I'm a different person, I can be around people; it makes all the difference in the world, no longer self-conscious	5	12
Clothing	I have gone wild on bras and bathing suits; I don't have to worry about clothes; I can wear a bra without it hurting	5	12

*Reconstruction had not started or it was too soon after initial reconstruction to have the women assess the results in seventeen cases. Seven women were in phased reconstruction and the results were not determinable. These twenty-four women were not included in the tallies.
†Percentage is based on a total of 41 women whose reconstruction had been completed or was close to completion.

Along with positive affect, the women tended to be pleased with their appearance and were satisfied with the results. Some women believed that their husbands were pleased, and three of them felt that their sex life had become more relaxed.

These findings are analogous to those reported for women experiencing augmentation mammaplasties. It has been reported that augmentation procedures result in feelings of self-enhancement, positive affect, and general satisfaction with the results.[3,4,6,7] There is need for caution in interpreting these results, however. First, according to the principle of cognitive dissonance, positive feelings would be experienced because the woman is heavily invested emotionally in the procedure and expects positive results. In order to justify her time, effort, and energy, results must be experienced as positive. Second we do not know anything about the permanency of these reactions, since no long-term follow-up studies are available.

Negative reactions to reconstruction

These forty-one women were asked specifically to detail any negative reactions to breast reconstruction. Eleven of the women stated that they had no negative comments to make. An equal number omitted any negative comments during discussions about their reactions. The remaining nineteen women had complaints about the amount of pain experienced; the length of time the process itself took, with one woman stating that she had given a year of her life to reconstruction; the length of the hospital stay; having to wait too long for appointments.

Complaints about the results of the surgery had to do with appearance factors. Eight women stated dissatisfaction with the size of the breasts (too small), the appearance of the nipple, or the site and size of scar tissue. Three of these women characterized the results as being unsuccessful or disappointing.

Several negative comments were made about communication. The general tenor of the remarks revolved about not being given a sufficient amount of information, the need to devote more time to the decision-making process, and feelings that information was being withheld.

It should be pointed out, however, that negative and positive evaluations often were associated. Thus, for example, several women who were pleased with the results and liked their appearance had negative comments to make about the unanticipated pain involved or the length of hospitalization. Similarly women who experienced poor communication pointed out that positive results superseded any other disappointments they had. Three women felt that the results were unacceptable, and they hoped for later improvement.

SUMMARY AND CONCLUSIONS

Unstructured and open-ended psychologic interviews were conducted with sixty-five women who were in the process of having their breasts reconstructed.

They were asked to share their experiences and feelings about breast cancer, mastectomy, and reconstruction.

Reactions to experiencing mastectomy were solicited because of possible relations between these experiences and the search for breast reconstruction. Most of the women did not emphasize concerns about cancer possibly because of manifested faith in the physician who performed the mastectomy or possibly because they had been reassured that reconstruction would not be available to them if there was a strong probability of the recurrence of the cancer.

Reactions to breast loss typically involved several reactions, with the predominant responses revolving about dissatisfactions with body contour and with the self as a person. Breast loss heightened feelings of self-consciousness, which appeared to be related to appearance. Some women continued to experience depressive-like or angry feelings, and a few had some form of contact with mental health professionals. No evidence was presented, however, which would link directly the need for psychotherapy with the mastectomy.

In general husbands were preceived to be supportive in helping the women both to face their anxieties about cancer and to face the uncertainties of reactions to having lost a breast. Despite the supportiveness of the husbands, however, a number of marital relationships were reported to be relatively poor. Many of these poor marriages, however, were impoverished before the mastectomy took place.

Although some physicians take the point of view that the search for restitution represents an adaptive failure, because the woman has not adjusted to her appearance status, little evidence could be presented to support such a position. On the contrary the women in this study appeared to be reality oriented and the drive for restitution could be considered an effort to achieve a normalcy through the rejection of a physical disability that may be remedial. Women did not seek restitution, for the most part, to solve an inner problem or emotional turmoil. The drive was clearly restorative.

The gains of breast reconstruction are reflected in positive feelings about a restored appearance status, greater self-enhancement, and loss of self-consciousness. Secondary benefits were obtained because the husband was pleased with the result. Negative results were minimal, and very few women were completely dissatisfied. The women, however, when given the opportunity, did emphasize problems of communication about the surgery and expressed a desire to have more extensive consideration given to their need for information and their need for more extended conversations.

Finally four women experienced reconstruction immediately after mastectomy. None of the usual negative psychologic sequelae associated with mastectomy were reported by these women. Whereas there are too few women to use as a source of generalization or prediction, these preliminary findings are intriguing and should be explored more extensively and more rigorously.

The findings emanating from these interviews should be considered suggestive rather than definitive. As a first approximation, the interviews should be considered a first step in developing more adequate research protocols. Despite the methodological limitations, however, it is clear that many of the negative psychologic consequences posited simply do not take place with any degree of intensity. Equally it is clear that the burden of proof lies with the investigator proposing a psychologic consequence. Women experiencing mastectomy and reconstruction should not be burdened further by naive speculation about their motivations, their rationalizations, their defense mechanisms, or their ability to cope with reality effectively.

ACKNOWLEDGMENT

I wish to express my appreciation to Dr. Nicholas G. Georgiade for encouraging this study and for providing opportunities to interview his patients.

REFERENCES

1. American Cancer Society: Women's attitudes regarding breast cancer, Occup. Health Nurs. **22:**20-23, February 1974.
2. Asken, M. J.: Psychoemotional aspects of mastectomy: a review of recent literature, Am. J. Psychiatry **132:**56-59, 1975.
3. Baker, J. L., Kolin, I., and Bartlett, E.: Psychosexual dynamics of patients undergoing mammary augmentation, Plast. Reconstr. Surg. **53:**652-659, 1974.
4. Gifford, S.: Emotional attitudes toward cosmetic breast surgery: loss and restitution of the "ideal self." In Goldwyn, R. M., editor: Plastic and reconstructive surgery of the breast, Boston, 1976, Little, Brown and Co.
5. Goldsmith, H. S., and Alday, E. S.: Role of the surgeon in the rehabilitation of the breast cancer patient, Cancer **28:**1672-1675, 1971.
6. Grossman, A. R.: Psychological and psychosexual aspects of augmentation mammaplasty, Clin. Plast. Surg. **3:**167-170, 1976.
7. Hoopes, J. E., and Knorr, N. J.: Psychology of flat-chested women. In Masters, F. W., and Lewis, J. R., Jr., editors: Symposium on aesthetic surgery of the face, eyelid and breast, St. Louis, 1972, The C. V. Mosby Co.
8. Katz, J. L., Weiner, H., Gallagher, T. F., and Hellman, L.: Stress, distress and ego defenses: psychoendocrine response to impending breast tumor biopsy, Arch. Gen. Psychiatry **23:**131-142, 1970.
9. Kent, S.: Coping with sexual identity crises after mastectomy, Geriatrics **30:**145-146, 1975.
10. Maguire, P.: The psychological and social sequelae of mastectomy. In Howells, J. G., editor: Modern perspectives in the psychiatric aspects of surgery, New York, 1976, Brunner/Mazel, Inc.
11. Schain, W.: Psychological impact of the diagnosis of breast cancer on the patient. In Vaeth, J. M., editor: Breast cancer, Basel, 1976. S. Karger.
12. Snyderman, R. K., and Guthrie, R. H.: Reconstruction of the female breast following radical mastectomy, Plast. Reconstr. Surg. **47:**565-567, 1971.
13. Sutherland, A. M.: Psychological observations in cancer patients, Int. Psychiatry Clin. **4:**75-92, 1976.

CHAPTER 3

Surgical anatomy of the breast

Donald Serafin

During the last decade considerable attention has been directed to the reconstruction of the female breast. This is reflected both in the voluminous literature and in multiple presentations and panel discussions at national meetings. Many operative procedures have been advocated and subsequently abandoned because of the poor esthetic result and associated high tissue morbidity. It has become increasingly apparent that the blood supply to the nipple-areolar complex and the preservation of sensation are extremely important as reconstructive surgeons become more discerning.

With changing concepts toward earlier reconstruction following mastectomy and preservation of the nipple-areolar complex, a thorough knowledge of the surgical anatomy of the breast is indispensable.

EMBRYOLOGY

Early in the sixth week of gestation the mammary ridges can be identified on the ventral surface of the developing embryo extending bilaterally from the axilla to the groin (Fig. 3-1, *A*). These ridges, which are epithelial derivatives, continue their development in the pectoral region as the remaining regions disappear. These epithelial cells proliferate, become bulbous, and grow downward into the underlying mesenchymal tissue. By the end of the fifth month of gestation, fifteen to twenty solid cords can be identified. These cords continue to grow downward and branch, then slowly acquire lumina by hollowing. At maturation these become the lactiferous ducts, whose terminal portions become the acini (Fig. 3-1, *B*). Developmentally these acini are thought to be homologous to the apocrine sweat glands.

The originally elevated flat surface of the developing nipple develops a depression, into which these lactiferous ducts empty. At birth or later this area is elevated to form the nipple as a result of the underlying proliferating mesenchyme.

The areola can be identified by the fifth month as a circular pigmented area of skin about the nipple containing the rudimentary apocrine glands of Montgomery.[1]

GENERAL ANATOMY AND PHYSIOLOGY

The majority of breast parenchyma is located between the third and seventh intercostal spaces. The nipple-areolar complex in the young adult is frequently

35

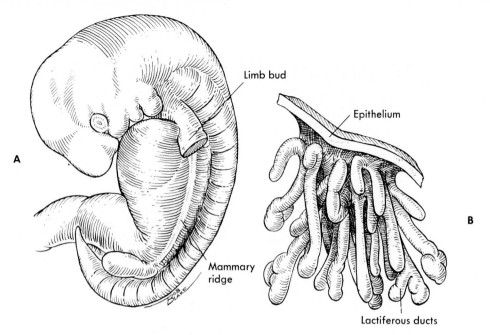

Fig. 3-1. A, Mammary ridges in 6-week-old embryo. **B,** Developing lactiferous ducts and acini. (From Serafin, D.: Anatomy of the breast. In Georgiade, N. G., editor: Reconstructive breast surgery, St. Louis, 1976, The C. V. Mosby Co., p. 18.)

located 1 to 2 cm lateral to the midclavicular line, frequently in the fourth to fifth intercostal space. With advancing age and obesity the nipple-areolar complex may descend a variable degree.

The breast, being an ectodermal derivative, is closely adherent to the skin and more loosely adherent posteriorly to the pectoralis fascia (Fig. 3-2). It is generally thought to be contained in a fascial envelope, continuous above with the superficial cervical fascia and continuous below with the superficial abdominal fascia (fascia of Camper).[8] The anterior layer (superficial layer of the superficial fascia) is poorly developed, whereas the posterior layer (deep-layer superficial fascia) is better developed, lying in part on the pectoralis fascia. The upper outer quadrant of the breast, the tail of Spence, exits through a fascial defect, Langer's foramen, to lie deep in the axillary fascia. The anterior fascial envelope and skin are linked to the posterior fascia by the ligaments of Cooper, fibrous and elastic prolongations that divide the gland into multiple septa and give suspensory support (Fig. 3-3).

Stiles[33] demonstrated that the breast parenchyma follows these suspensory ligaments of Cooper to their attachment to the corium and that to remove all of the breast tissue one ". . . must either sacrifice a large amount of skin or keep so close to it in dissecting it off the mamma as to run some risk of sloughing" (p. 13).[14]

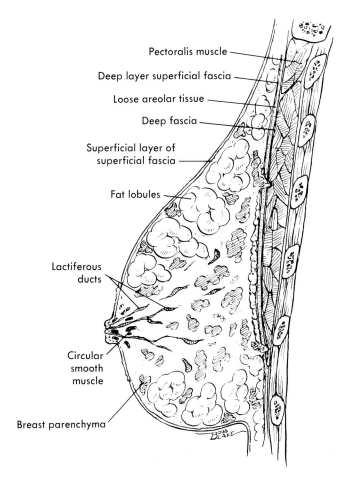

Pectoralis muscle

Deep layer superficial fascia

Loose areolar tissue

Deep fascia

Superficial layer of
superficial fascia

Fat lobules

Lactiferous
ducts

Circular
smooth
muscle

Breast parenchyma

Fig. 3-2. Sagittal anatomy of breast. Note close adherence of breast parenchyma to dermis anteriorly and penetration into pectoralis posteriorly. (From Serafin, D.: Anatomy of the breast. In Georgiade, N. G., editor: Reconstructive breast surgery, St. Louis, 1976, The C. V. Mosby Co., p. 19.)

The deep layer of the superficial fascia is fixed posteriorly to the pectoralis fascia by fascial projections. Breast parenchyma accompanies these fibrous processes into the substance of the pectoralis major muscle itself.[33] Thus adequate removal would necessitate excision of the pectoralis fascia and a layer of muscle as well.

It is important to appreciate the extensive penetration of breast parenchyma anteriorly along the Cooper ligaments to the corium and posteriorly into the pectoralis muscle and into the axilla as the tail of Spence. When performing both simple[12,16] and subcutaneous mastectomies[7] for either benign or premalignant disease, 5% to 15% of breast tissue, by necessity, is left behind.

The glandular tissue is embedded in subcutaneous tissue of varying amounts,

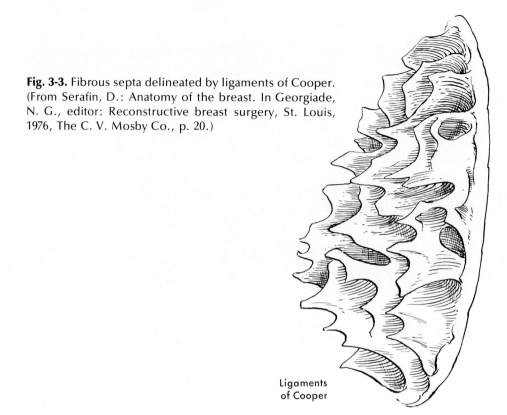

Fig. 3-3. Fibrous septa delineated by ligaments of Cooper. (From Serafin, D.: Anatomy of the breast. In Georgiade, N. G., editor: Reconstructive breast surgery, St. Louis, 1976, The C. V. Mosby Co., p. 20.)

Ligaments
of Cooper

greatest laterally and diminishing progressively to the nipple cone where there is none. The epithelial parenchyma is made up of fifteen to 20 lobes, each of which empties into a secretory duct at the nipple (Fig. 3-1, *B*). Each lobe consists of multiple lobules, each of which is made up of ten to a hundred acini grouped around a collecting duct.

In childhood both ductal and alveolar cells consist of a two-celled basal layer of epithelium. Under estrogen influence, the alveolar epithelium proliferates, becomes multilayer, and differentiates into: (1) superficial (luminal) A cells; (2) basal B cells (chief cells); and (3) myoepithelial cells (Fig. 3-4). It is suggested that the clear basal cells may be precursors to both the luminal (dark) A cells and the myoepithelial cells. Luminal dark cells contain a high ribosome content and are believed to be actively involved in milk synthesis and secretion during lactation. The myoepithelial cells are located adjacent to the basement membrane of alveoli and the small ducts. Being ten to twenty times more sensitive to oxytocin than uterine smooth muscle, they contract during the stimulus of sucking, ejecting milk secretions into the larger ducts[36] (Fig. 3-5).

Estrogen and progesterone are the principal hormones that act on the glandular epithelium of the breast. Receptor sites for steroid hormones have been

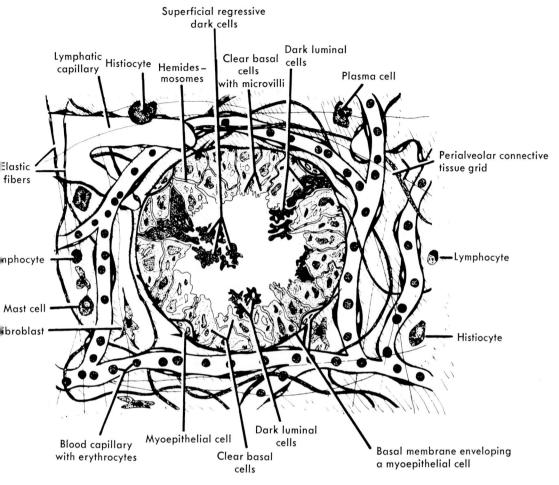

Fig. 3-4. Microanatomy of acini under estrogen influence. (Reprinted with permission of Vorherr, H.: The breast: morphology, physiology, and lactation, New York, 1974, Academic Press, Inc., p. 42.)

demonstrated in the cytosol of the responding cell. Both hormones are secreted by the ovary, although a small amount may be secreted by the adrenal cortex. Prolactin, from the anterior pituitary, is a peptide whose receptor is located on the membrane of the breast epithelial cell.

Estradiol, progesterone, and prolactin are all responsible for breast development. At puberty, rising levels of estradiol result in increased RNA, DNA, and protein synthesis. Although prolactin levels remain the same, estradiol binding[19,31] and RNA synthesis are probably enhanced.[5]

In nonpregnant, menstruating females, the breast undergoes cyclic volumetric changes. In the proliferative phase cellular hyperplasia and proliferation

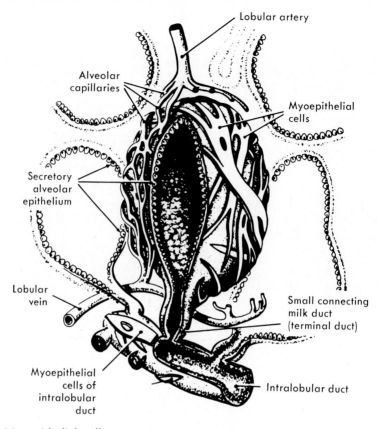

Fig. 3-5. Myoepithelial cell arrangement around alveoli and small ducts. (Reprinted with permission of Vorherr, H.: The breast: morphology, physiology and lactation, New York, 1974, Academic Press, Inc., p. 46.)

are induced by estrogens. Mammary ducts become dilated under the influence of progesterone, and alveolar cells differentiate into secretory cells. Enhanced water retention results in lobular edema and contributes to volumetric increase.

In the luteal phase of the menstrual cycle, breast volume is further increased, as is blood flow.[9,36] The breast is characterized by nodularity, increased turgor, fullness, and pain. Increased connective tissue water is evident, resulting in interlobular edema, probably the result of an estrogen-induced histamine effect on the microcirculation.[36,38]

With menstruation, secretory activity is apparent and "epithelial regression" becomes evident.

Postmenstrually cellular regression continues and tissue edema disappears. A minimum of breast volume is noted.

ARTERIAL BLOOD SUPPLY

According to Maliniac,[21] Manchot[24] laid the foundation for poorly conceived mammaplasty operations by an inaccurate description of the arterial blood

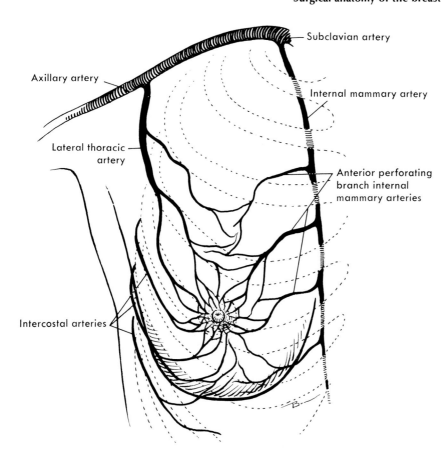

Subclavian artery

Axillary artery

Internal mammary artery

Lateral thoracic
artery

Anterior perforating
branch internal
mammary arteries

Intercostal arteries

Fig. 3-6. Principal arterial pathways to breast. (From Serafin, D.: Anatomy of the breast. In Georgiade, N. G., editor: Reconstructive breast surgery, St. Louis, 1976, The C. V. Mosby Co., p. 21.)

supply. These incorrect anatomic descriptions were further expounded by Kaufmann[18] with disastrous results. They both advocated, based on anatomic dissections, that the lateral thoracic artery had no important role in supplying the breast and nipple-areolar complex. Biesenberger[3] based his lateral glandular resection on this principle with a high incidence of breast and nipple necrosis.

According to Maliniac,[23] Rouvière[29] strongly criticized this concept, basing this criticism on the presence of significant lymphatic pathways to the axilla and their constant accompaniment with venous and arterial supply. He believed (as did Cooper[6] and Testut[34]) that the lateral thoracic artery contributed significantly to the blood supply of the breast. Later Salmon,[30] Gitis and Livshits,[11] and Marcus,[25] using a roentgenographic technique and dissection, confirmed these observations.

Considering these observations, Maliniac[21,23] concluded that there were three main sources of arterial blood supply to the breast: (1) internal mammary artery, (2) lateral thoracic artery, and (3) intercostal arteries (Fig. 3-6).

The internal mammary artery, a branch of the first portion of the subclavian artery, supplies the medial aspect of the breast by anterior and posterior perforating arteries. Its contributions were represented in 100% of all the breasts studied. The second and third anterior perforating arteries, exiting in their respective intercostal spaces at the costo-chondral junction, are, by far, the most significant. The first and fourth are less constant. The posterior penetrating arteries exit more laterally from the intercostal space and supply the posterior aspect of the breast especially by the fourth branch.

Being cutaneous arteries, these anterior perforating branches lie within the subcutaneous layer of tissue adjacent to the parenchyma of the breast. Depending on the thickness of this subcutaneous layer, these arteries may be found 0.5 to 1.0 cm from the medial surface of the breast. They course inferiorly and laterally to affect anastomoses with the lateral thoracic and intercostal arteries.

The lateral thoracic artery arises from the second part of the axillary artery (or from the thoracoacromial or subscapular arteries). It then courses inferiomedially within the subcutaneous tissue of the lateral breast to anastomose freely in the areolar area with the branches of the internal mammary and intercostal arteries. Because the lateral breast tissue frequently has more subcutaneous tissue than medially, the artery is often found 1 to 2 cm from the skin surface. As the areola is approached, all of these vessels become more superficial. Maliniac's[21,23] review revealed that this artery is absent 30% of the time but that it may be the only source of blood supply to the nipple 13% of the time. Thus operative procedures designed to sacrifice extensive breast tissue laterally may result in nipple necrosis a certain percentage of the time.

The intercostal arteries are the least important of the arteries supplying blood to the breast. They take origin from the aorta posteriorly and course anteriorly in the intercostal spaces, terminating in an anastomotic plexus in the lower quadrants of the breast with the lateral thoracic and internal mammary arteries. The fourth or fifth intercostal arteries are usually dominant.

The blood supply to the nipple has, for a long time, been the focus of attention for surgeons operating on the breast. Cooper[6] described anterior and posterior branches from the arterial arcade as they approach the nipple. Schwarzmann[32] popularized the dermal pedicle flap and emphasized the importance of the dermal blood supply in maintaining the viability of the nipple. Marcus and Maliniac[21] described three major types of periareolar plexuses (Fig. 3-7): (1) circular with maximum blood supply to the nipple, present in 70% to 74% of cases studied: (2) loop, less direct blood supply to the nipple with branches of the lateral thoracic looping above and below the nipple to affect anastomoses, present in 20% of cases; and (3) radial without obvious plexus, both internal mammary and lateral thoracic branches going directly to the nipple, present in 6% of cases. In describing these plexuses, the authors suggested that a deep periareolar incision in a certain percentage of cases (especially breasts with a radial plexus) could result in nipple necrosis by the interruption of the only blood

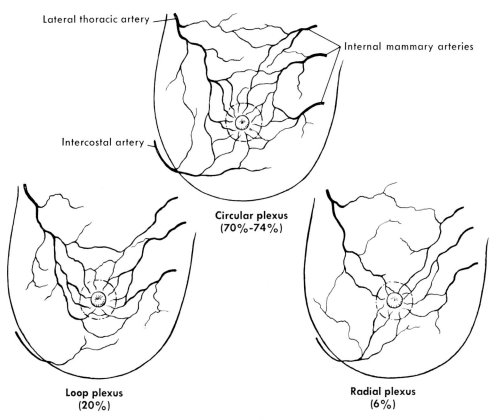

Lateral thoracic artery

Internal mammary arteries

Intercostal artery

Circular plexus
(70%-74%)

Loop plexus
(20%)

Radial plexus
(6%)

Fig. 3-7. Principal arterial plexuses to nipple-areolar complex. (From Serafin, D.: Anatomy of the breast. In Georgiade, N. G., editor: Reconstructive breast surgery, St. Louis, 1976, The C. V. Mosby Co., p. 23.)

supply. It is easy to see how this conclusion could be reached particularly if one examines closely the operative procedures advocated at this time.[20,22] In these operative porcedures not only was the areolar-nipple complex separated from its dermal blood supply, but the breast parenchyma was isolated as well. Thus the periareolar plexus was violated and its direct communication to the lateral thoracic, internal mammary, and intercostal vessels, which are predominantely subcutaneous in their course and distribution, was interrupted.

Montagna[27] reviewed the cutaneous blood supply and noted that the patterns of cutaneous vascular beds differed considerably. Regularities were, in fact, an exception. These vascular beds were determined by the kind of skin perfused, the thickness of the dermal layer, the number of appendages, and the relationship to underlying structures. Segmental vessels were noted to give off perforating arteries (musculocutaneous arteries), which passed through muscles supplying them and then terminated in cutaneous branches (Fig. 3-8). Skin was also

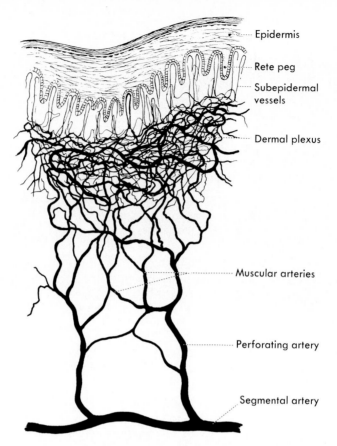

Epidermis

Rete peg

Subepidermal vessels

Dermal plexus

Muscular arteries

Perforating artery

Segmental artery

Fig. 3-8. Musculocutaneous arterial blood supply to breast. Note that direct cutaneous arteries exist as well, that is, branches of lateral thoracic artery. (From Serafin, D.: Anatomy of the breast. In Georgiade, N. G., editor: Reconstructive breast surgery, St. Louis, 1976, The C. V. Mosby Co., p. 24.)

supplied by a few direct cutaneous vessels. Montagna dispelled the concept that blood is distributed to the dermis by separate plexuses, which ". . . are interconnecting vessels of different sizes at all levels of the dermis" (p. 144).[27] Many cross communications exist as arteriovenous shunts. Precapillary sphincters determine the relative perfusion of capillary beds (Fig. 3-9).

Arterioles and venules arch in a perpendicular direction from this dermal plexus. The relative number and distribution of these arches are influenced in part by the number and size of the rete pegs. It is unlikely that this excessive vascularity represents solely nutrient flow. It also serves to regulate blood pressure and thermoregulatory functions.[37]

In summary to ensure viability of both the nipple and glandular tissue: (1) an intact dermal blood supply of the nipple-areolar complex attached to adjacent

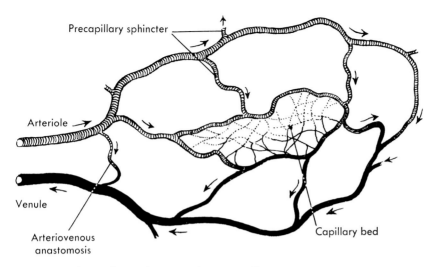

Precapillary sphincter

Arteriole

Venule

Arteriovenous anastomosis

Capillary bed

Fig. 3-9. Dermal capillary plexus with precapillary sphincters. (From Serafin, D.: Anatomy of the breast. In Georgiade, N. G., editor: Reconstructive breast surgery, St. Louis, 1976, The C. V. Mosby Co., p. 24.)

skin is essential; and (2) the underlying glandular tissue and dermal pedicle should remain in continuity to the cutaneous blood supply.

VENOUS BLOOD SUPPLY

The venous return of the breast has both a superficial and deep system. The superficial veins of the breast can be located just posterior to the superficial layer of the superficial fascia and can be readily seen with infrared photography. Using such a system, Massopust and Gardner[26] (Fig. 3-10) classified these veins into: (1) those coursing transversely across the breast toward the midline (91%); and (2) those directed in a longitudinal direction toward the suprasternal notch (9%). A small percentage of patients demonstrated the superficial venous plexus of Heller around the nipple and areola.

The superficial plexus empties into the deeper system (usually associated with a corresponding artery of the same name) via several communications (Fig. 3-11): (1) Transverse superficial veins empty directly into the midline internal mammary veins or into perforating branches and then into this same system. More inferiorly, drainage may be via the superficial epigastric tributaries. (2) The longitudinal veins empty in the region of the suprasternal notch into the jugular system. (3) Laterally these superficial veins may empty into the lateral thoracic vein or one of its tributaries (for example, thoracoepigastric vein) and then into the axillary vein. (4) Inferiorly (and from the posterior aspects of the gland) drainage may be into the intercostal system. From these intercostal veins flow is directed posteriorly into the vertebral and azygos system and then into the superior vena cava. Since this system is without valves, in the larger vessels the

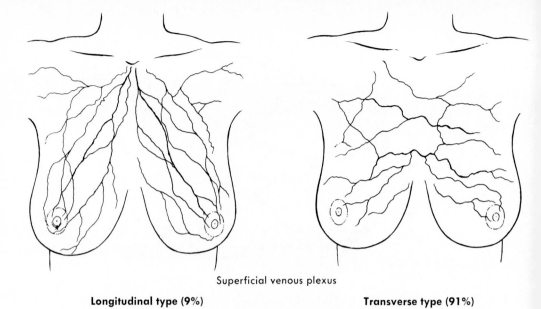

Superficial venous plexus

Longitudinal type (9%)   **Transverse type (91%)**

Fig. 3-10. Common patterns of superficial venous plexus. (From Serafin, D.: Anatomy of the breast. In Georgiade, N. G., editor: Reconstructive breast surgery, St. Louis, 1976, The C. V. Mosby Co., p. 25.)

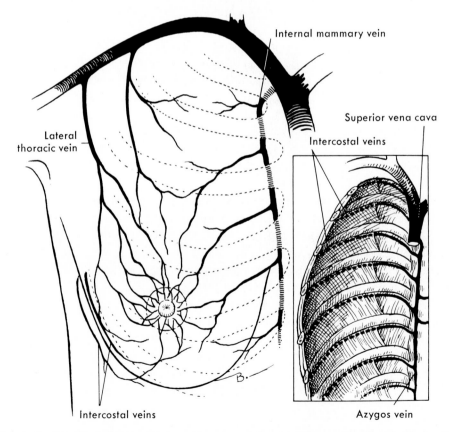

Internal mammary vein

Superior vena cava

Lateral thoracic vein

Intercostal veins

Intercostal veins

Azygos vein

B.

Fig. 3-11. Principal deep venous pathways of breast. Note azygos communication with variable blood flow. (From Serafin, D.: Anatomy of the breast. In Georgiade, N. G., editor: Reconstructive breast surgery, St. Louis, 1976, The C. V. Mosby Co., p. 26.)

flow may be quite variable depending on intrathoracic and intra-abdominal pressure relationships. Batson[2] described the importance of this system in the transportation of malignant cells to distant foci in the pelvis, vertebral column, and base of the skull.

The microvenous circulation is similar to that previously described for the arterial supply of the skin.

INNERVATION

The breast, being an ectodermal derivative, has, as would be expected, segmental sensory innervation following the distribution of the intercostal nerves. It will be recalled that the intercostal nerve, shortly after leaving the vertebral foramen, divides into an anterior and posterior nerve ramus. The latter provides the cutaneous innervation to the skin of the back (Fig. 3-12). The anterior ramus courses laterally in the intercostal space to about the level of the anterior axillary line, where, after piercing the anterior serratus muscle, it gives rise to a lateral

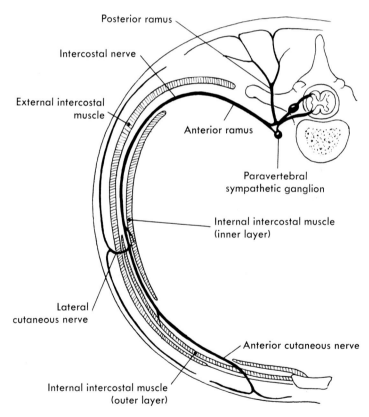

Fig. 3-12. Surgical anatomy of intercostal nerve. (From Serafin, D.: Anatomy of the breast. In Georgiade, N. G., editor: Reconstructive breast surgery, St. Louis, 1976, The C. V. Mosby Co., p. 27.)

cutaneous branch. The main ramus then continues anteriorly and terminates in the midline as the anterior branch.

Because of the developing limb bud, several modifications of this segmental pattern occur. The superior aspect of the breast is supplied by the supraclavicular nerves, branches C_3 and C_4 of the cervical plexus.

The first three intercostal nerves are irregular.[13] The first intercostal nerve has no cutaneous representation on the anterior chest wall, having neither a lateral nor an anterior cutaneous branch. The lateral branch of the second intercostal nerve (intercostobrachial nerve) crosses the axilla to innervate the medial posterior aspect of the upper arm. The anterior branch pierces the pectoralis major muscle and supplies a cutaneous distribution medially. The lateral branch of the third intercostal nerve (brachiocutaneous nerve) supplies the medial aspect of the upper arm to the elbow, the anterior branch supplying medial cutaneous innervation to the anterior chest wall.

Sensory fibers in the lateral cutaneous branches of the fourth to the sixth intercostal nerves supply the majority of the breast, including the nipple-areolar complex (Fig. 3-13). These lateral cutaneous branches further divide into ante-

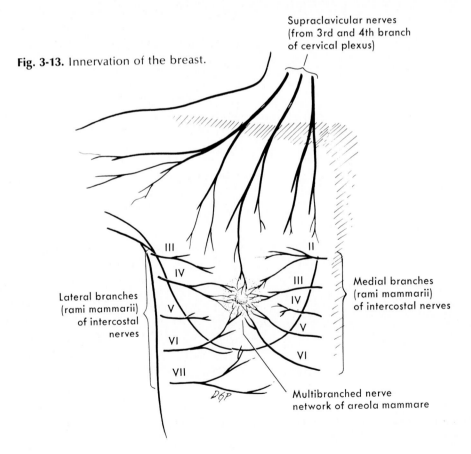

Fig. 3-13. Innervation of the breast.

Supraclavicular nerves (from 3rd and 4th branch of cervical plexus)

Lateral branches (rami mammarii) of intercostal nerves

Medial branches (rami mammarii) of intercostal nerves

Multibranched nerve network of areola mammare

rior and posterior branches that course in the superficial fascia. The anterior branches of the lateral cutaneous nerves innervate the lateral portion of the breast and nipple-areolar complex by the lateral rami mammarii. The medial aspect of the breast is innervated by the medial rami mammarii from the anterior cutaneous branches of the second through sixth intercostal nerves. These medial rami supply the skin after first penetrating the pectoralis major muscle medially.

The epidermis of the nipple-areolar complex is poorly innervated as is evidenced by poor sensory discrimination.[7;36] Light touch, stereognosis, and two-point discrimination are diminished. The deeper portions of the dermis and skin appendages are well innervated.[4] Mammary responsiveness to mechanical stimuli is thought to be mediated predominantly by Krause and Ruffini-like receptors located in the dermis of the nipple-areolar complex. Stimulation induces release of adrenohypophyseal prolactin and neurohypophyseal oxytocin via an afferent sensory reflex arc. Following delivery this results in milk synthesis and secretion into the alveoli and milk ejection through lactiferous ducts.

The smooth muscle present in blood vessels and in the nipple-areolar complex receives its innervation from the sympathetic nervous system (Fig. 3-14). Connector cells of the intermediolateral column of the spinal cord send medulated postganglionic fibers via the anterior nerve roots and white rami communicans to cell stations of the paravertebral ganglia. From these ganglia postganglionic fibers pass via gray rami communicans to the second through sixth intercostal nerves and thence to their final distribution.[13] Mechanical stimulation of the var-

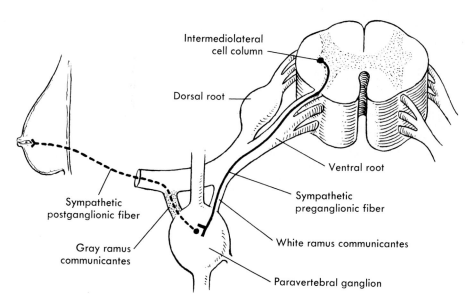

Fig. 3-14. Sympathetic innervation of nipple-areolar complex. (From Serafin, D.: Anatomy of the breast. In Georgiade, N. G., editor: Reconstructive breast surgery, St. Louis, 1976, The C. V. Mosby Co., p. 27.)

ious end-organs in the nipple-areolar complex can initiate neural transmission through the afferent limb of the reflex arc and then through the efferent sympathetic limb may bring about smooth muscle contraction and nipple erection.

LYMPHATICS

There are no lymphatics present in the epidermis. The dermis, however, has two plexuses.[14] A superficial dermus plexus without valves sends branches around the rete pegs. It is connected to a deeper, more substantial, dermal plexus with valves. From this deep dermal plexus communications exist with the subdermal lymphatics.

There are four principal lymphatic pathways draining the breast: (1) axillary; (2) internal mammary; (3) posterior intercostal; and (4) cutaneous.[10,15] Of these pathways the axillary and internal mammary are most important, accounting for more than 95% of the total lymphatic flow.[17,35] The posterior intercostal and

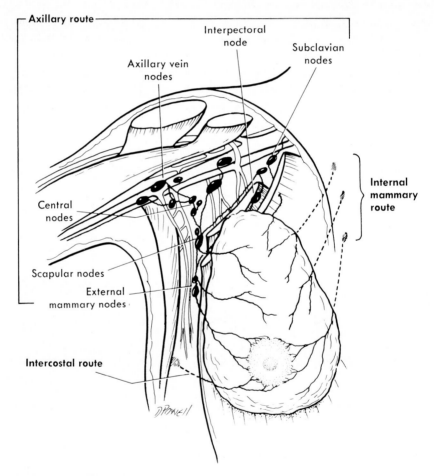

Fig. 3-15. Principal lymphatic pathways of breast.

cutaneous pathways account for only a small percentage of total lymphatic flow and assume greater importance only when the dominant systems are obstructed (Fig. 3-15).

Turner-Warwick[35] demonstrated that the axillary lymphatic pathway was predominant, accounting for 75% of the lymph flow, with the remainder draining into the internal mammary chain. In addition all quadrants of the breast drained into both the axillary and the internal mammary nodes.

Rouvière's[28] concept of centripetal lymph flow into a subareolar plexus and thence into large subcutaneous lateral and medial lymphatic channels is probably not correct. Turner-Warwick[35] found that lymph flow is centrifugal, minimizing the importance of the subareolar plexus. Lymphatics course upward and laterally through the substance of the breast predominantly to the central group of axillary nodes. Some lymphatic channels emerge from the posterior surface of the breast, through the pectoralis major muscle, and thence superiorly between the pectoralis major and minor muscles to the axillary vein or subclavicular group of nodes.[15]

CONCLUSION

In this chapter attention has been directed to the anatomy of the breast, particularly with regard to how this information influences the reconstructive surgeon. Significant operative morbidity from ill-conceived operative procedures can be avoided by a thorough knowledge of the surgical anatomy.

REFERENCES

1. Arey, L. B.: Developmental anatomy, Philadelphia, 1965, W. B. Saunders Co., pp. 449-453.
2. Batson, O. V.: The function of the vertebral veins and their role in the spread of metastases, Ann. Surg. **112:**138, 1940.
3. Biesenberger, H.: Deformitäten und kosmetische operationen der weiblichen brust, Wien, 1931, Verlag W. Mandrich, pp. 155-181.
4. Cathcart, E. P., Gairns, F. W., and Garven, H. S. D.: The innervation of the human quiescent nipple, with notes on pigmentation, erection, and hyperneury, R. Soc. Edinb. Trans. **61:**699, 1948.
5. Chomczynski, P., and Topper, Y. J.: A direct effect of prolactin and placental lactogen on mammary epithelial nuclei, Biochem. Biophys. Res. Commun. **60:**56, 1974.
6. Cooper, A. P.: Anatomy of the breast, London, 1840, Longman Group, Ltd.
7. Courtiss, E. H., and Goldwyn, R. M.: Breast sensation before and after plastic surgery, Plast. Reconstr. Surg. **58:**1, 1976.
8. Cramer, L. M., and Lapayowker, M. S.: Applied anatomy of the female breast: Surgical, radiographic and thermographic. In Masters, F. W., and Lewis, J. R., Jr., editors: Symposium on aesthetic surgery of the face, eyelid and breast, St. Louis, 1972, The C. V. Mosby Co., pp. 130-138.
9. Dabelow, A.: Die milchdrüse. In Bargmann, W., editor: Handbook der mikroskopischen anatomie des menschen, Berlin, 1957, Haut and Sinnesorgane, Springer-Verlag, vol. 3, part 3, pp. 277-485.

10. Edwards, E. A.: Surgical anatomy of the breast. In Goldwyn, R. M., editor: Plastic and reconstructive surgery of the breast, Boston, 1976, Little, Brown and Co.
11. Gitis, M. K., and Livshits, D. L.: Arterial supply of the female breast, Sovet. Khir. **6:**981, 1936.
12. Goldman, L. D., and Goldwyn, R. M.: Some anatomical considerations of subcutaneous mastectomy, Plast. Reconstr. Surg. **51:**501, 1973.
13. Grant, J. C.: A method of anatomy, Baltimore, 1958, The Williams & Wilkins Co., p. 90.
14. Haagensen, C. D.: Diseases of the breast, Philadelphia, 1956, W. B. Saunders Co.
15. Haagensen, C. D.: Diseases of the breast, ed. 2, Philadelphia, 1971, W. B. Saunders Co., pp. 1-54.
16. Hicken, N. F.: Mastectomy: clinical pathological study demonstrating why most mastectomies result in incomplete removal of the mammary gland, Arch. Surg. **40:**6-14, 1940.
17. Hultborn, K. A., Larsson, L. G., and Ragnhult, I.: The lymph drainage from the breast to the axillary and parasternal lymph nodes, studied with the aid of colloidal Au[198], Acta Radiol. **43:**52, 1955.
18. Kaufmann, R.: Artéres de la gland mammaire chez la femme, Ann. Anat. Pathol. **10:**925, 1933.
19. Leung, B. S., and Sasak, G. H.: Prolactin and progesterone effect on specific estradiol binding in uterine and mammary tissues in vitro, Biochem. Biophys. Res. Commun. **55:**1180, 1973.
20. Maliniac, J. W.: Assymetrical breast deformities, Ann. Surg. **99:**743, 1934.
21. Maliniac, J. W.: Arterial blood supply of the breast, Arch. Surg. **47:**329, 1943.
22. Maliniac, J. W.: Two stage mammaplasty in relation to blood supply, Am. J. Surg. **68:**55, 1945.
23. Maliniac, J. W.: Breast deformities and their repair, New York, 1950, Grune & Stratton, Inc., pp. 14-38.
24. Manchot, C.: Die hautarterien des menschlichen körpers, Leipzig, 1889, F. C. W. Vogel.
25. Marcus, G. H.: Untersuchungen über die arterielle blutversorgung der mamilla, Arch. Klin. Chir. **179:**361, 1934.
26. Massopust, L. C., and Gardner, W. D.: Infrared photographic studies of the superficial thoracic veins in the female, Surg. Gynecol. Obstet. **91:**717, 1950.
27. Montagna, W., and Parakkal, P. F.: The structure and function of skin, New York, 1974, Academic Press, Inc., pp. 142-155.
28. Rouvière, H.: Anatomie des lymphatiques de l'homme, Paris, 1932, Masson et Cie Editeurs.
29. Rouvière, H.: In discussion of Kaufmann before the Anatomical Society of Paris, 1933.
30. Salmon, M.: Les artères de la peau, Paris, 1936, Masson et cie Editeurs.
31. Sawin, C. T.: Endocrine physiology and pathophysiology of the breast. In Goldwyn, R. M., editor: Plastic and reconstructive surgery of the breast, Boston, 1976, Little, Brown and Co.
32. Schwarzmann, E.: Über eine neue methode der mammaplastic, Wien. Med. Wochenschr. **86:**100, 1936.
33. Stiles, H. J.: Contributions to the surgical anatomy of the breast, Edinburgh Med. J. **37:**1099, 1892.
34. Testut, J .L.: Traite' d' anatomie humaine, ed. 8, Paris, 1928-1931, Doin Editeiurs.
35. Turner-Warwick, R. T.: The lymphatics of the breast, Br. J. Surg. **46:**574, 1959.

36. Vorherr, H.: The breast, New York, 1974, Academic Press, Inc., pp. 38-50.
37. Winkelmann, R. K., Scheen, S. R., and associates: Cutaneous vascular patterns in studies with injection preparation and alkaline phosphatase reaction. In Montagna, W., and Ellis, R. A., editors: Advances in biology of skin, blood vessels and circulation, Oxford, 1961, Pergamon Press, Inc., vol. 2, pp. 1-19.
38. Zeppa, R.: Vascular response of the breast to estrogen, J. Clin. Endocrinol. Metab. **29:**695-700, 1969.

CHAPTER 4

Mammography in the diagnosis of breast cancer

Robert McLelland

Surgeons are in a particularly fortuitous position to detect asymptomatic, if not minimal, breast cancer and materially effect survival from this dreaded disease. Optimum mammography in combination with careful palpation can detect in excess of 90% of breast cancers including most minimal lesions. It can therefore be reasonably stated that mammography is an essential part of the preoperative work-up of all patients undergoing breast surgery.[14]

Furthermore mammography in women over 35 years of age without breast symptoms or signs (screening), including those having surgery for other reasons, has demonstrated an increasingly important role in the detection of breast cancer, especially in higher risk groups such as those with a past personal or family (mother and/or sisters) history of breast cancer and possibly those fulfilling Wolfe's mammography criteria which will be discussed later. The rarity of breast cancer in women under 35 years of age indicates that screening mammography has no role in this age-group.

Breast cancer is the most frequent, most feared, most treated, most costly, and leading cause of cancer death in women. The mortality rate has not changed in over 50 years, and less than half of the patients have localized disease when first diagnosed. Nevertheless, the 5-year and longer survival rates have improved[1] for a variety of reasons, including the increased use of mammography, more frequent and better self-examination, earlier contact with a physician when symptoms are present, and more effective therapeutic procedures including less mutilating surgery. Some of this represents a shift of 5-year survivors into the 10-year group, from the 10-year group into the 15-year group, etc. Some of our success is undoubtedly related to the extremely variable if not bizarre natural history of this disease. The numerous 5-, 10-, and even 25-year and longer "cures" that succumb to metastatic breast cancer document this. Survival is related to the size of the primary lesion[11] and the status of the regional lymph nodes, but the tumor cell type and host resistance may be even more important factors.[13] Smaller lesions have less lymph node involvement, which means improved survival and cure rates (lesions less than 1 cm in size with negative axillary nodes have a 95%-plus 10-year survival rate[17]). Consequently the major diagnostic thrust today is early detection, hopefully when the primary lesion is small and confined to the breast, and mammography plays a major role in this effort.

Over 90% of breast cancers are first detected by the patient; consequently regular careful self-examination remains a cornerstone in detection. However, our experience has taught us that very few women do this properly or regularly and that lesions detected in this manner are often large with more frequent involvement of regional lymph nodes. Lesions detected by physicians are often smaller, but nonpalpable breast cancer can only be detected by mammography. There is no way of knowing how many nonpalpable but mammographically detectable cancers lurk in breasts that have not had mammography before a benign lesion has been surgically removed. One can appreciate the enormous relief that this initial result provides, but we must also recognize the potentially tragic false sense of security that may result from this course of action.

In situations in which mammography and physical examination of asymptomatic women (screening) are done independently, such as at the Duke Breast Cancer Detection Demonstration Project, a higher percentage of lesions are detected by mammography (65%) than by physical examination (56%).[9] Nevertheless mammography and physical examination are clearly complementary diagnostic procedures (combined accuracy 90%-plus) with many lesions being detected by both examinations. A positive result with either examination dictates biopsy, and a negative result in the other modality should not deter this course of action. Equivocal results necessitate careful followup.

Ultrasound has proved useful[32] in differentiating solid from cystic lesions whether detected by mammography, physical examination, or both. The role of thermography (infrared photography of heat patterns) is less clearly defined because of its nonspecificity, rather high false-positive rate, and not insignificant false-negative rate.[6,10] There has been limited experience with computerized axial tomography (CAT), which has detected a few lesions not detected by other means, but it is prohibitively expensive and mammography is more reliable.

MAMMOGRAPHY

Mammography has been proved important in the detection, diagnosis, and management of breast cancer.[23] As has been mentioned, the indications for mammography include women with breast symptoms and/or signs, women at higher risk, breasts difficult to examine, and screening purposes. There are still too many breast biopsies being done without prior mammography and too many treated breast cancer patients being followed with physical examination alone. This is hard to reconcile with the fact that 32% of our breast cancers were found only by mammography (nonpalpable), whereas 22% were found only by palpation. No one would advocate a breast biopsy without palpation, yet this is often less accurate than mammography in the detection of cancer, especially when it is small.

Mammography is a demanding diagnostic procedure not only in terms of the interpretation of the images but also technically with the end results being directly proportional to the proficiency of both radiologists and technologists working in concert. This is especially true of nonpalpable lesions, for which mammography is the sole opportunity for detection. There are a variety of x-ray imaging systems available that are effective under optimum conditions. We have chosen the Xerox system because in our experience the images are easier to interpret, greater structural detail of the breast is afforded, and there is less fatigue in viewing and comparing large numbers of studies.[19]

The breast parenchyma is normally replaced with fat as women age, and this process is accelerated with parity. However, dense dysplastic changes (fibrocystic disease, adenosis, secretory disease, etc.) are extremely common. Mammography is most reliable and cancer is more readily detected in the fatty low-density breast. However, most cancers are in dense dysplastic breasts, which places greater demands on mammography. The mammographic signs of malignancy are:

1. A dominant mass, most often stellate (10% or less are well circumscribed and ultrasound can be quite helpful in evaluating these) or of mixed configuration. They are often considerably larger on physical examination than on the mammograms as a result of extension of the tumor into the surrounding soft tissues and lymphatics as well as desmoplastic reaction in adjacent tissue.

2. Microcalcifications may be benign or malignant. They can be distinguished in a high percentage of instances.[20] Malignant microcalcifications tend to be smaller and more difficult to see with the unaided eye (a magnifying glass is often necessary to detect them, whereas benign calcifications are usually readily seen with the naked eye). They are more irregular with branching, "broken needle tip" and comma patterns, and there is greater clustering, often in association with a malignant mass or some architectural distortion but not necessarily so.

3. Architectural distortion, which refers especially to focal stellate areas but also to focal densities.

4. Secondary changes including skin and/or nipple thickening and/or retraction, dilated veins, and lymphadenopathy are usually late or nonspecific manifestations of malignancy.

5. Finally Wolfe[35] has proposed a classification of risk to develop breast cancer on the basis of the mamographic appearance:

N1   normal; mainly fat; *lowest risk* (patient #3, p. 61)
P1   Prominent ducts (1 to 4 mm) in one fourth or less of the breast; *low risk (patient #4, p. 62)*
P2   more prominent ducts in more than one fourth of the breast (coalescence); *high risk* (patient #5, p. 63)
DY   general increased density with or without duct prominence; *highest risk* (patients #1 and #2, pp. 58 and 60)

He has concluded that persons in the DY category have a significantly increased risk of developing breast cancer. This claim has been disputed.[7,24,28] We have designed a statistically unbiased study to reexamine the issue.[15] Some of the mammograms were difficult to classify, suggesting an element of subjectivity and/or a need for other methods of classification (combining N1-P1 and P2-DY or subdividing the P2 and DY categories). To be useful and widely applicable, the method optimally should be simple and reproducible. Our results including statistical analyses are:

	N1	P1	P2	DY	Total
Breast cancer patients	12	26	58	75	171
Asymptomatic controls	29	40	62	40	171
Risk estimates*	1.0	1.5	2.7	7.2	

*Relative to N1, age stratified: $P < 0.0001$

Our findings support Wolfe's assertions and indicate that ductal prominence and dysplasia as determined by mammography are significantly related to risk of breast cancer, possibly only exceeded by a personal history of breast cancer.

Another Duke study[21] of the contralateral breast of previously treated breast cancer patients has revealed 12% unsuspected cancers (physical examination and mammography were negative for cancer). The average size of these cancers was 3 mm; one was invasive and the others were not. A statistically significant finding was the association of certain ductal epithelial hyperplasias with the study group and absence of this association with previously suspected lesions such as gross cystic disease and sclerosing adenosis.

These findings raise mammographic and other considerations that merit and are receiving further study.

Obviously nonpalpable lesions are the special province of mammography. The radiologist has an important role in the localization of these bothersome areas for biopsy and verification of their resection with biopsy specimen roentgenograms. A simple mammography technique that we have found useful is as follows: the biopsy site is first localized on the mammograms by quadrant and distance from the areola, skin surface, and/or chest wall; then a fine-gauge needle (21 gauge or less with its length predetermined by the depth of the lesion) is aseptically inserted to its hub (to minimize dislodgement prior to surgery) with the needle tip as close to the lesion as possible and taped in place; check mammograms are made to determine the results and adjustments are made accordingly (localization within a centimeter or so usually suffices as long as the surgeon is adequately informed of these relationships). The surgeon cuts down on the needle to its tip and takes a small, nonmutilating biopsy, which is immediately roentgenogrammed to determine whether the suspect lesion is in the biopsy specimen or not. When the lesion is detected, the optimum site for histologic sectioning is localized for the pathologist. This or an equivalent biopsy procedure with biopsy specimen roentgenograms[12,16,34] is essential in nonpalpable or surgically nonvisualized lesions and demands wider application.

The following patients illustrate the role of mammography in the detection, diagnosis, and management of breast cancer:

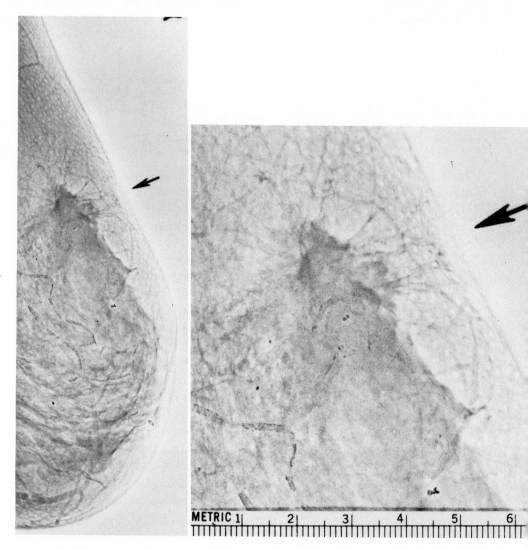

Fig. 4-1. A, Classical 1- to 2-cm stellate carcinoma blending with dysplastic breast tissue inferiorly and distended lymphatics extending to thickened and retracted overlying skin. **B,** Magnification demonstrates irregular fine punctate and linear microcalcifications with a tendency toward branching within the lower portion of this mass. There is marked duct prominence with coalescence and increased breast density (Wolfe DY). Note extensive arterial calcifications and scattered coarse benign calcifications elsewhere in this breast and how easily they are seen in comparison with malignant calcifications.

Patient #1: a classical stellate carcinoma of the breast

A 52-year-old multipara with a readily palpable 4- to 5-cm mass and minimal overlying skin changes in the upper outer quadrant of the left breast. Mammography (Fig. 4-1) revealed a classical 1- to 2-cm stellate carcinoma and dense dysplastic breasts (Wolfe DY).

Comment. This patient did not present any diagnostic difficulty either on physical examination or by mammography. It is shown as a classical mammographic example of carcinoma but also illustrates the discrepancy in size between physical examination and mammography and the apparent increased risk of developing cancer in markedly dysplastic breasts of this sort.

Patient #2: carcinoma of the breast obscured by dense dysplastic disease

A 55-year-old multipara with a long-standing history of lumpy, tender, and at times painful breasts difficult to examine. Mammography (Fig. 4-2) revealed a 1.5 cm stellate mass very suspicious of carcinoma in the left breast and dysplastic changes (Wolfe DY). Surgery revealed an infiltrating scirrhous ductal carcinoma (seventeen axillary lymph nodes were negative).

Comment. Comparison of the images of each breast as well as with previous studies accentuates any asymmetry. This illustrates the common problem of a carcinoma obscured by extensive dysplastic disease.

Patient #3: palpable carcinoma in one breast and nonpalpable carcinoma in the other breast

A 74-year-old nullipara with a palpable 3-cm mass in the upper part of the right breast. Mammography (Fig. 4-3) revealed fatty, low-density breasts (Wolfe N1) and a 1.5-cm stellate mass (smaller than on palpation) on the right but also revealed a smaller 1-cm nonpalpable stellate mass in the other breast. These were infiltrating ductal carcinomas (twenty right and ten left axillary lymph nodes were all negative).

Comment. This patient demonstrates the importance of mammography in asymptomatic as well as symptomatic breasts. Prior to the advent of mammography, the traditional approach would have been to biopsy the right breast (nothing else if the biopsy was benign) with subsequent mastectomy, and the lesion in the left breast would have been missed!

Patient #4: focal stellate architectural distortion

A 60-year-old asymptomatic multipara. Screening mammography (Fig. 4-4) revealed some duct prominence (Wolfe P1) and a subtle 8- to 9-mm stellate area of architectural distortion deep in the right breast near the chest wall suspicious of malignancy. This proved to be an infiltrating ductal carcinoma (nineteen axillary lymph nodes were negative).

Comment. This is the goal of mammography, namely to detect minimal lesions of this sort.

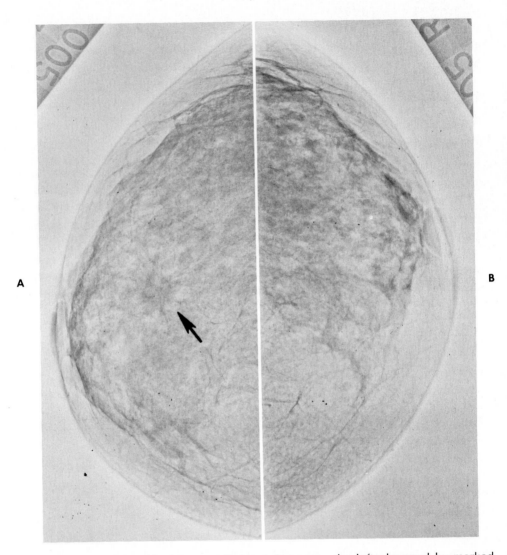

Fig. 4-2. A, Nonpalpable 1.5-cm stellate carcinoma on the left obscured by marked coalescent duct prominence and extensive breast density (Wolfe DY). **B,** This is more evident on comparison with the opposite breast.

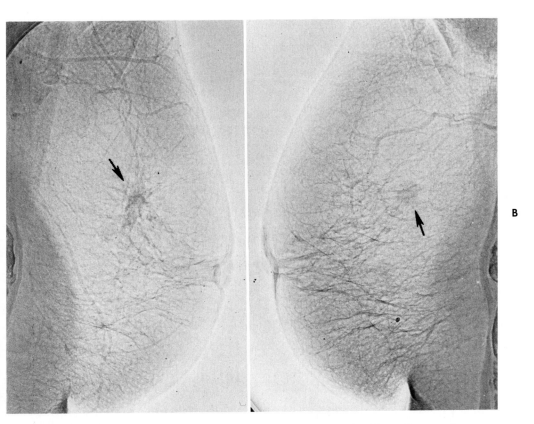

Fig. 4-3. A, Fatty low-density breasts (Wolfe N1) and 1.5-cm palpable stellate carcinoma on the right and, **B,** smaller 1-cm nonpalpable stellate carcinoma in other breast.

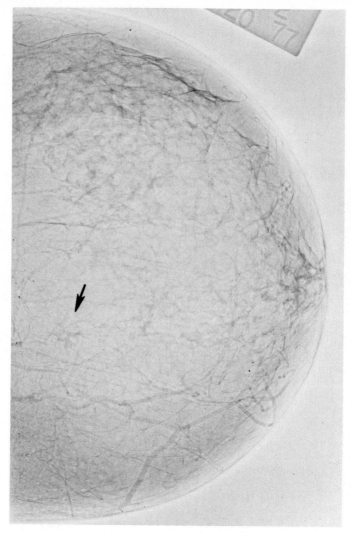

Fig. 4-4. Nonpalpable 8- to 9-mm stellate area of architectural distortion that proved to be carcinoma near the chest wall. There is some minimal duct prominence (Wolfe P1).

Patient #5: role of mammography in detection and management of nonpalpable lesions

A 45-year-old asymptomatic nullipara. Screening mammography (Fig. 4-5, *A* and *B*) revealed marked duct prominence (Wolfe P2), some suggestive architectural distortion, and some microcalcifications (best seen with magnification, Fig. 4-5, *B*) very suspicious of malignancy. Biopsy with preoperative mammography needle localization (Fig. 4-5, *C*) of the suspicious microcalcifications was

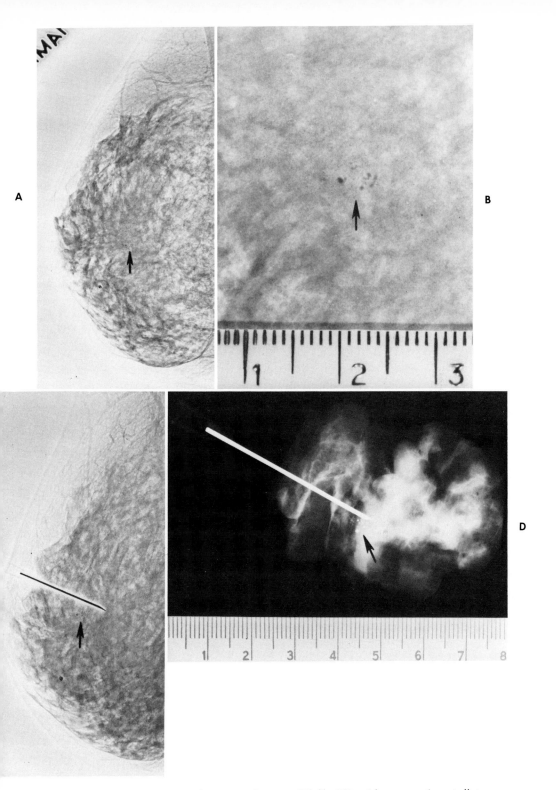

Fig. 4-5. A, Marked coalescent duct prominence (Wolfe P2) with suggestive stellate architectural distortion. **B,** Magnification better demonstrates small group of clustered, irregular microcalcifications in this stellate area. **C,** Prebiopsy mammography needle localization and, **D,** roentgenography of biopsy specimen that proved to be minimal duct carcinoma. (From McLelland, R.: Mammography in the detection, diagnosis and management of carcinoma of the breast, Surg. Gynecol. Obstet. **146:**735-740, May 1978. Reprinted by permission of Surgery, Gynecology, and Obstetrics.)

recommended as well as roentgenography of the biopsy specimen (Fig. 4-5, *D*) to verify that they had been resected. This was done and proved to be a minimal infiltrating ductal carcinoma and extensive fibrocystic disease (eleven axillary lymph nodes were negative).

Comment. The radiologist has an important role in the detection but also the diagnosis and management of asymptomatic, minimal lesions such as in this patient and patient #4.

Regarding benefits and risks of mammography,[18,33] it is important to realize that the controversy is in regard to annual screening mammography[31] of asymptomatic women under age 50 years (not symptomatic women, those at higher risk regardless of age, or those over age 50 years). This point is not widely appreciated by patients and physicians alike. Of the one third of our breast cancer patients in the screening setting, (Duke Breast Cancer Detection Demonstration Project) who are under age 50 years, about half of their cancers were detected by mammography alone and over 80% of these patients were free of axillary node metastases. There has been a similar experience with the other breast screening projects throughout the country and elsewhere. With earlier detection there will be increasing numbers of women in the younger age-group. The hypothetical risks of mammography[2,4,27] pale in comparison with these facts.[22,36] They are based on a combined breast screening experience with physical examination and less than optimum mammography about 15 years ago[29] and debatable if not improper extrapolations[5,8] from radiation exposures far in excess[3] of those delivered with current optimum mammography. This does not mean that radiation exposure should not be kept to a minimum. There are extensive ongoing efforts to do just that, but not at the expense of diagnostic information. In the meantime, this controversy has distracted if not confused some physicians, and frightened, if not prevented some women who should have mammography from having it done.

SUMMARY

Breast cancer is a staggering problem, and the main diagnostic effort is detection when the primary lesion is small, if not nonpalpable. Mammography, which has a major role and is essential in this effort, should be more widely applied. Although mammography is at least as important as palpation and the only means of detecting nonpalpable lesions, both examinations are most effective as complementary procedures.

Breast surgery for suspected cancer should never be done without preoperative mammography. Mammographic needle localization and biopsy specimen roentgenography are extremely useful, if not essential, in the surgical management of nonpalpable lesions.

Regarding screening, asymptomatic women should have a base-line mammogram at about 40 years of age but certainly by age 45 years. Depending on the mammographic appearance (Wolfe) and other risk factors (personal or family history of breast cancer), they should have mammography at 1- to 3-year intervals until 50 years of age and annually thereafter until some better detection procedure is available. It is beyond the scope of this presentation to discuss economic, personnel, and equipment limitations that currently prevent this.

REFERENCES

1. Axtell, L. M., and associates: End results in cancer (report no. 4): female breast, End Results Section, Biometry Branch, National Cancer Institute, 1972, pp. 99-105.
2. Bailar, J. C.: Mammography: a contrary view, Ann. Intern. Med. **84**(1): 77-84, 1976.
3. Beebe, G. W., and Kato, H.: Biological effects E: cancer other than leukemia, in review of thirty years study of Hiroshima and Nagasaki atomic bomb survivors, J. Radiat. Res. (Tokyo) (Suppl.) **16:** 97-107, 1975.
4. Breslow, L., Thomas, L. B., and Upton, A. C.: Final reports of National Cancer Institute Ad Hoc Working Groups on Mammography Screenings for Breast Cancer and a Summary Report of their Joint Findings and Recommendations, DHEW Publications No. (NIH) 77-1400, March 1977.
5. Bulletin 43, National Council of Radiation Protection and Measurements, 1975.
6. Dodd, G. D.: Present status of thermography, ultrasound and mammography in breast cancer detection, Cancer **39:**2796-2805, 1977.
7. Egan, R. L., and Mosteller, R. C.: Breast cancer mammography patterns, Cancer **40:**2087-2090, 1977.
8. Feig, S. A.: Can breast cancer be radiation induced? In Logan, W. W., editor: Breast carcinoma: the radiologist's expanded role, 1977, John Wiley & Sons, Inc., pp. 5-14.
9. Feig, S. A., and associates: Analysis of clinically occult and mammographically occult breast tumors, Am. J. Roentgenol. **128:**403-408, 1977.
10. Feig, S. A., and associates: Thermography, mammography and clinical examination in breast cancer screening, Radiology **122:**123-127, 1977.
11. Fisher, B., and associates: Cancer of the breast: size of neoplasm and prognosis, Cancer **24:**1071-1080, 1969.
12. Frank, H. A., and associates: Preoperative localization of non-palpable breast lesions demonstrated by mammography, N. Engl. J. Med. **295:**259-260, 1976.
13. Gardner, B.: Editorial: breast cancer revisited, J.A.M.A. **232:**742-743, 1975.
14. Gershon-Cohen, J., Hermel, M. B., and Murdock, M. G.: Priorities in breast cancer detection, N. Engl. J. Med. **283:**82-85, 1970.
15. Hainline, S., and associates: Mammographic patterns and risk of breast cancer, Am. J. Roentgenol. Radium Ther. Nucl. Med. **130:**1157-1158, 1978.
16. Horns, J. W., and Arndt, R. D.: Percutaneous spot localization of nonpalpable breast lesions, Am. J. Roentgenol. Radium Ther. Nucl. Med. **127:**253-256, 1976.
17. Leis, H. P.: The diagnosis of breast cancer, CA **27**(4):209-232, 1977.
18. Lester, R. G.: A radiologist's view of the benefit/risk ratio of mammography. In Breast carcinoma: the radiologist's expanded role, New York, 1977, John Wiley & Sons, Inc.
19. Martin, J. E.: Xeromammography, an improved diagnostic method: a review of 250 biopsied cases, Am. J. Roentgenol. **117**(1):90-96, 1973.
20. Martin, J. E.: Breast calcifications, benign or malignant? Scientific Exhibit, American Roentgen Ray Society Meeting, Washington, D. C., September 21-24, 1976.
21. McCarty, K. S., Jr., Kesterson, G. H. D., and Georgiade, N.: Histopathologic study of subcutaneous mastectomy specimens from patients with carcinoma of the contra-lateral breast, Surg. Gynecol. Obstet. **147:**682-688, November 1978.

22. McLelland, R.: Editorial: mammography in the diagnosis of breast cancer, N.C. Med. J. **37**(10):553-554, 1976.
23. McLelland, R.: Mammography in the detection, diagnosis and management of breast cancer, Surg. Gynecol. Obstet. **146:**735-740, 1978.
24. Mendell, L., Rosenbloom, M., and Naimark, A.: Are breast pattens a risk index for breast cancer? A reappraisal, Am. J. Roentgenol. **128:**547, 1977.
25. Moskowitz, M., and associates: Breast cancer screening: benefit and risk for the first annual screening, Radiology **120:**431-432, 1976.
26. Moskowitz, M., and associates: Lack of efficacy of thermography as a screening tool for minimal and stage I breast cancer, N. Engl. J. Med. **295**(5): 249-252, 1976.
27. National Research Council Advisory Committee on the Biological Effects of Ionizing Radiation, The Effects on Populations of Exposure to Low Levels of Ionizing Radiation: Report, National Academy of Sciences—National Research Council, 1972.
28. Peyster, R. G., Kalisher, L., and Cole, P.: Mammographic parenchymal patterns and the prevalence of breast cancer, Radiology **125:**387-391, 1977.
29. Shapiro, S.: Evidence on screening for breast cancer from a randomized trial, Cancer **39:**2772-2782, 1977.
30. Shapiro, S., and associates: Changes in five year breast cancer mortality in a breast cancer screening program, Seventh National Cancer Conference, Proceedings, Philadelphia, 1973, J. B. Lippincott Co.
31. Strax, P.: Control of breast cancer through mass screening, J.A.M.A. **235:**1600-1602, 1976.
32. Teixidor, H. S., and Kazam, E.: Combined mammographic-sonographic evaluation of breast masses, Am. J. Roentgenol. Radium Ther. Nucl. Med. **128:**409-417, 1977.
33. Thier, S. O.: Editorial: Breast cancer screening: a view from outside the controversy, N. Engl. J. Med. **297**(19):1063-1065, 1977.
34. Threatt, B., and associates: Percutaneous needle localization of clustered mammary microcalcifications prior to biopsy, Am. J. Roentgenol. **121:**839-843, 1974.
35. Wolfe, J. N.: Breast patterns as an index of risk for developing breast cancer, Am. J. Roentgenol. **126:**1130-1139, 1976.
36. Wolfe, J. N.: Editorial: mammography—a radiologist's view, J.A.M.A. **237**(20):2223-2224, 1977.

CHAPTER 5

Clinical significance of histopathologic lesions observed in subcutaneous mastectomy specimens

Kenneth S. McCarty, Jr., Gregg H. D. Kesterson, and Nicholas G. Georgiade

The earliest descriptions of the clinical and pathologic features of what we now call fibrocystic disease of the breast were provided from 1880 to 1892 by Reclus,[22] Brissaud,[2] and Schimmelbusch.[23] In their essays attention was directed toward the cystic dilation of the duct systems, whereas little emphasis was placed on the epithelial and stromal proliferative components present in the tissues. When Konig[10] added his descriptions in 1893, he expressed the belief that the breast changes observed were inflammatory in nature, and the term chronic cystic mastitis was added to further extend our misconceptions of the disease processes involved. Over the past 60 years the terms cystic mastitis complex, fibrocystic disease, cystic disease, fibrocystic mastopathy, and similar designations have been employed in studies attempting to correlate these entities with the risk of mammary carcinoma in prospective and retrospective studies.[18]

An association of breast cancer with "fibrocystic disease" and "cystic mastitis complex" have been drawn by some[4] and refuted by others.[3] Much of the disparity between the results of various studies can be traced to imprecise definition of terms. In many centers, a biopsy containing varying degrees of deviation from the nulliparous "normal" breast, but not found to contain carcinoma or a specific benign lesion such as fibroadenoma, will be called "fibrocystic mastopathy" or "cystic mastitis complex." When a careful examination of biopsy specimens is coupled with more precise classification (Table 5-1) of the changes observed within the tissues, a basis for communication and comparison of clinical-pathologic correlations of the various "benign" lesions of the breast is set. The first such study was published by MacCarty in 1913.[12] Numerous groups[26] have refined the techniques of tissue examination and classification while drawing together several lines of evidence to attempt to identify "premalignant" lesions of the breast[1] and distinguish them from "simple mastopathies."

The purpose of the present discussion is to demonstrate pathologic changes associated with various clinical findings in patients who have undergone sub-

Table 5-1. Classification of benign lesions of the breast*

I. Intraductal epithelial hyperplastic lesions
    Papillary hyperplasia
    Solid hyperplasia
    Cribriform hyperplasia
    Papillary/solid hyperplasia within focal area of single duct
    Papillary/cribriform hyperplasia within focal area of single duct
    Solid/cribriform hyperplasia within focal area of single duct
II. Persistent lobules in otherwise atrophic breast (focal/multifocal)
III. Lobular epithelial hyperplastic lesions
    Lobular hyperplasia
    Small cell lobular hyperplasia
IV. Metaplastic lesions
    Apocrine
    Squamous
V. Cystic duct dilation
    Microcystic change
    Macrocystic change
VI. Myoepithelial, stromal proliferations/adenosis
    Sclerosing adenosis
    Blunt duct adenosis
    Fibroadenomatous change (focal/multifocal)
    Interlobular stromal fibrosis
    Intralobular fibrosis (nonsclerosing)
VII. Inflammatory and/or degenerative changes
    Lymphocytic inflammation (focal/multifocal)
    Plasma cell mastitis
    Fat necrosis
    Scarring from previous trauma and/or biopsy
    Acute mastitis (focal/multifocal)

---

*Each category identified as to quadrant, subareola. Each category classified as mild, moderate, severe; atypia grades 1 to 5. Each category classified as to location in mammary ducts—terminal alveoli A to D.

cutaneous mastectomies for various specific indications other than overt malignancy (these indications are outlined in other chapters contained in this volume).

FAT NECROSIS

Whereas fat necrosis provides no difficulty histopathologically (Fig. 5-1), fat necrosis may present clinically as a palpable, firm to hard mass.[11] In instances in which there has been hemorrhage, calcification may become apparent as the hemorrhage is resorbed. This pattern may provide a lesion that is mammographically suspicious for carcinoma. In our experience the patient rarely recalls antecedent trauma unless a surgical procedure such as a biopsy has been previously performed.

The importance of this lesion is underscored when it is realized that fat necro-

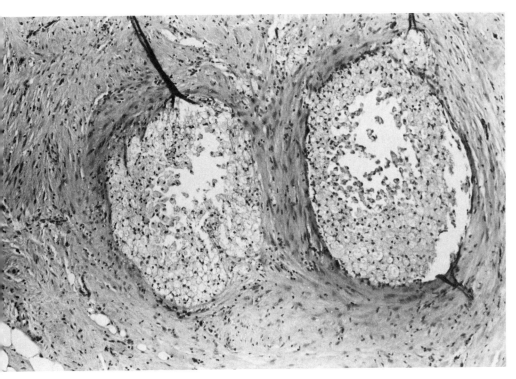

Fig. 5-1. Fat necrosis. Dissolution and fusion of individual fat cells accompanied by fibroblast and epithelioid cell cuffing is seen. There is a large concentration of histiocytes present. The lesion appeared grossly as an area of firm discolored tissue (H & E; 160X).

sis, to a greater or lesser extent, accompanies any biopsy of the breast. The granulomatous changes with their component fibrosis and histiocytic reaction (Fig. 5-1) may make the physical (and mammographic) examination of the multiply biopsied patient exceedingly difficult. Several subcutaneous mastectomy specimens in our series have contained evidence of multiple previous biopsies with resulting fat necrosis immediately proximal to a malignant tumor. The areas were no longer suspected because the changes observed were believed to be secondary to the previous biopsies. The subcutaneous mastectomy procedure, while providing corrective measures to the multiply scarred breast, provides an adequate specimen to assess changes that may be masked by these scars.

CYSTIC DUCT DILATION

Gross cystic duct dilation is a frequent source of palpable masses of the breasts. Multiple grapelike clusters of cysts or a single large cyst may provide the palpable mass. These structures tend to be pliable to fluctuant, but, when deep in the parenchyma, may be firm to palpation. The cysts tend to wax and wane with the menstrual cycle and are most prominent during the luteal phase (second half) of the cycle. A newly discovered cyst in a normally cycling young woman followed for 2 to 3 months often demonstrates its hormonally induced variation in consistency and size.[21]

If a prominent cyst continues to enlarge, aspiration may prove helpful to reassure the patient.[19] One difficulty with this procedure is the (rare) induction of inflammatory changes from hemorrhage or cyst fluid leaked from the cyst. This inflammation may lead to mastodynia or the development of a firm scar. Additionally, aspiration does not resolve the question of the presence of proliferative changes among the cyst complexes.

Some have suggested that the presence of gross cysts is associated with an increased risk of carcinoma.[6] No good evidence for the association of simple cystic change with its usual apocrine metaplasia (Fig. 5-2) with either a simultaneous or a subsequent increased risk of malignancy exists. The finding of cystic change in a breast with extensive intraductal epithelial hyperplasia represents a different category.[15] In the latter instance the epithelial proliferative change may obstruct the ducts with inspissation of secretions and dilation of ducts. The finding of intraductal epithelial hyperplasia does have a close association with cancer risk.[9,15]

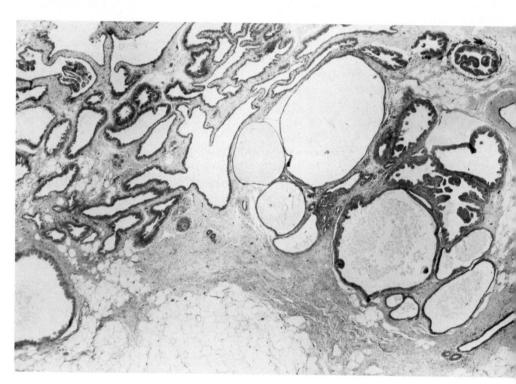

Fig. 5-2. Cystic duct dilation with apocrine metaplasia. Normal cuboidal epithelium lining ductule is replaced by larger columnar cells with characteristic eosinophilic cytoplasm and small, basal nuclei. This change is most often seen with cystic dilation of the ducts (H & E; 25X).

In the premenopausal woman cystic change should be carefully examined and the size or sizes of the cysts recorded. The patient may then be reexamined after three normal menstrual cycles (reexamination should be performed during the follicular phase of the menstrual cycle) and the lesion sizes carefully documented. If the changes are persistent despite normal menstrual cycling (anovulatory cycles are often associated with persistent proliferative changes) or if aspiration fails, histopathologic evaluation is indicated. This histopathologic examination is optimally performed during the early follicular phase of the menstrual cycle. If severe intraductal epithelial hyperplasia is present, a glandular extirpation may be preferred over repeated biopsies of the cystic complexes. More often, however, the histopathologic finding in the premenopausal patient during this phase of the cycle is simple cystic (Fig. 5-2). The finding of multiple microcysts or apocrine metaplasia is of no clinical significance.[13]

Cystic masses in the distinctly postmenopausal patient (who may have unopposed estrogen from peripheral conversion of adrenal androstenedione)[24] should be approached more aggressively in terms of seeking a histopathologic diagnosis. In the setting of unopposed estrogen, cysts are often associated with epithelial proliferative changes. The finding of simple cystic change (as in Fig. 5-2) is likely to reflect an androgen-progestin stimulation of estrogen-primed ducts and is not closely associated with cancer. Cystic change may be managed conservatively unless the patient has other risk factors for carcinoma and multiple biopsies become a part of the problem.

FIBROADENOMA

Two aspects of the fibroadenoma make it a lesion of particular interest to the clinician. It is frequently observed and produces a distinct mass lesion. In the United States the fibroadenoma is the third most common breast tumor in women.[5] It shows a propensity for youth, being the tumor most often encountered in women under the age of 25.[25] Because of the solid tumorous nature of the lesion, needle aspirations are unsuccessful in reducing or diagnosing the mass and biopsy is often required.

An area of fibroadenomatous change can offer a variety of signs. Most frequently this lesion presents a small (2- to 3-cm diameter) unilateral, painless tumor that is firm, yet resilient. The tumor grows slowly, usually taking months to double in size, is freely movable in the surrounding breast stroma, and is often seemingly encapsulated. These tumors do not produce retraction signs. Fibroadenomas may appear anytime after puberty (usually before age 25 years). Large adenofibromas may occur in perimenopausal, middle-aged women (age 40 to 50 years) who are often experiencing anovulatory cycles. Multifocal fibroadenomas sometimes occur as multiple bilateral masses, either developing at the same general time period or appearing recurrently.[20]

A specimen of breast tissue containing a fibroadenoma gives a characteristic gross and microscopic appearance. The lesion has a sharply delimited, nonfixed focus of neoplasia easily separated from the surrounding tissue. While still *in situ* the mobility of the area suggests an encapsulated mass. The specimen usually reveals no true capsule but rather a compressed nonreactive stroma encircling the tumor. The cut surface may vary from glistening white to dull brown in color, reflecting the glandular epithelial content and/or stromal cellularity. Microscopically areas of fibroadenomatous change display a lobulated, circular to ovoid tumor consisting primarily of proliferative fibrous tissue with a frequently hyperplastic glandular epithelium, often compressed into cords by the proliferation of the connective tissue (Fig. 5-3).

Carcinoma of either the alveolar or ductal epithelium is rarely found associated with fibroadenoma. The adenofibroma may, however, show hyaline change and/or dystrophic calcification, which can create worrisome mammographic signs. Infarction of the larger tumors may create central areas of necrosis providing a more ominous macroscopic appearance. Although not associated with malignancy, the mass effect of recurrent or multiple fibroadenomas often precipitates repeated biopsy, providing the difficulties associated with the multiply biopsied breast.

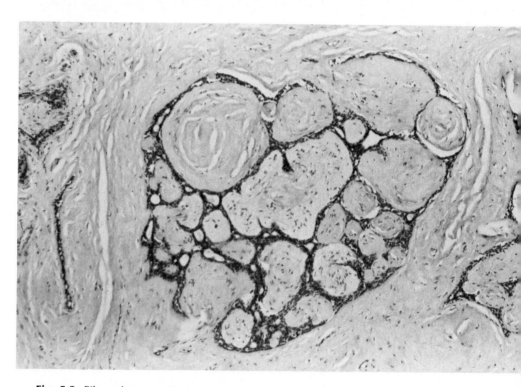

Fig. 5-3. Fibroadenoma. Lesion appears grossly as a firm, encapsulated nodule. Cut surface is grey white. Microscopically two components are present—branching tubular ducts, which usually comprise a double layer of inactive appearing epithelial cells, and dense, variably cellular stroma (H & E; 25X).

MASTITIS

True mastitis, focal or multifocal, is often associated with mastodynia. Mastitis may be either acute or chronic; the tissue-containing plasma cells or other mononuclear cell infiltrates in the periductal stroma, often perineurally. The lesion may be the result of reaction to cystic fluid expressed from dilated ducts or may be secondary to infection of ductal secretions, often with anaerobes. In the latter instance a response to a broad-spectrum antibiotic may be gratifying. In instances in which the inflammatory change and mastodynia are chronic and refractory to conservative management, glandular mastectomy with reconstruction may provide a satisfactory means of achieving relief. Mastitis per se has no association with carcinoma.

SCLEROSING ADENOSIS

Sclerosing adenosis is of major clinical significance because of its gross and microscopic resemblance to carcinoma.[16] This lesion has no increased association

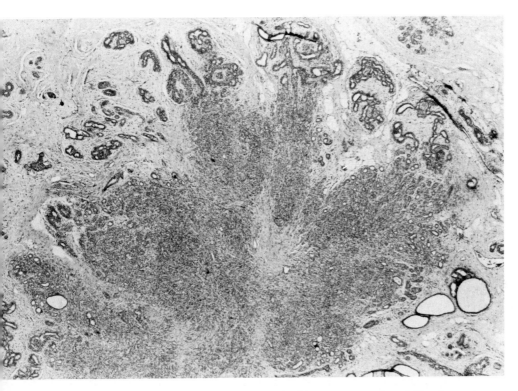

Fig. 5-4. Sclerosing adenosis. Presence of a palpable mass or of multifocal poorly delimited firm areas make this lesion grossly similar to carcinoma. Microscopic characteristics of marked myoepithelial proliferation combine with fibrous scarring to modify typical alveolar formation, producing a pattern of parenchymal cells resembling superficially the pattern of an invasive malignancy (H & E; 25X).

with the presence of, or risk of developing, carcinoma.[14] An area of sclerosing adenosis frequently is seen as a palpable mass. Such an area is often firm, but less so than most palpable carcinomas. These lesions appear relatively circumscribed, or they may be diffuse with coarse margins. Mammograms of breasts containing areas of sclerosing adenosis provide difficulty in interpretation, particularly when the pattern of the lesion is that of slightly separated lobules contracting in the center (Fig. 5-4). In many instances the lesion presents as a contracted mass density in a relatively fatty stroma (Fig. 5-5). A disconcerting picture on mammography is also seen when subepithelial calcifications are present (Figs. 5-6 and 5-7). The experienced mammographer, however, readily recognizes the dystrophic calcification (see Chapter 9).

The microscopic pattern of sclerosing adenosis is variable (Figs. 5-4 to 5-7). A prominent element in these lesions is the proliferation of the myoepithelial cells.[7] In the postmenopausal, estrogen-deficient patient, a predominance of fibrotic change is noted in the lesion, as opposed to the more florid epithelioid

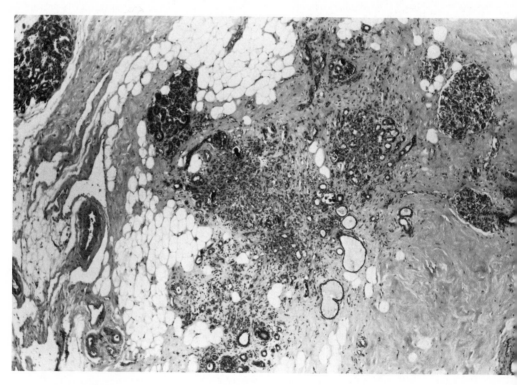

Fig. 5-5. Sclerosing adenosis. Disorganized epithelial pattern of sclerosing adenosis is seen in association with dilated ducts that produce a macroscopic appearance of a firm brown-tan retracted area with numerous blue-domed cysts. Focal areas of dystrophic calcification in a subepithelial location are noted (H & E; 25X).

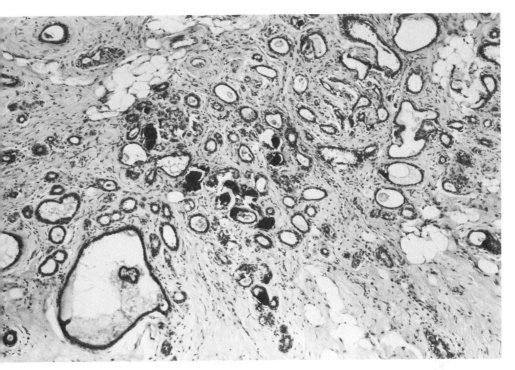

Fig. 5-6. Sclerosing adenosis. Pattern is dominated by myoid cell elongation and proliferation. Extensive subepithelial calcification is present. The complex is associated with cysticly dilated ducts (H & E; 63X).

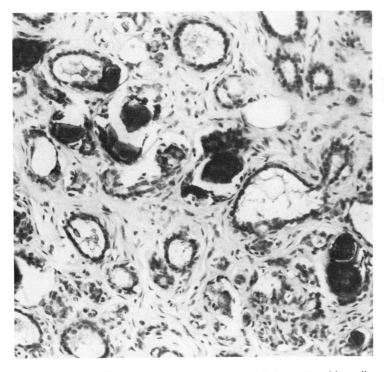

Fig. 5-7. Subepithelial calcifications. Ductules contained deposits of lamellar calcification located between basement membrane and epithelial cells. Several ducts contain inspissated secretions, which have calcified intralumenally (H & E; 320X).

(Fig. 5-4) lesions seen in younger women or those treated with estrogenic steroids.[8] Sclerosing adenosis may persist apparently unchanged through the menopause and is observed in postmenopausal patients.

LOBULAR HYPERPLASIA AND PERSISTENT LOBULES

Lobular hyperplasia has no distinct clinical presentation. It is a change observed in premenopausal patients or patients on estrogenic hormones. It may be seen in women who have galactorrhea. The degree of hyperplasia often has distinct variation with the menstrual cycle. The observation of prominent lobular hyperplasia in a postmenopausal woman should prompt a search for a source of estrogens. A common source for exogenous estrogen in postmenopausal patients is cosmetic creams containing pregnenolone or similar estrogen precursors. There is often significant absorption of the hormone applied by this route. No increased association of lobular hyperplasia with breast cancer is seen. The postmenopausal "persistent" lobular hyperplasia seen in the absence of exogenous or endogenous hormone stimulation has been suggested to have greater significance in relation to carcinoma, although this remains to be proved.

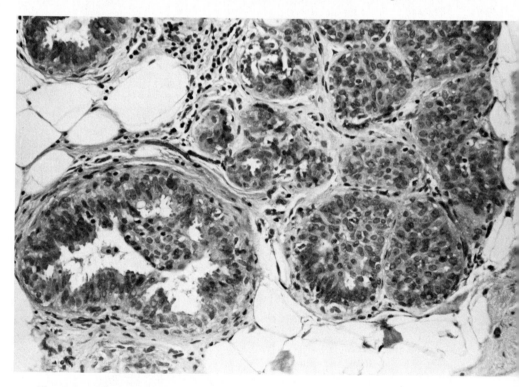

Fig. 5-8. Early epithelial proliferative change. Glandular epithelial lining of alveoli assumes a papillary pattern (lower left field) and a solid pattern (upper right field) as it encroaches on lumenal space; normal columnar cell type is lost in hyperplastic ingrowth (H & E; 320X).

INTRADUCTAL EPITHELIAL HYPERPLASIAS

The intraductal epithelial hyperplasias rarely are seen as distinct clinical entities but are more often found in biopsy material obtained because another lesion was observed clinically. Intraductal papillomatosis may be associated with a bloody nipple discharge, and the discharge may lead to a biopsy being performed.

The intraductal epithelial hyperplasias comprise a whole spectrum of degrees of proliferative change. These lesions have a significant association with carcinoma.[15,17] Indeed in some specimens the "benign" intraductal proliferative changes blend imperceptibly with *in situ* or invasive malignant components. The early forms of proliferative change (Fig. 5-8) often vary with ovarian function, whereas the more severe forms are associated with prolonged noncyclic estrogens or are not hormonally responsive. The proliferative forms in which a cribriform pattern is assumed (Fig. 5-9 and 5-10) most closely resemble intra-

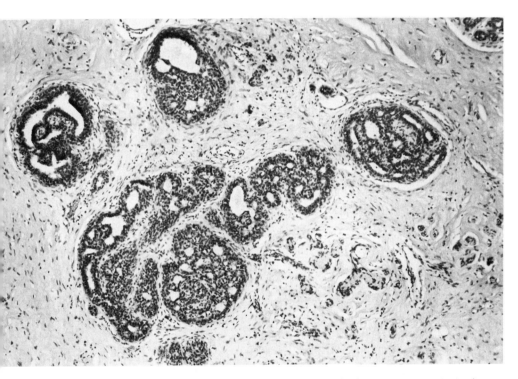

Fig. 5-9. Intraductal epithelial hyperplasia, papillary and cribriform patterns. A single duct is sectioned at different angles through its tortuous course and displays nearly complete occlusion by proliferative epithelium. Lesion presents both papillary (upper left and right fields) and cribriform (lower center field) patterns, suggesting steady ingrowth of parenchyma progressing from papillary to cribriform. The stromal stalks of the papillae are evident at their base (H & E; 80X).

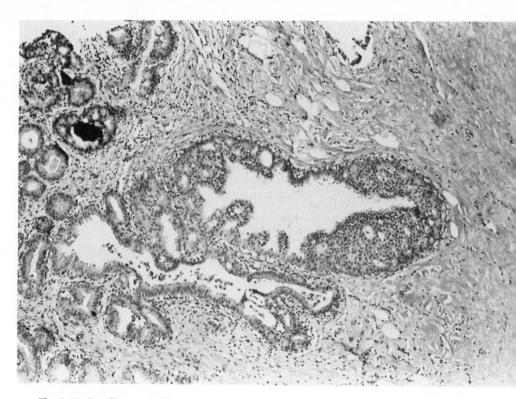

Fig. 5-10. Papillary, cribriform intraductal epithelial hyperplasia with microcalcifications. Ductal epithelium is seen to form an amorphous mass of cells with pseudogland formation (cribriform pattern) as it proliferates into lumen. Two areas of calcification are noted in the upper left field *(arrows)* (H & E; 126X).

ductal carcinoma (Fig. 5-11). The solid and cribriform patterns are both closely associated with carcinoma.[17] It is these lesions that warrant the most intense scrutiny to discern if they indeed represent "premalignant lesions."

CARCINOMA

Carcinoma has been found in 6% of the nearly 600 subcutaneous mastectomy specimens in our series. Of these, all but one (Fig. 5-12) have been *in situ* or minimally invasive lesions of histologic grade I or II. The average size of the tumors has been 0.3 cm³ (3 mm³), reflecting the careful screening that the patients undergo prior to the election of the subcutaneous mastectomy procedure. The means of processing the breast tissue to allow adequate examination of the glandular mastectomy specimen is outlined in Chapter 9.

The role of subcutaneous mastectomy in overt cancer is controversial at best. In the tumor-bearing patients in our series, however, the procedure has provided the opportunity to diagnose lesions at an early stage as well as to provide

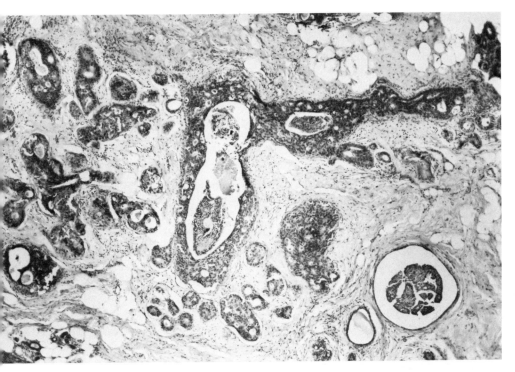

Fig. 5-11. Intraductal carcinoma. Photograph includes total extent of this lesion (0.2 cm maximum diameter), which displays classic findings of intraductal malignancy—cells stain darkly basophilic, high nuclear/cytoplasmic ratio, central necrosis, and cribriform arrangement of epithelium. Occasional bizarre mitoses are seen (H & E; 80X).

resection of the "minimal" tumors without major mutilation. Careful 10- and 15-year follow-up of this population is needed to confirm the effectiveness of this approach.

CONCLUSIONS

The majority of commonly observed lesions of the breast are clinically important because of the production of symptoms of severe mastodynia or because of their resemblance to malignant tumors. A classification of breast lesions in which epithelial proliferative lesions are distinguished from stromal proliferative, simple cystic, and involutional lesions provides much greater prognostic acumen to the clinician. Several of the lesions are associated with specific clinical findings. Examples of such lesions are shown in Figs. 5-1 to 5-10. Tumors found in our subcutaneous mastectomy specimens have, for the most part, been small lesions and noninvasive (see Figs. 5-11 to 5-15). The careful preoperative screening of the patient is emphasized so that the optimal procedure may be selected

Text continued on p. 84.

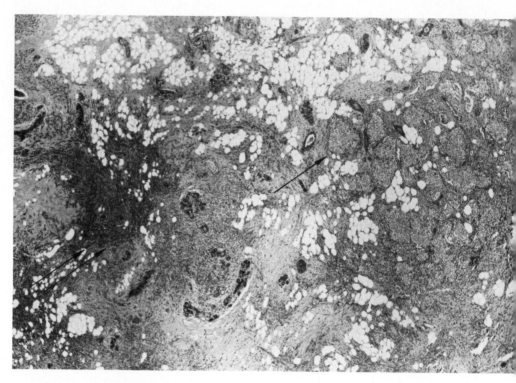

Fig. 5-12. In situ and infiltrating lobular carcinoma. Alveoli are replaced by "in situ" component of lobular carcinoma *(single arrow)*. Stroma is diffusely invaded by linearly arranged cells *(double arrows)* typical of invasive lobular carcinoma (H & E; 25X).

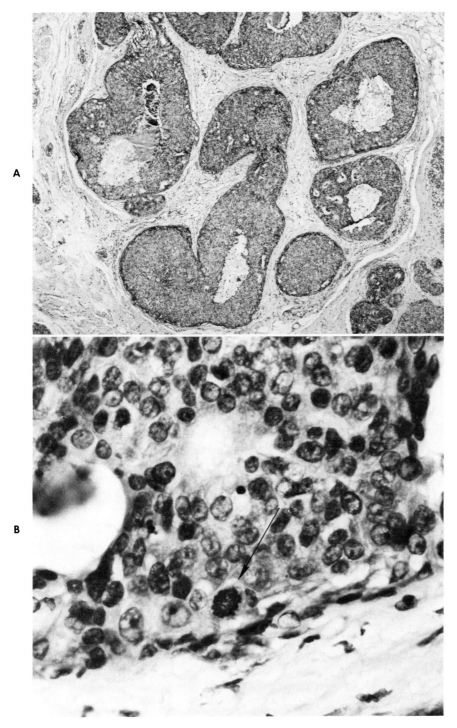

Fig. 5-13. Intraductal comedocarcinoma. **A,** This malignant lesion measured 3 mm³ in toto. Ducts are occluded by pleomorphic basophilic epithelial cells. There is central necrosis. **B,** High-power inset illustrates disorganized cellular pattern and example of one of many atypical mitotic figures seen *(arrow)* (H & E; **A,** 40X; **B,** 100X).

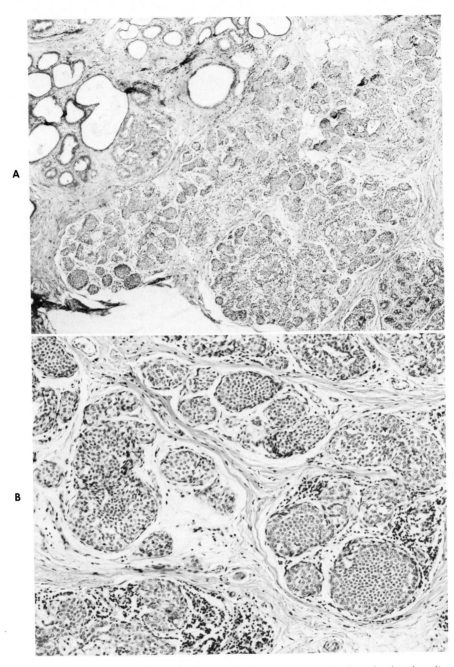

Fig. 5-14. A, Lobular carcinoma in situ. Lobule composed of multiple alveoli, each distended by homogeneous sheets of epithelial cells that are one and one half to twice the size of normal alveolar epithelial cells. This is characteristic of lobular carcinoma in situ. **B,** Uniform cell type present in alveoli; alveolar basal lamina is intact (H & E; **A,** 40X; **B,** 100X).

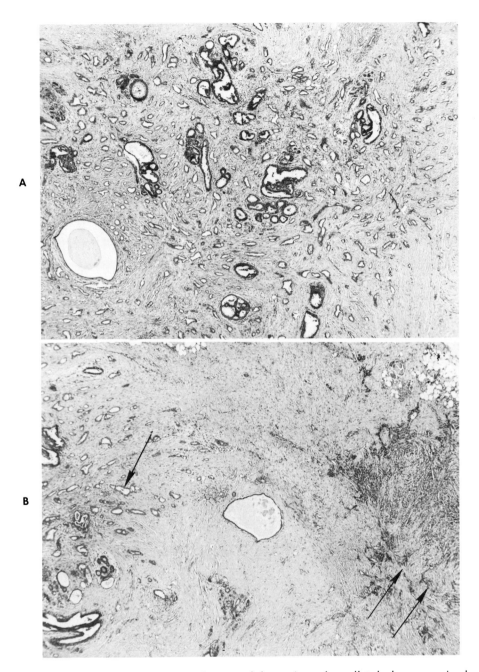

Fig. 5-15. A, Tubular carcinoma. Structural formation of small tubules comprised of single layer of pleomorphic small cells invading fibrous stroma (H & E; 40X). **B,** Tubular carcinoma in close proximity to deposition of hemosiderin pigment. *Double arrows,* Area of tubular carcinoma; *single arrow,* foci of hemosiderin pigment, mononuclear inflammatory response, and dense fibrosis produced by previous biopsy of the site. Small size of carcinoma (2.5 mm³) and biopsy scar combined to prevent detection of lesions until breast was removed and carefully sectioned (H & E; 25X).

preoperatively. Certain lesions are recognized as of greater potential significance than others (Figs. 5-9 and 5-10).

ACKNOWLEDGMENT

These studies supported by National Cancer Institute NO1-CB-63996 and NO1-CB-84223.

REFERENCES

1. Black, M. M., and associates: Association of atypical characteristics of benign breast lesions with subsequent risk of breast cancer, Cancer **29:**338-343, 1972.
2. Brissaud, E.: Anatomic pathological de la malade kystique des mamells, Arch. Physiol. Norm. Pathol. **3:**98, 1884.
3. Davis, H. H., Simons, M., and Davis, J. B.: Cystic disease of the breast relationship to carcinoma, Cancer, **17:**957-978, 1964.
4. Donnelly, P. K., Balner, K. W., Carney, J. A., and O'Fallon, W. M.: Benign breast lesions and subsequent breast carcinoma—in Rochester, Minnesota, Mayo Clin. Proc. **50:**650-656, 1975.
5. Haagensen, C. D.: Adenofibroma of the breast, Haagensen, C. D., editor: Diseases of the breast, ed. 2, Philadelphia, 1971, W. B. Saunders Co., pp. 212-226.
6. Haagensen, C. D.: Cystic disease of the breast. In Haagensen, C. D., editor: Diseases of the breast, ed. 2, Philadelphia, 1971, pp. 155-175.
7. Hamperl, H.: Uber die myothelien (myo-epithelialen elements) der brustchuse, Virchows Arch. [Pathol. Anat.] **305:**171-215, 1939.
8. Huseby, R. A., and Thomas, L. B.: Histological and histochemical alterations in the normal breast tissues of patients with advanced breast cancer being treated with estrogenic hormones, Cancer **7:**54-74, 1954.
9. Jensen, H. M., Rice, J. R., and Wellings, S. R.: Preneoplastic lesions in the human breast, Science **191:**295-299, 1976.
10. Konig, F.: Mastitis chronica cystica, Controlbl. Chir. **20:**49, 1893.
11. Kuzma, F. J.: Breast. In Anderson, W. A. D., and Kissane, J. M., editors: Pathology, ed. 7, St. Louis, 1977, The C. V. Mosby Co., vol. 2, pp. 1780-1781.
12. MacCarty, W. C.: The histogenesis of cancer (carcinoma) of the breast and its clinical significance, Surg. Gynecol. Obstet. **17:**441-459, 1913.
13. Marcuse, P. M.: Fibrocystic disease of the breast; correlation of morphologic features with the clinical course, Am. J. Surg. **103:**428, 1962.
14. McCarty, K. S., Jr., Kesterson, G. H. D., and Georgiade, N.: Rationale for subcutaneous mastectomy of the contralateral breast in patients with breast carcinoma. In Georgiade, N. G., editor: Reconstructive breast surgery, St. Louis, 1978, The C. V. Mosby Co.
15. McCarty, K. S., Kesterson, G. H. D., and Georgiade, N.: Histopathology of subcutaneous mastectomy specimens from patients with carcinoma of the contralateral breast, Surg. Gynecol. Obstet. **147:**682-688, 1978.
16. McDivitt, R. W., Stewart, F. W., and Berg, J. W.: Tumors of the breast, ed. 2, Atlas of tumor pathology, No. 2, 1968, pp. 133-137.
17. Nizze, H.: Fibrous mastopathy and epitheliosis in the opposite breast of mammary carcinoma patients, Oncology **28:**319-330, 1973.
18. Nomura, A., Cornstock, G. W., and Tanascia, J. A.: Epidemologic characteristics of benign breast disease, Am. J. Epidermiol. **105:**505-512, 1977.
19. Olch, I. Y.: On the treatment of gross cysts of the breast by aspiration, International Union against Cancer, **15:**1145, 1962.

20. Oliver, R. L., and Major, R. C.: Cyclomastopathy: a physiopathological conception of some benign breast tumors with an analysis of 400 cases, Am. J. Cancer **21:**1, 1934.
21. Patey, D. H., and Nurick, A. W.: Natural history of cystic disease of the breast treated conservatively, Br. Med. J. **1:**15, 1953.
22. Reclus, P.: La maladie kystigue des mamelles, Rev. Chir. **3:**761, 1883.
23. Schimmelbusch, C.: Das cystadenom der Mamma, Arch. Klin. Chir. **44:**117, 1892.
24. Vermeulen, A.: The hormonal activity of the postmenopausal ovary, J. Clin. Endocrinol. Metab. **42:**247-253, 1976.
25. Walsin, J. H.: Large breast tumors in adolescent females, Ann. Surg. **152:**151, 1960.
26. Wellings, S. R., Jensen, H. M., and Marcu, R. G.: An atlas of subgross pathology of the human breast with special reference to possible precancerous lesions, J. Natl. Cancer Inst. **55:**231-243, 1975.

CHAPTER 6

Surgical management of fibrocystic disease of the breast

Nicholas G. Georgiade and Ronald Riefkohl

HISTORY

Adenomammectomy or subcutaneous mastectomy has been performed for many years. Thomas,[35] in *On the Removal of Benign Tumors of the Mamma without Mutilation of the Organ,* published in 1882, discussed his rationale for the removal of benign tumors of the mammary gland through an inframammary incision. Bartlett[1] in 1917 further expounded on the total excision of the glandular tissue through an inframammary incision. He restored the breast contour by filling the resultant defect with an excess of adipose tissue since he believed that there was a definite psychologic need for restoration of a reasonable breast form. Lexer[18] employed a thoracomammary incision to extirpate the total glandular tissue and rotated axillary fatty tissue to reconstruct the breast. Rosenauer[29] used free fat transplants to restore breast contour, but in his two cases there was considerable absorption of the implanted fatty tissue. Berson[2] formed the breast contour by transplantation of derma-fat-fascia and claimed that this reduced the degree of absorption. Maliniac,[22] Marino,[24] Longacre,[19,20] Letterman and Schurter,[16] and De Cholnoky[5] reconstructed breast contour following total en bloc excision of the glandular tissue of the breast by utilizing a variety of dermal-fat pedicle flaps and dermal-fat fascia transplants. Malbec[21] inserted a hollow acrylic mold into the breast defect to establish breast contour.

Freeman[7] was the first to recommend that a subcutaneous mastectomy be performed through a submammary incision with immediate or delayed insertion of a prosthesis to restore the breast contour. Zbylski[37] modified this technique by applying the dermal-pedicle technique of Strombeck to reposition the nipple Later Marino and Solian[23] reported a similar approach. Goulian and McDivitt[12], Georgiade and Hyland,[9] and Weiner and associates[36] described combining subcutaneous mastectomies with dermal pedicle flaps, simultaneously correcting breast ptosis and/or hypertrophy of the breast. Horton, Adamson, Mladick, and Carraway[15] and Rubin[31] advocated using the nipple-areolar complex as a free graft in reconstruction of the breasts following subcutaneous mastectomy. Since these studies there have been numerous reports in the literature regarding subcutaneous mastectomy and breast reconstruction.*

The surgical technique for the resection of benign, possibly premalignant breast tissue including the so-called cystic mastitis complex is currently widely practiced. Technical improvements have made possible the removal of a maximum amount of breast tissue with minimal resultant deformity.

The selection of patients for subcutaneous mastectomy is controversial and probably will remain so for many years until sufficient data pertaining to this patient population have been accumulated. Nevertheless, certain criteria such as the following have been used to determine a reasonable basis for selection of patients who are considered to be in the higher risk group for carcinoma.

1. Histologic evidence of extensive dysplastic changes, particularly atypia and intraductal solid or cribiform epithelial hyperplasia
2. Lobular carcinoma *in situ*
3. Papillomatosis with atypia
4. Cytosarcoma phylloides
5. A family history for breast carcinoma (especially bilateral)
6. A combination of multi-risk factors in a patient with epithelial proliferative fibrocystic disease
7. Postmenopausal persistent breast nodularity and/or persistent epithelial proliferative changes in the postmenopausal patient not taking exogenous estrogens
8. Management of the contralateral breast postablative surgery for carcinoma of one breast, particularly in patients with lobular or multifocal intraductal carcinoma
9. Patients having multiple previous biopsies revealing epithelial proliferative lesions who subsequently develop scarring that prevents adequate physical or mammographic examination
10. Severe mastodynia associated with fibrocystic disease
11. Patients with true mastitis with recurrent infection of cysts that are not responsive to conservative management
12. Cancerphobia in patients with severe fibrocystic disease

PREOPERATIVE EVALUATION

The preoperative selection of patients is extremely important. The principles governing this evaluation are based on the previously outlined indications. Thus patients who are candidates for the subcutaneous procedure are selected, whereas those who would best be followed for a period of time and those who have evidence of invasive malignancy are eliminated. The identification of patients with clinically overt malignancy permits the general surgeon member of the

*See references 3, 6, 8, 11, 13, 26, 27, and 32.

breast team to apply more conventional extirpative surgery to these patients in consultation with the reconstructive surgeon.

The preoperative evaluation includes examination of the breast by at *least two experienced* examiners in addition to the referring obstetrician, surgeon, or internist. The examination is performed in all standard positions for breast examination and includes careful attention to the axillae and supraclavicular region. The examination is augmented by the use of xeromammography and mammograms. All previous biopsy material is obtained, and the histopathology is reviewed with careful attention to the temporal course of these biopsies in relation to medications and menstrual status.

The family history with respect to breast disease is carefully pursued, as is the patient's endocrinologic status and history. The emphasis is placed on menstrual history, thyroid and pituitary status, age at birth of first child, and parity.

OPERATIVE PROCEDURE

The subcutaneous tissues at the periphery of the breast are infiltrated with 0.5% lidocaine (Xylocaine) containing 1:200,000 epinephrine in order to minimize small vessel bleeding and thus blood loss during the operative procedure.

Fiberoptic illumination and optical magnification have been found to be indispensable for visualizing the breast parenchyma and maximizing the excision of breast tissue.

The curvilinear submammary incision has been employed for approximately

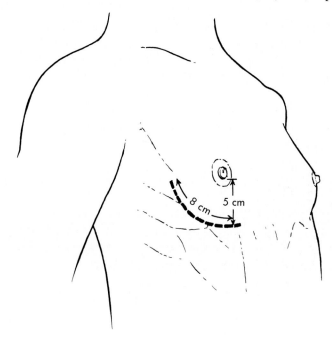

Fig. 6-1. Curvilinear submammary incision, which is used on 85% of our subcutaneous mastectomies.

85% of our 900 subcutaneous mastectomies. The incision is extended 8 to 10 cm laterally along a 5- to 5½-cm line drawn vertically from the inferomedial aspect of the nipple (Fig. 6-1). The incision is deepened directly to the pectoralis major muscle, establishing the initial plane of dissection, which is then extended superiorly to the superior border of the pectoralis major muscle in a relatively avascular plane.

The second phase of the glandular excision is initiated inferiorly utilizing *sharp dissection* to separate the glandular tissue at the fatty-subdermal level. This layer of fat varies in thickness with the individual female. Dissection is continued superiorly, excising the ligaments of Cooper as encountered. In order to facilitate the dissection, the breast excision is started at the medial aspect

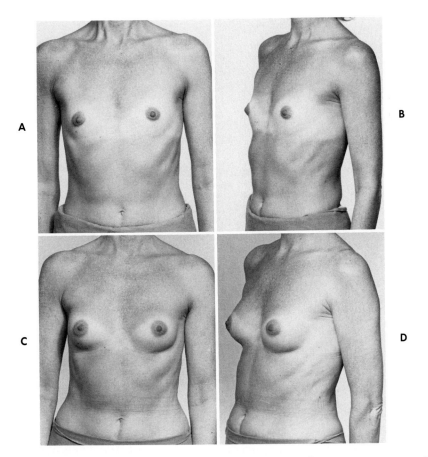

Fig. 6-2. A, Preoperative front view of 42-year-old patient with recurrent masses of the breasts necessitating biopsies. A bilateral subcutaneous mastectomy was performed with simultaneous augmentation with a 165-ml gel-filled prosthesis. **B,** Preoperative lateral view of same patient. **C,** Nineteen-month postoperative front view of same patient. **D,** Nineteen-month postoperative lateral view of same patient.

of the glandular tissue and with *sharp dissection* the mammary tissue medial to the nipple-areolar complex is released. The dissection is then started along the lateral aspect of the breast and directed medially; however, the upper outer quadrant of the breast is not excised at this time. A 3-0 silk suture is placed through the tissue at the base of the nipple during the excision of the breast tissue in order to identify this area for special pathologic evaluation by the pathologist in the breast team. Only a small layer of breast tissue, approximately 0.5 cm in thickness, is left beneath the nipple-areolar complex. The remaining breast is excised by dissecting the superior and lateral segment of the mammary tissue, including the tail of Spence, which extends to the axillary region. The

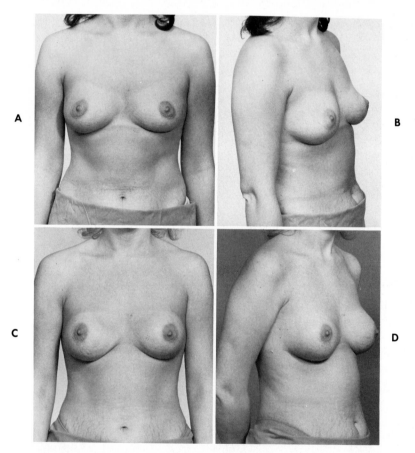

Fig. 6-3. A, Preoperative front view of 27-year-old patient with 10-year history of fibrocystic disease of the breasts necessitating multiple biopsies. At the time of surgery this patient had multiple cysts with severe mastodynia. A bilateral subcutaneous mastectomy was carried out with the immediate insertion of 225-ml gel-filled Georgiade Surgitek prostheses. **B,** Preoperative lateral view of same patient. **C,** Three-year postoperative front view of same patient. **D,** Three-year postoperative lateral view of same patient.

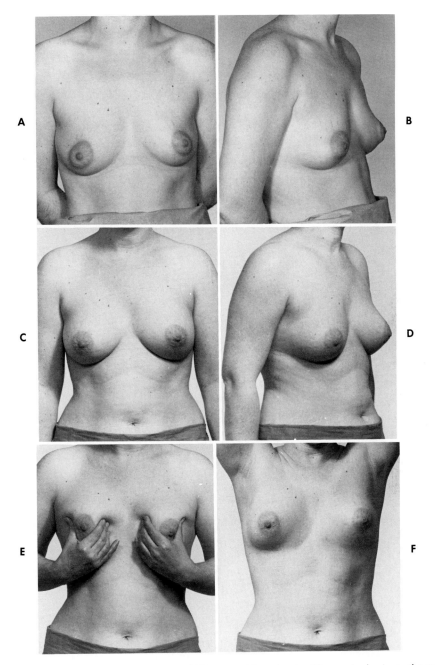

Fig. 6-4. A, Preoperative front view of 27-year-old patient with mastodynia and severe fibrocystic disease of the breasts. A bilateral subcutaneous mastectomy was performed with simultaneous augmentation. **B,** Preoperative lateral view of same patient. **C,** Four-year postoperative front view of same patient. **D,** Four-year postoperative lateral view of same patient. **E,** Four-year postoperative view to show softness of breasts and lack of capsular formation. **F,** Four-year postoperative view to show excellent contour and motion of breasts.

specimen is removed and the axillary tail of the breast is always labeled for proper orientation in the subsequent gross, subgross, and histologic evaluation.

After meticulous hemostasis is obtained with electrocautery, the breast envelope and parameters of excision are carefully examined for any small residual remnants of ligaments of Cooper or breast tissue, which are removed while preserving the fatty layer.

The resultant cavity is irrigated with bacitracin solution (50,000 U/500 ml of normal saline). Through a small stab wound 2 cm inferior to the incision at its lateral aspect, a suction drain is inserted and placed into the lateral most dependent area and axilla. A suitably sized teardrop-shaped prosthesis is inserted superficially to the pectoralis major muscle and oriented so that the apex aligns with the axillary tail area. We prefer a Georgiade Surgitek* 185- or 225-ml gel-filled Silastic† prosthesis. A 3-0 plain catgut suture is used to approximate the midlateral border of the pectoralis major muscle and the lateral skin flap. This suture prevents the lateral displacement of the prosthesis. The incision is then approximated with 4-0 white nylon sutures in the deepest layer, followed by 5-0 Vicryl‡ sutures in the dermal layer and interrupted 6-0 Prolene‡ sutures for the skin edges (Figs. 6-2 to 6-4).

Subpectoral implantation

In approximately 25% of the standard subcutaneous mastectomies, the subcutaneous fatty layer is so thin that the viability of the nipple-areolar complex or even the breast skin envelope may be in question. The operator at this point must decide whether to insert a prosthesis at all. If a delayed insertion, 2 to 3 months later, is preferable, immediate insertion of a thin Silastic† sheet designed to maintain a portion of the pocket may be considered.

The subpectoral implantation opens an additional operative plane, and it may be advisable to defer subpectoral augmentation until the subgross and microscopic evaluation of the breast specimen, which has been serially sectioned, has been completed by the pathologist. By the third postoperative day it is usually possible to proceed with the placement of the prosthesis at the subpectoral-subserratus muscle level, if the histopathologic findings indicate that it is feasible. Access to the subpectoral plan is best accomplished through an incision 6 to 8 cm in length and 4 to 5 cm inferior and lateral to the infralateral border of the pectoralis major muscle, directly on the sixth rib (Fig. 6-5). The dissection is carried out carefully superiorly under the serratus anterior muscle, along the rib cage, and under the pectoralis major muscle. The dissection is extended in this plane superiorly to the inferior clavicular area and laterally above the pectoralis minor muscle, incising the lateral attachments of this muscle. This muscle then re-

*Medical Engineering Corp., Racine, Wis.
†Dow Corning Corp., Midland, Mich.
‡Ethicon, Sommerville, N.J.

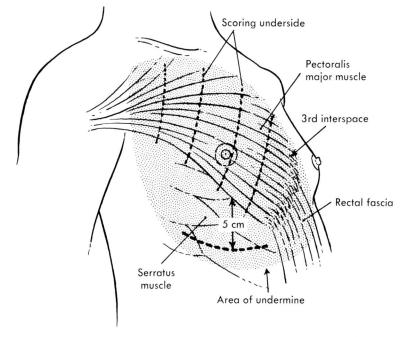

Fig. 6-5. Surgical incision utilized for access to subpectoral plane. Note that approach to subpectoral area is via a 6-cm incision through serratus muscle. Dotted area shows area of undermining. Dotted lines designate incisions that are placed partially through pectoralis muscle to allow additional projection of prosthesis when inserted.

mains as the floor on which the prosthesis will be placed. An important surgical maneuver is to extend the sharp dissection inferiorly 6 cm into the lateral rectus sheath and also release the medial attachments of the pectoralis major muscle to their fascial attachment superior to the level of the third intercostal interspace, but still leaving the sternal attachments of the pectoralis muscle. A Deaver type retractor is particularly helpful in exposing the pectoralis major muscle medial attachments as well as the perforating branches of the internal mammary vessels, which are coagulated as encountered. If the pectoralis major muscle resists forward projection, several incisions placed partially through the muscle across its width will further release the muscle and allow additional projection of the prosthesis when inserted (Fig. 6-5). Thorough hemostasis is secured with the electrocautery, and the operative area is again irrigated with a normal saline and bacitracin solution (50,000 bacitracin per 500 ml normal saline). A suction drain is inserted through a stab wound inferior to the skin incision as previously described. Following this a Georgiade double lumen Surgitek prosthesis of appropriate size is filled with a solution containing 10 mg of methylprednisolone sodium succinate (Solu-Medrol) and 30 to 40 ml of saline in the outer compartment. The amount of solution added to the outer envelope depends on the size

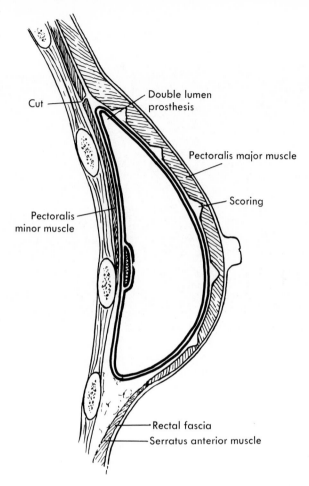

Fig. 6-6. Anatomic placement of double-lumen prosthesis subpectorally. Note scoring of undersurface of pectoralis muscle.

of the prosthesis desired. (The usual amount is 225 to 265 ml.) The prosthesis is inserted and carefully positioned with the greater projection of the prosthesis slightly below the nipple. The cut edges of the serratus anterior muscle are joined and sutured over the inferior portion of the prosthesis with 4-0 white nylon, thus completely covering the prosthesis with this muscle layer (Fig. 6-6). This is followed by a second layer of 4-0 white nylon sutures approximating the deep layer of the skin incision. Interrupted 5-0 Vicryl sutures are placed in the dermal layer and 5-0 or 6-0 Prolene sutures are used to approximate the skin edges. The same procedure is repeated on the opposite side.

The characteristic looseness of the skin that is invariably seen is redraped into the desired position, utilizing a skin adherent and paper tape for 10 to 14 days.

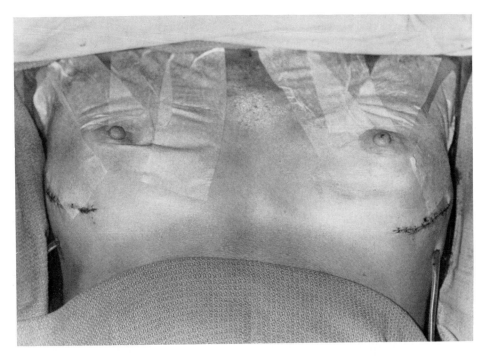

Fig. 6-7. Redraping of skin utilizing skin-adherent paper tape.

This will allow the slightly ptotic breast to be positioned in a more suitable location (Figs. 6-7 and 6-8).

A large bulky dressing with mechanic's waste is used to surround each breast mound, and rolls of 10-inch stockinette cut on the bias are then applied in a figure eight to stabilize the breasts, (Fig. 6-9). The dressing is split on the first postoperative day to inspect the breasts for possible hematoma formation or pending skin necrosis. The drains are maintained until a maximum of 30 ml/day drainage is attained, usually 3 to 4 days. Ambulation is started once the drains have been removed. The patient is discharged on the sixth or seventh postoperative day, at which time the skin sutures are removed but not the tape used to elevate the breast skin.

Subcutaneous mastectomy—hypertrophied breast

The management of the hypertrophied breast in those patients who are candidates for subcutaneous mastectomy usually presents a multitude of problems such as performing an adequate subcutaneous mastectomy and reduction mammaplasty, with satisfactory breast contouring, correction of the existing ptosis, and finally the simultaneous augmentation mammaplasty.

To attain these goals accurate measurements of the breasts must be obtained

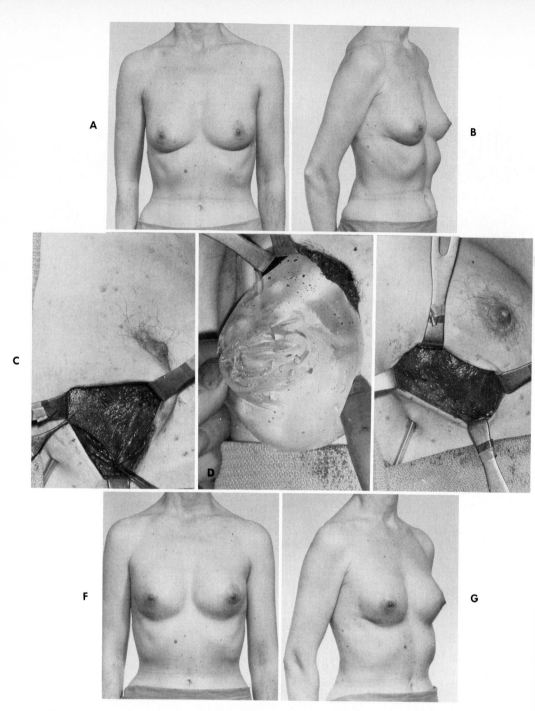

Fig. 6-8. A, Preoperative front view of 40-year-old patient who had had multiple biopsies over the past 12 years. Xeromammograms were consistent with severe dysplastic changes. Patient's mother had died of breast cancer at 63 years of age. A bilateral subcutaneous mastectomy was performed. Because of thinness of subcutaneous fatty layer, prostheses were inserted subpectorally. Georgiade double-lumen Surgitek prostheses consisting of an inner compartment filled with 185 ml of gel and an exterior compartment filled with 20 ml of normal saline containing 10 mg of methylprednisolone sodium succinate (Solu-Medrol)) were utilized. **B,** Preoperative lateral view of same patient. **C,** Serratus anterior muscle layer is exposed. **D,** Double-lumen prosthesis was inserted below pectoralis major muscle. **E,** Serratus anterior muscle is sutured over inserted prosthesis, thus completely covering prosthesis. **F,** One-year postoperative front view of same patient. **G,** One-year postoperative lateral view of same patient.

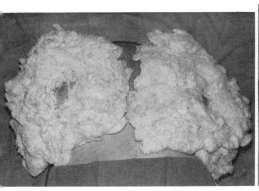
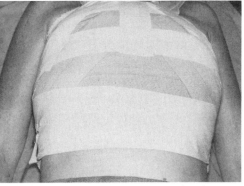

B

Fig. 6-9. A, Mechanic's waste positioned over reconstructed breasts. **B,** Large bulky dressing covering mechanic's waste consists of rolls of 10-inch stockinette cut on the bias and applied in a figure eight manner to stabilize the breasts.

preoperatively with the patient in a standing position. The desired key points for the new location of the nipples can be correctly judged and the size of the breast flaps established.

A number of surgical techniques have been described. The most successful of these techniques involves a dermal pedicle, interposed from any number of directions, separating the skin flaps and skin closure from the prosthesis.

The use of an inferiorly based dermal fat flap in larger breasts is an acceptable method[16,17] (Fig. 6-10). Spira[33] has also described the use of an inferiorly based dermal flap that is attached to the inferior border of the pectoralis muscles after placing the prosthesis in the subpectoral area (Fig. 6-11). Our preference, and the procedure utilized most frequently, involves a wide, vertical dermal fat pedicle flap that is as wide as possible yet still conforms to the final outline form of the breast. The prosthesis is usually placed above the pectoralis and serratus anterior muscles. The dermal pedicle flap originally described for a reduction mammaplasty has been modified to meet the surgical requirements of a subcutaneous mastectomy.[4,25,28] This type of dermal flap will allow the largest area of protection between the skin flaps and implant and still allow viability of the nipple-areolar complex. In the very large hypertrophied breast the nipple-areolar complex is removed as a free graft and then replaced after the new breast mound has been created following resection of breast tissue with the implant being placed either suprapectorally or infrapectorally, depending on the thickness of the subdermal fatty layer.[31]

Surgical technique. Preoperatively the measurements are outlined in brilliant green dye with the patient in a standing position. The new nipple site is located along the midclavicular line approximately 22 cm from the sternal notch (Fig. 6-12). Adjustments in configuration or measurements are made according to the

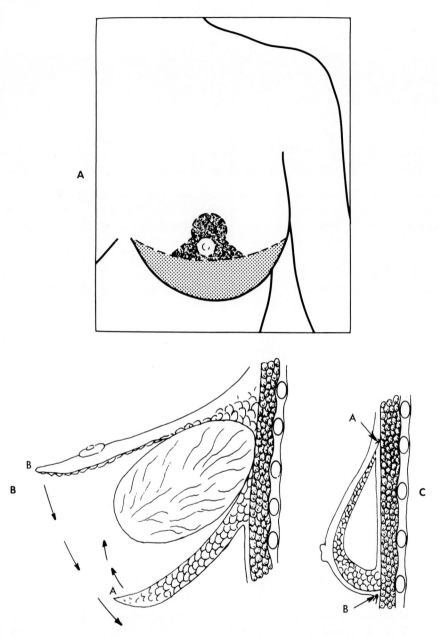

Fig. 6-10. A, Periareolar shaded area represents dermal flaps to be used in maintaining vascularity of nipple. Dotted zone inferior to this dotted line represents inferior dermal flaps, which will be transferred superiorly. **B,** Flap designated *A* represents inferior dermal flap shown in **A** from side view and is moved superiorly. Flap designated *B* and carrying areola is brought inferiorly outside of dermal flap *A*. **C,** Final positions of dermal flaps *A* and *B* are shown around prostheses.

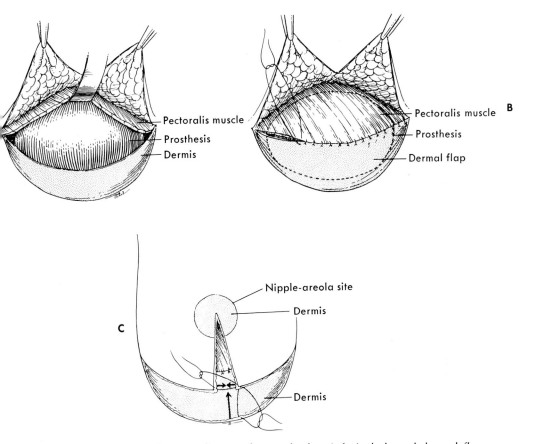

Fig. 6-11. A and **B,** Use of pectoralis muscle attached to inferiorly based dermal flap protecting prosthesis. **C,** Skin flaps are positioned over dermal pectoralis muscle flap. Free nipple-areolar graft is then placed in its proper location.

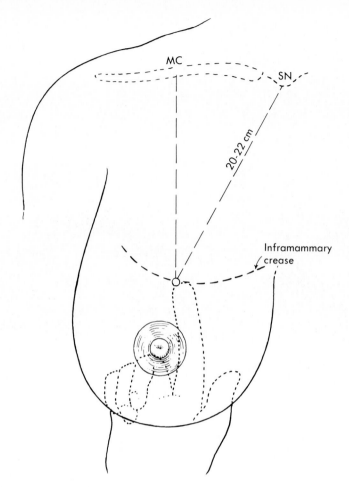

Fig. 6-12. Determination of new nipple site in recontouring of hypertrophied breast. Most superior portion of new areola is usually located at level of inframammary crease. Position of new areola is at bisection of midclavicular line.

projection of the inframammary crease. The proper distance between the skin flaps is judged by the ability to approximate redundant breast in the inferior areolar area and also at points 5 cm inferiorly (Fig. 6-13). The width at the base usually varies from 10 to 14 cm. The skin between the markings subsequently will be partially deepithelialized. A small, flexible, preformed, steel wire loop with centimeter markings on the limbs allows the surgeon to quickly outline the new areolar circumference as well as mark the vertical limbs of the new breast flaps, usually 5 cm in length (Fig. 6-14). The remaining tissue in the inframammary area

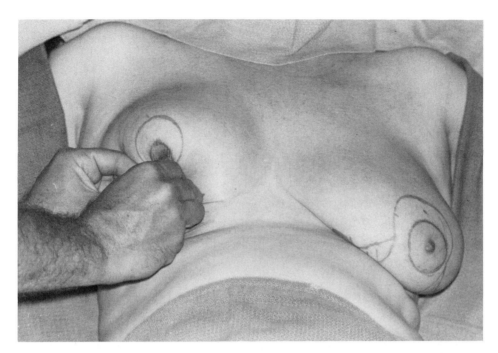

Fig. 6-13. Determination of proper distance between skin flaps is judged by ability to approximate redundant breast tissue comfortably for approximately 6 cm inferior to nipple. The points are then marked at the points considered to yield a satisfactory breast cone, and width of one breast at the base is compared to width of the other breast.

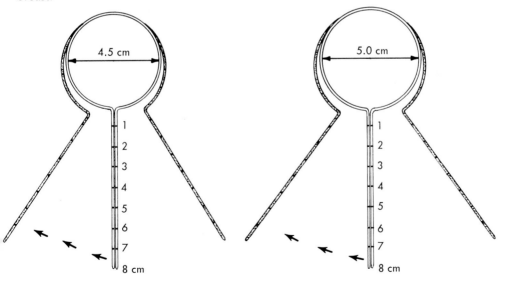

Fig. 6-14. Diagram of flexible steel loop wires available in two areolar diameters to mark position and circumference of new areola and borders of breast flaps. Arms of wires are serrated in centimeters in order to mark new flap length accurately.

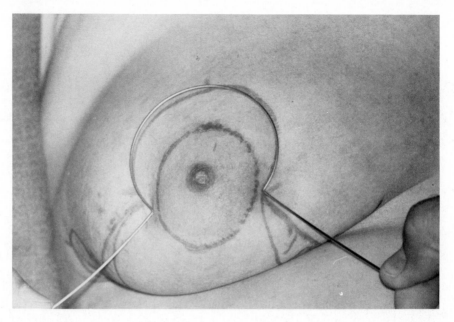

Fig. 6-15. Utilization of flexible wire loop to expedite outlining new areolar circumference in relation to previously determined width. Length of flaps (usually 5 cm) is then marked from wire arms.

is marked for excision to within 1 cm of the inframammary crease (Fig. 6-15). The inferior dermal pedicle is designed with as wide a base as possible. If the length of the inferior flap exceeds the width by 50%, another type of procedure should be considered in which a free nipple-areolar complex graft is utilized, such as the procedure described by Rubin.[30]

Operative procedure. Under general orotracheal anesthesia and in a supine position, the patient's outstretched arms are slightly adducted and contained in a special steel frame. The entire shoulders, chest, and upper abdominal areas are prepared with three layers of povidone-iodine (Betadine) surgical scrub followed by povidone-iodine solution. The chest is then draped as a sterile field and the drapes are secured in place with skin sutures.

The previously outlined breast pattern, including the lateral flaps, is reinforced with brilliant green (Figs. 6-16 and 6-17). Sutures are placed on the superior and inferior ends of the flaps. A thick split-thickness of skin is then excised within the outline, resulting in the appropriate dermal pedicles (Fig. 6-18). Through a lateral incision that extends the length of the vertical dermal pedicle and approximately 2 cm along the areolar border, the lateral skin flaps are developed and separated from the breast tissue (Fig. 6-19). The dermal fatty layer should be preserved to minimize the chance of nipple-areolar necrosis and skin necrosis. The dissection is extended to the pectoralis major muscle and then superiorly and medially. A second vertical incision is made along the medial

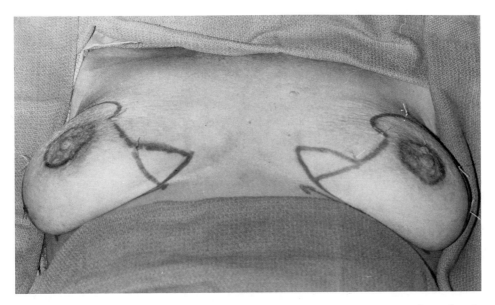

Fig. 6-16. Markings of breast flaps are shown. Note sutures at corners of previously marked new breast flaps.

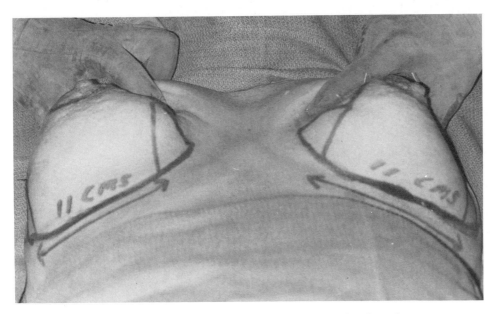

Fig. 6-17. Width of breast dermal flaps to be developed.

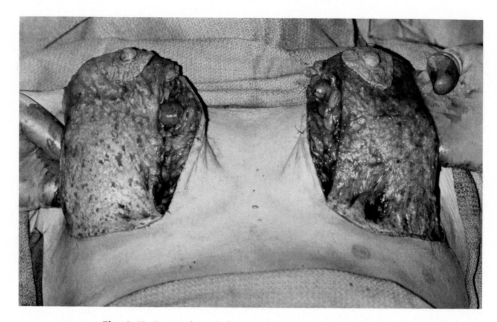

Fig. 6-18. Dermal pedicle nipple-areolar bearing flaps.

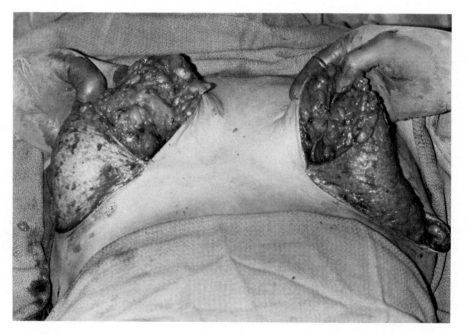

Fig. 6-19. Medial and lateral skin flaps dissected free from breast tissue.

aspect of the vertical dermal pedicle in a similar manner, and the breast tissue is separated from the skin flaps and from the dermal pedicle flap. About 0.5 cm of breast tissue is allowed to remain at the base of the nipple-areolar complex. The corresponding area on the specimen of the nipple base is marked with a suture for separate histopathologic evaluation. The final dissection is carried superiorly to the axilla, freeing the tail of Spence, which is tagged for proper orientation. After hemostasis by coagulation has been attained, the operative area is inspected utilizing magnification and fiberoptic illumination to ascertain that no visible remnants of breast tissue are present. A suction drain is inserted through a stab wound 2 cm inferior to the incision.

The skin flaps are now approximated accurately in respect to the previously placed marking sutures. A suitably sized breast prosthesis is inserted, usually a 185- or 225-ml Georgiade Surgitek gel-filled prosthesis. The dermal edges are incised lightly and approximated with 3-0 and 4-0 white Vicryl sutures (Fig. 6-20). The final step in tailoring the breast involves the medial and lateral portions of the skin flaps. If there is considerable redundancy remaining in these areas, a V-type of closure is carried out in order to minimize extension of the incisions and resultant scars toward the midline. This type of closure is also carried out laterally. The skin is sutured with interrupted and running 5-0 Prolene. A dressing of mechanic's waste gauze is placed over and around the breast

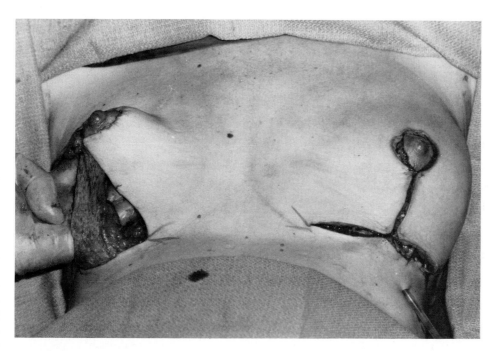

Fig. 6-20. Approximation of breast dermal flaps following insertion of suitably sized breast prosthesis.

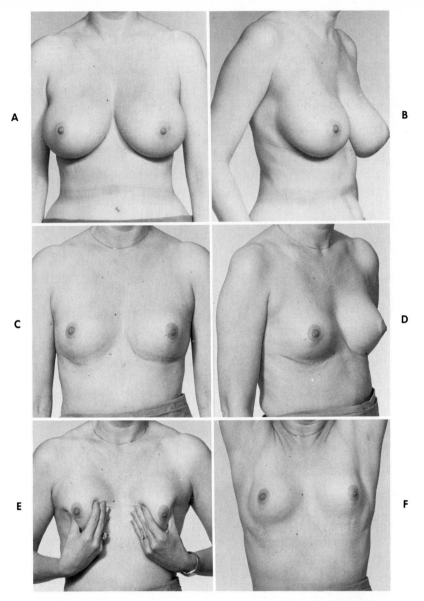

Fig. 6-21. A, Preoperative front view of 40-year-old patient with macromastia, masto-dynia, and severe fibrocystic disease of the breasts. A reduction mammaplasty utilizing bipedicle vertical flaps, correction of ptosis, and bilateral subcutaneous mastectomy with immediate insertion of 225-ml Georgiade Surgitek gel-filled prostheses was per-formed. **B,** Preoperative lateral view of same patient. **C,** Twenty-two–month post-operative front view of same patient. **D,** Twenty-two–month postoperative lateral view of same patient. **E,** Twenty-two–month postoperative view of same patient illustrating lack of capsular contracture and softness of breasts. **F,** Twenty-two–month postopera-tive view of same patient illustrating excellent contour and motion of recontoured breasts.

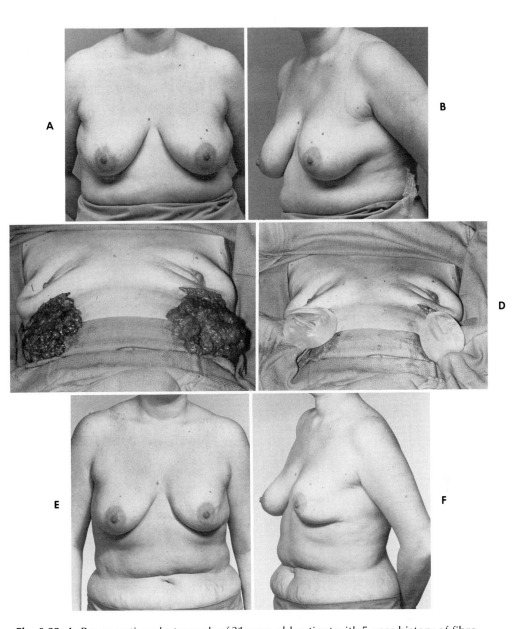

Fig. 6-22. A, Preoperative photograph of 31-year-old patient with 5-year history of fibrocystic disease of the breasts with severe mastodynia. Patient had familial history of breast cancer. A bilateral subcutaneous mastectomy was performed with simultaneous augmentation mammaplasty with insertion of 260-ml prostheses. **B,** Preoperative lateral photograph of same patient. **C,** Breast specimens that were removed by sharp dissection. **D,** Prostheses prior to insertion. **E,** Three-year postoperative photograph of same patient exhibiting capsular contracture and ptosis. **F,** Three-year postoperative lateral photograph of same patient.   *Continued.*

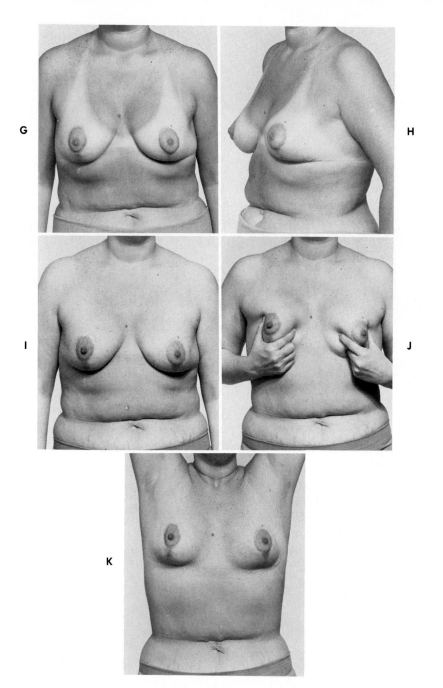

Fig. 6-22, cont'd. G, Front view of patient 3 months after correction of ptosis and release of capsular contractures with removal of prostheses and insertion of 185-ml gel-filled Georgiade Surgitek prostheses. **H,** Lateral view of patient 3 months after correction of ptosis and release of capsular contractures. **I, J,** and **K,** Postoperative views of patient 1 year after correction of ptosis and release of capsular contractures. Breasts are soft and have an excellent contour.

mounds, and rolls of 10-inch stockinette cut on a bias are used as a figure eight to add sufficient support and snugness, minimizing the possibility of prosthesis displacement. The breasts are exposed in 24 hours for inspection for possible hematoma formation and for nipple-areolar viability. The dressing is reapplied and maintained for 7 days, after which time the sutures are removed and the patient is given a brassiere, preferably a Warner* model style 1078 (Figs. 6-21 to 6-25).

Moderate hypertrophy with associated ptosis

The simplest technique to correct the ptotic breast with some hypertrophy involves the marking of the new areolar position in the usual manner, utilizing the preformed loop wire, which is available in two areolar diameters, 4.5 and 5 cm (Fig. 6-14). Once the circumference of the new areola is outlined in brilliant green, the amount of redundant skin in the inferior areola is determined by approximating sufficient skin to create a satisfactory cone as described previously (Fig. 6-26, *A*). Partial deepithelialization of this entire outlined area is now carried out (Fig. 6-26, *B* and *C*).

A semicircumscribed incision is made 5 cm below the inferior areolar area for a distance of 8 cm. Through this incision the subcutaneous mastectomy is completed. A suction drain is inserted in the lateral inferior aspect through a skin stab wound. A Georgiade Surgitek 185-ml prosthesis is then inserted under the dermal fat flap and skin envelope. If this skin dermal fat flap is considered to be too thin, subpectoral implantation should be considered. The dermal flaps are approximated and the nipple-areolar complex is sutured in position with interrupted 5-0 Prolene sutures. The skin edges of the dermal flap are approximated with interrupted subcuticular 4-0 Vicryl sutures. The skin closure is completed with interrupted 5-0 Prolene sutures for the vertical limb and a continuous suture for the inframammary component.

This technique is excellent for correction of ptosis that does not necessitate greater than a 2-cm lift (Fig. 6-27). When the nipple-areolar complex is elevated only with difficulty, incising and creating a wedge-shaped dermal flap at least 5 to 6 cm in length facilitates elevation of the nipple-areolar complex yet still allows adequate approximation of the dermal components that form a layer of dermis between the skin flaps and the prosthesis (Figs. 6-28 and 6-29).

DISCUSSION

Technically the objective of a subcutaneous mastectomy is to remove all breast tissue except for an approximately 0.5-cm button underlying the nipple and areolar complex. The glandular tissue removed must be carefully oriented and marked with the base of the nipple-areolar complex appropriately identified for the pathologic evaluation. It is mandatory that the entire glandular specimen

*Warnaco Inc.

Text continued on p. 117.

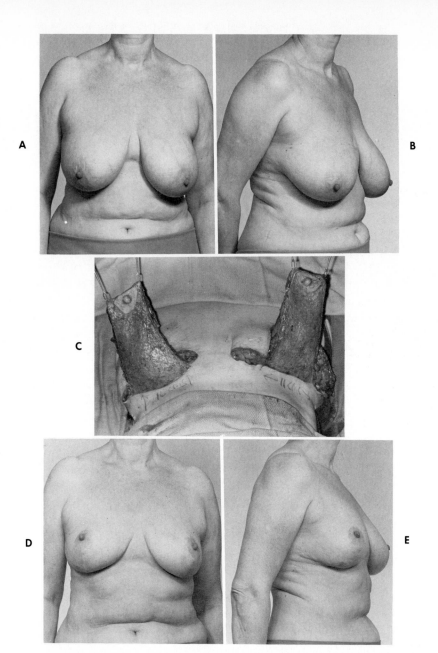

Fig. 6-23. A, Preoperative front view of 46-year-old patient who had 20-year history of fibrocystic disease of the breast. She had had palpable nodules in upper outer quadrant of left breast for 1 year. A reduction mammaplasty and subcutaneous mastectomy with simultaneous augmentation were performed. A wide inferior pedicle flap was utilized in performing the reduction mammaplasty, at which time 420 g of breast specimen was removed from left breast and 450 g from right breast. **B,** Preoperative lateral photograph of same patient. **C,** Operative photograph of bipedicle flap with wide-based inferior pedicle flap. **D,** One-year postoperative front view of same patient. **E,** One-year postoperative lateral view of same patient.

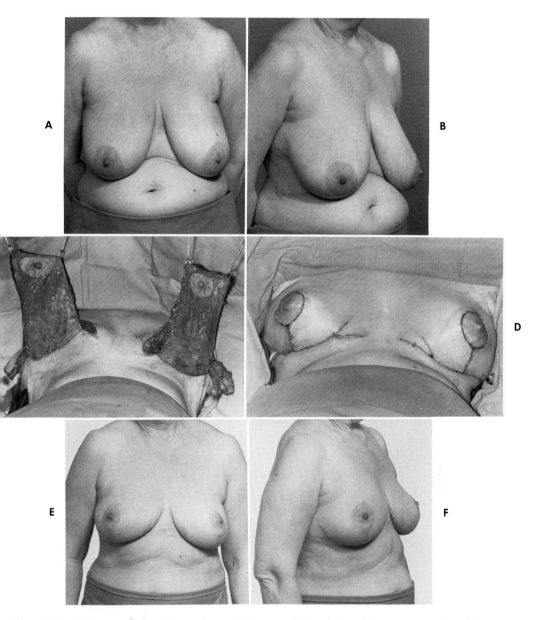

Fig. 6-24. A, Preoperative front view of 64-year-old patient with macromastia with severe fibrocystic disease of the breasts. A reduction mammaplasty utilizing vertical broad-based inferior pedicle flaps was carried out simultaneously with a subcutaneous mastectomy and immediate augmentation. **B,** Preoperative lateral view of same patient. **C,** Operative view showing bipedicle flap with wide-based inferior pedicle. **D,** Operative view showing immediate postoperative closure of newly contoured breasts. **E,** Ten-month postoperative front view of same patient. **F,** Ten-month postoperative lateral view of same patient.

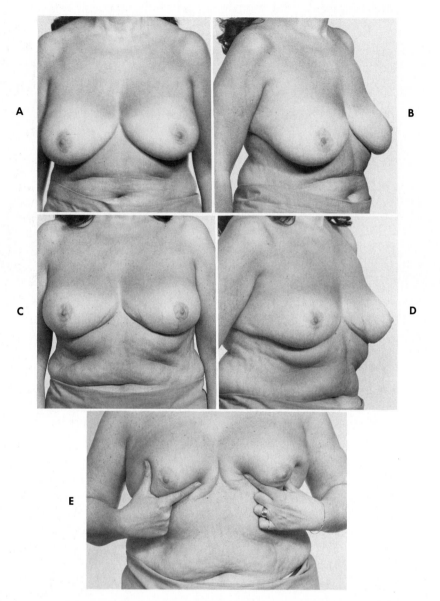

Fig. 6-25. A, Preoperative front view of 47-year-old patient who had a 10-year history of fibrocystic disease of the breasts with multiple biopsies and a familial history of breast cancer. A reduction mammaplasty was carried out utilizing vertical dermal pedicle flaps and simultaneous subcutaneous mastectomy with augmentation using 140-ml gel-filled Georgiade Surgitek prostheses. **B,** Preoperative lateral view of same patient. **C,** Ten-month postoperative view of same patient. **D,** Ten-month postoperative lateral view of same patient. **E,** Seventeen-month postoperative view of same patient illustrating softness of patient's breasts.

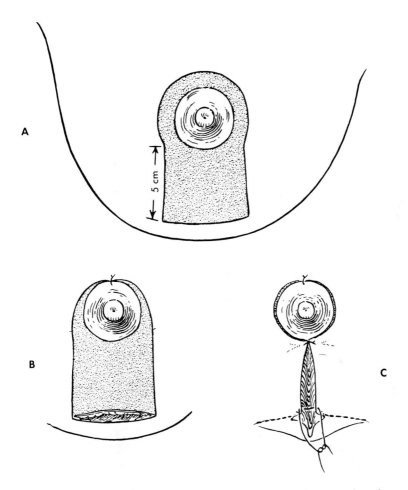

Fig. 6-26. Correction of simple ptosis of breast in conjunction with subcutaneous mastectomy with less than 3 cm elevation of areola. Shaded areas represent location of split-thickness skin removed. Closure is accomplished by using remaining dermal layer inferiorly as an added layer between prosthesis and outer skin layer.

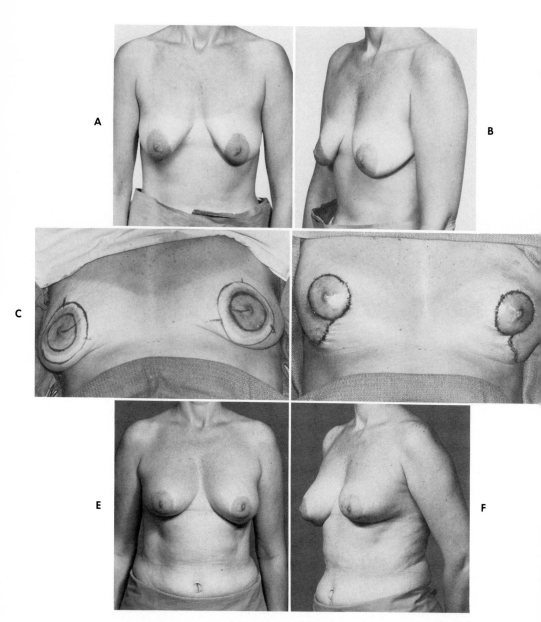

Fig. 6-27. A, Preoperative front view of 34-year-old patient with ptotic breasts and multiple nodules in deeper surfaces of the breasts. A ptosis procedure and bilateral subcutaneous mastectomy were carried out with simultaneous insertion of 100-ml gel-filled prostheses. **B,** Preoperative lateral view of same patient. **C,** Preoperative markings utilized for ptosis procedure. **D,** Skin closure of breasts immediately following surgery. **E,** Three-year postoperative front view of same patient. **F,** Three-year postoperative lateral view of same patient.

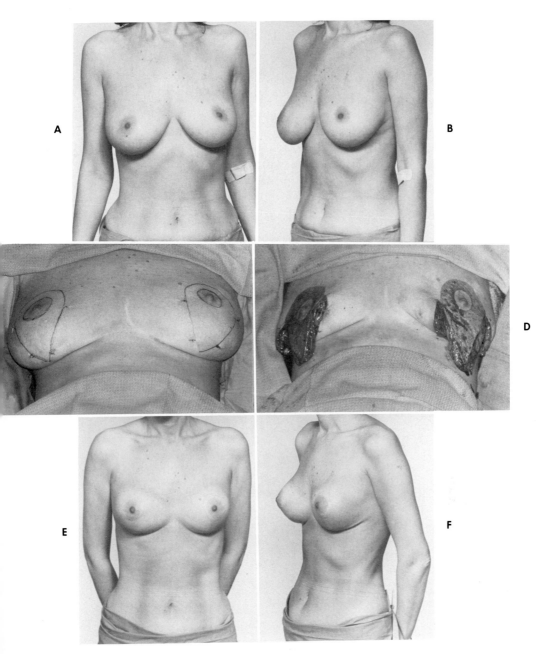

Fig. 6-28. A, Preoperative front view of 35-year-old patient with ptosis and severe fibrocystic disease of the breasts who had had multiple biopsies beginning 12 years ago. The
patient had a ptosis procedure and simultaneous bilateral subcutaneous mastectomy
performed with immediate insertion of a 185-ml Georgiade Surgitek gel-filled prosthesis. **B,** Preoperative lateral view of same patient. **C,** Operative view showing marking
of flaps for ptosis procedure. Note suture marking limits of new flap width. **D,** Operative view of partially deepithelialized flap area that will be advanced superiorly when
areola is sutured in its new position. **E,** Two and one half year postoperative front view
of same patient. **F,** Two and one half year postoperative lateral view of same patient.

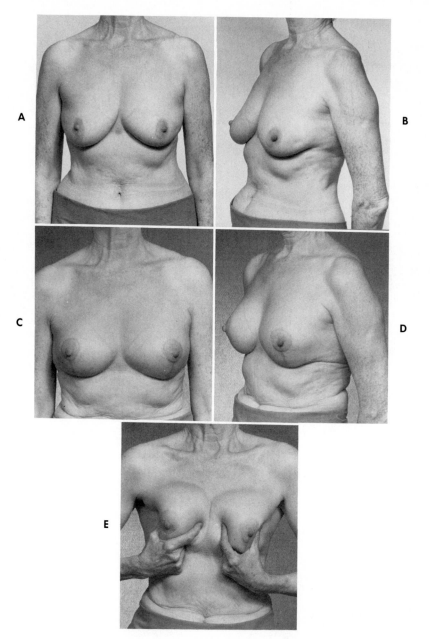

Fig. 6-29. A, Preoperative front view of 58-year-old woman with extensive fibrocystic disease of the breasts who had four biopsies of her breasts over the last 15 years. A correction of ptosis of the breasts and subcutaneous mastectomy with immediate insertion of a 185-ml gel-filled Georgiade Surgitek prosthesis was carried out. **B,** Preoperative lateral view of same patient. **C,** Six-month postoperative front view of same patient. **D,** Six-month postoperative lateral view of same patient. **E,** Six-month postoperative view illustrating softness of breasts.

be serially evaluated as discussed in Chapter 5. If the histopathologic findings demonstrate sparing of the subareolar region from epithelial proliferative changes, one can feel reasonably secure about retaining the nipple-areolar complex. However, in spite of all efforts, the surgeon must accept the fact that there remains a small percentage of breast tissue, ranging from 5% to 10%.

The findings of Stiles,[34] Hicken,[14] and Goldman and Goldwyn[10] suggest that small remnants of breast tissue remain in scattered minute segments after a radical mastectomy, a modified radical mastectomy, or a subcutaneous mastectomy. These remnants of breast tissue are particularly common in the axillary tail and inframammary areas. Prolongations of breast parenchyma are found in the ligaments of Cooper, the pectoral fascia, and, in some cases, medially into the epigastric space and even beyond. Thus, although the majority of the breast tissue has been removed, the patient should have routine follow-up breast examinations, including mammography.

The use of a free nipple-areolar graft routinely is not advisable since most of the patients who have had a subcutaneous mastectomy are in the 30- to 40-year-old age-group and wish to avoid complete loss of sensation of the nipple as part of their postsubcutaneous mastectomy disability.

The use of the larger subpectoral pockets with double lumen prostheses has dramatically improved the results in the group of patients who previously yielded the poorest results. Interestingly enough, these implants placed subpectorally seem smaller immediately postoperatively than 6 months later, when the breasts have improved in appearance.

Undesirable results

Hematoma. This usually occurs within the first 24 hours postoperatively and necessitates exposure and inspection of the breasts on the first postoperative day. If a hematoma is present, the prosthesis is removed, the hematoma is evacuated, and hemostasis is established. The prosthesis is then reinserted after the wound has been thoroughly irrigated. This can be carried out with local anesthesia supplemented with intravenous meperidine (Demerol) and diazepam (Valium) (Fig. 6-30).

Ischemia of breast skin. Occasionally an area of ischemia may develop. If eventual necrosis is anticipated, the prosthesis should be removed immediately in order to minimize the tension under this area. This will quite often prevent subsequent necrosis. Replacement of the prosthesis at a later date will probably require subpectoral insertion because of the thin skin flaps. Subpectoral implantation a few days postoperatively can also be considered.

Necrosis of breast tissue. Removal of the breast implant is mandatory. The implant is then replaced subpectorally at a later date.

If the necrosis of the breast tissue is adjacent to an area where a flap can be transferred, then the necrotic tissue is excised and the flap transferred directly into the defect. Occasionally the prosthesis can be immediately reinserted

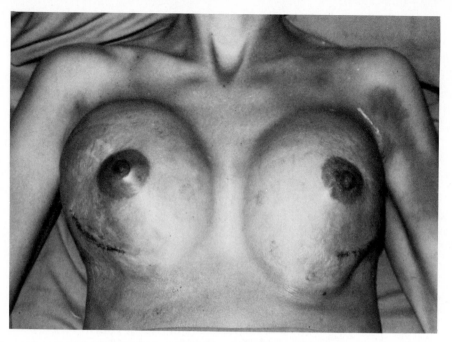

Fig. 6-30. Bilateral hematomas shown in a patient on second postoperative day prior to evacuation.

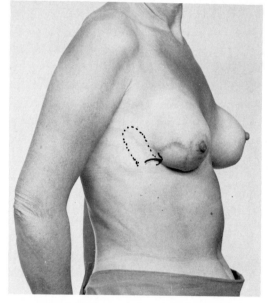

Fig. 6-31. Forty-two–year-old patient who had sustained necrosis of the lateral skin flap with exposure of the prosthesis following a subcutaneous mastectomy. A local flap, outlined by the dotted line, was utilized to reconstruct the breast area sustaining the necrosis. Dotted line shows area from which flap was obtained and transferred to breast mound. Patient is shown 6 months after transfer of flap.

(Fig. 6-31). If the necrosis involves the nipple-areolar area, the prosthesis must be removed and reconstruction of this area delayed until healing has occurred Figs. 6-32 and 6-33).

Capsular contracture with firmness and possible breast mound distortion. In the majority of the patients this occurs a number of months after subcutaneous masectomy. Release of the contractures can be carried out under local or general anesthesia. The incision is made through the previous incision, and the capsule is entered utilizing low-intensity cutting current to prevent damaging the prosthesis. The capsule is then incised circumferentially at its base and radially. Vertical incisions are made over the entire dome of the capsule down to the cut edges

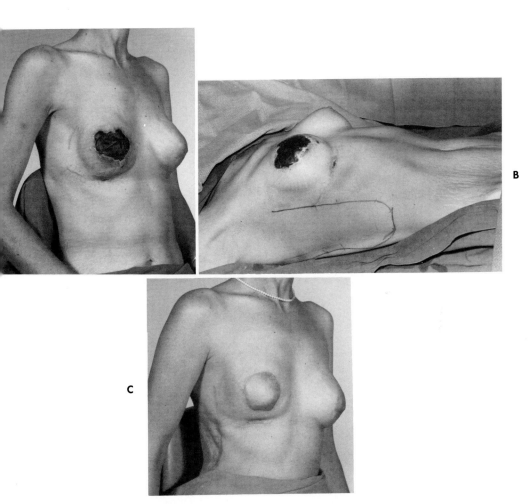

Fig. 6-32. A, This 39-year-old patient was referred to us because of sloughing of the right nipple areola and breast skin with resultant extrusion of prosthesis. **B,** Flap to be transferred to right breast area is marked. **C,** The patient 1 year after reconstruction of sloughed area with a flap.

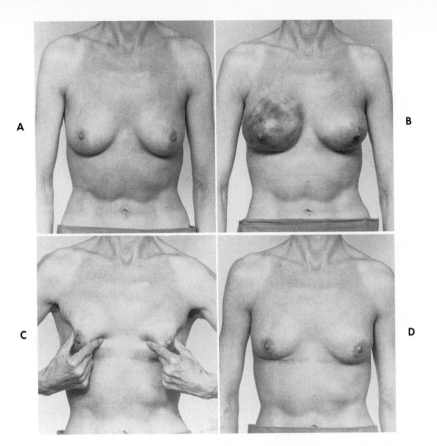

Fig. 6-33. A, Preoperative view of 39-year-old patient who had severe fibrocystic disease with associated mastodynia. Surgeon performed a bilateral subcutaneous mastectomy with immediate insertion of a 225-ml inflatable saline-filled prosthesis. **B,** Two weeks postoperatively patient had large hematoma of right breast and ischemia of nipple and areolar area of left breast. Patient was taken to operating room, at which time hematoma was evacuated, prostheses were removed, and double-lumen 185- to 225-ml Georgiade Surgitek prostheses were inserted subpectorally. Outer lumen of prosthesis was filled with 30 ml of dextran 70 containing 10 mg of methylprednisolone sodium succinate (Solu-Medrol). **C,** Postoperative view of same patient 5 months after placement of prostheses subpectorally. **D,** Five-month postoperative view illustrating softness of breasts.

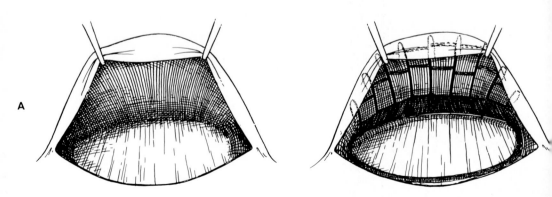

Fig. 6-34. For legend see opposite page.

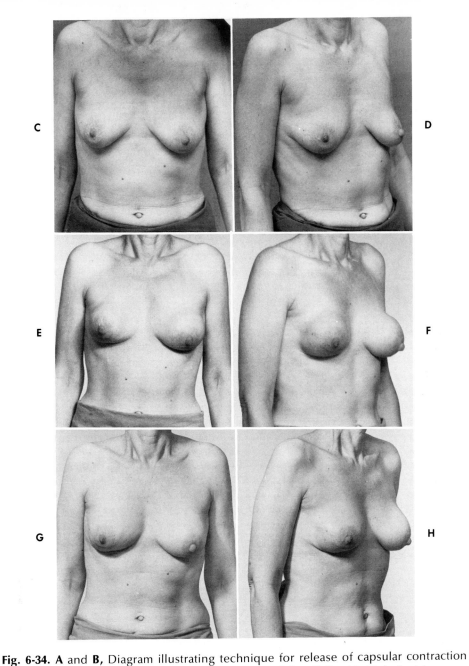

Fig. 6-34. A and **B,** Diagram illustrating technique for release of capsular contraction by incising capsule circumferentially at its base and radially. Multiple incisions are made over entire dome of capsule down to cut edges of base. Horizontal incisions are then carried out, further segmenting capsule. **C,** Preoperative front view of 49-year-old patient who had a 10-year history of fibrocystic disease of the breast with aspiration of cysts and biopsies 6 years previously. She had a familial history of breast cancer. A bilateral subcutaneous mastectomy with simultaneous augmentation with a 230-ml gel-filled prosthesis was carried out. **D,** Lateral preoperative view of same patient. **E,** Two and one half year postoperative front view of same patient, in which capsular contractures are evident in both breasts. **F,** Two and one half year postoperative lateral view of same patient exhibiting capsular contractures. **G,** Postoperative front view 16 months after removal of prostheses from both breasts and release of capsular contractures. Prostheses were replaced with smaller 185-ml Georgiade Surgitek gel-filled prostheses. **H,** Postoperative lateral view of same patient 16 months after release of capsular contractures. These photographs were taken 5 years after original subcutaneous mastectomy.

at the base. Horizontal incisions are then carried out, further segmenting the capsule. With a sufficient number of incisions through the capsule into the fatty tissue, the contracture will be released. Any area of excessive scarring is completely released, and undermining is carried out in all directions. Thorough hemostasis is then obtained with the coagulation current. A suitably sized prosthesis is inserted. The incision is closed with interrupted 4-0 white nylon sutures in the deeper layers followed by 5-0 Vicryl sutures subcutaneously and 5-0 Prolene sutures approximating the skin edge (Fig. 6-34).

The use of force over the breast prosthesis has been described as a suitable method for rupturing the capsule. In our opinion this is a technique fraught with many potential problems as a result of the considerable force rupturing the envelope of the prosthesis and disseminating the gel into the surrounding tissues. At best it is difficult to ascertain the effectiveness of this maneuver, and we do not recommend it.

REFERENCES

1. Bartlett, W.: An anatomic substitute for the female breast, Ann. Surg. **66:**208, 1917.
2. Berson, M. I.: Derma-fat-fascia transplants used in building up the breasts, Surgery **15:**451, 1944.
3. Bouman, F. G.: Reconstruction of the breast after subcutaneous mastectomy, Arch. Chir. Neerl. **XXVI-IV:**343, 1974.
4. Courtiss, E., and Goldwyn, R. M.: Reduction mammaplasty by the inferior pedicle technique, Plast. Reconstr. Surg. **59:**500, 1977.
5. De Cholnoky, T.: Mastectomies with simultaneous reconstruction of breasts, Surgery **44:**649, 1958.
6. Fredricks, S.: A 10 year experience with subcutaneous mastectomy, Clin. Plast. Surg. **2:**347, 1975.
7. Freeman, B. S.: Subcutaneous mastectomy for benign breast lesions with immediate or delayed prosthetic replacement, Plast. Reconstr. Surg. **30:**676, 1962.
8. Freeman, B. S.: Subcutaneous mastectomy. In Georgiade, N. G., editor: Reconstructive breast surgery, St. Louis, 1976, The C. V. Mosby Co.
9. Georgiade, N. G., and Hyland, W.: Technique for subcutaneous mastectomy and immediate reconstruction in the ptotic breast, Plast. Reconstr. Surg. **56:**121, 1975.
10. Goldman, L. D., and Goldwyn, R. M.: Some anatomical considerations of subcutaneous mastectomy, Plast. Reconstr. Surg. **51:**501, 1973.
11. Goldwyn, R. M.: Subcutaneous mastectomy, N. Engl. J. Med. **297:**503, 1977.
12. Goulian, D., and McDivitt, R. W.: Subcutaneous mastectomy with immediate reconstruction of the breasts using the dermal mastopexy technique, Plast. Reconstr. Surg. **50:**211, 1972.
13. Gynning, I., and associates: Subcutaneous mastectomy in 80 patients with breast tumors, Acta Chir. Scand. **141:**488, 1975.
14. Hicken, N. F.: Mastectomy—clinical pathologic study demonstrating why most mastectomies result in incomplete removal of the mammary gland, Arch. Surg. **40:**6, 1940.
15. Horton, C. E., Adamson, J. E., Mladick, R. A., and Carraway, J. H.: Simple mastectomy with immediate reconstruction, Plast. Reconstr. Surg. **53:**42, 1974.
16. Letterman, G. S., and Schurter, M.: Total mammary excision with immediate breast reconstruction, Am. Surg. **21:**835, 1955.

17. Letterman, G. S., and Schurter, M.: Inframammary based dermo-fat flaps in mammary reconstruction following a subcutaneous mastectomy, Plast. Reconstr. Surg. **55:**156, 1975.
18. Lexer, E.: Die gesamte wiederherstellung, chirurge, vol. 2, Leipzig, Johann Ambrosius Barth Verlagsbuchhandlung, p. 555.
19. Longacre, J. J.: The use of local pedicle flap for reconstruction of the breast after subtotal or total extirpation of the mammary gland and for the correction of distortion and atrophy of the breast due to excessive scar, Plast. Reconstr. Surg. **11:**380, 1953.
20. Longacre, J. J.: Correction of hypoplastic breast with special reference to reconstruction of "nipple type breast" with local dermofat pedicle flaps, Plast. Reconstr. Surg. **14:**431, 1954.
21. Malbec, E. F.: Gigantomastia unilateral por fibroadenoma; Reparación plástic Diá Méd. **19:**414, 1947.
22. Maliniac, J. W.: Breast deformities and their repair, New York, 1950, Grune & Stratton, Inc.
23. Marino, E., and Solian, J. A.: Benign mastopathies, Int. Surg. **47:**16, 1967.
24. Marino, H.: Glandular mastectomy: immediate reconstruction, Plast, Reconstr. Surg. **10:**204, 1952.
25. McKissock, P. K.: Reduction mammaplasty with a vertical dermal flap, Plast. Reconstr. Surg. **49:**245, 1972.
26. Molenaar, A.: Subcutaneous mastectomy, Clin. Plast. Surg. **1:**427, 1974.
27. Pennisi, V. R., Capozzi, A., and Perez, F. M.: Subcutaneous mastectomy data, Plast. Reconstr. Surg. **59:**53, 1977.
28. Robbins, T. H.: A reduction mammaplasty with the areola-nipple based on an inferior dermal pedicle, Plast. Reconstr. Surg. **59:**64, 1977.
29. Rosenauer, F.: Mammaer satzplastic nach radikaloperation wegen ca, Munch. Med. Wochenschr. **93:**890, 1951.
30. Rubin, L. R.: Surgical treatment of the massive hypertrophic breast. In Georgiade, N. G., editor: Reconstructive breast surgery, St. Louis, 1976, The C. V. Mosby Co.
31. Rubin, L. R.: The cushioned augmentation repair after a subcutaneous mastectomy, Plast. Reconstr. Surg. **57:**23, 1976.
32. Schurter, M., and Letterman, G.: Subcutaneous mastectomy, J. Am. Med. Wom. Assoc. **27:**463, 1972.
33. Spira, M.: Subcutaneous mastectomy in the large ptotic breast, Plast. Reconstr. Surg. **59:**200, 1977.
34. Stiles, H. J.: In Haagensen, C. D.: Diseases of the breast, ed. 2, Philadelphia, 1971, W. B. Saunders Co., p. 16.
35. Thomas, T. G.: On the removal of benign tumors of the mamma without mutilation of the organ, N.Y. Med. J. Obst. Rev. **35:**337, 1882.
36. Weiner, D. L., and associates: A single dermal pedicle for nipple transposition in subcutaneous mastectomy, reduction mammaplasty or mastopexy, Plast. Reconstr. Surg. **51:**115, 1973.
37. Zbylski, J. R., and Parsons, R. W.: A method of adenectomy and breast reconstruction for benign disease, Plast. Reconstr. Surg. **37:**38, 1966.

CHAPTER 7

Surgical treatment of cancer of the breast (extirpation) and how it relates to reconstruction; team relationship: adjuvant therapy and its relation to surgery

H. F. Seigler and Nicholas G. Georgiade

The therapeutic regimens available to physicians treating breast cancer patients include surgery, chemotherapy, radiation, hormonal therapy, and immunotherapy. Many features must be taken into account before proper selection of the treatment regimen can be made, such as predisposing family and medical history, age, size of the primary tumor, cellular differentiation, mitotic index, level of invasion, cell type, hormonal receptor, and lymph node status. Careful evaluation by a team of specialists can permit selection of patients whose disease makes them favorable candidates for modified surgical intervention to eradicate macroscopic disease. Afterward they are given adjuvant systemic therapy, if indicated, for possible microscopic disease, followed by early breast reconstruction.

HISTOLOGIC TYPES OF BREAST CANCER

By far the most common breast cancer is that of duct cell origin. This type accounts for approximately half of all breast cancers. When compared with other tumor types there is a greater likelihood that this lesion will have a high mitotic index with lymphatic invasion. Medullary carcinoma of the breast may exhibit a large primary lesion that is grossly circumscribed. The host response to this tumor cell type is typified by a striking lymphocytic infiltrate. Lymphatic involvement is less common than ductal carcinoma, and the long-term prognosis is improved. Lobular carcinoma may be *in situ,* multifocal, or frankly invasive. This lesion has been described by numerous authors as having a high instance of bilateralism.[5,10] Intraductal carcinoma may be masked in its premalignant form as intraductal papillary growths. Such growths are not uncommon and usually are associated with a bloody nipple discharge. When promptly and adequately treated, this disease is associated with a prolonged, disease-free interval and a favorable long-term prognosis.[3,8] Paget's disease of the breast, or epidermal malignant changes of the nipple, comprises less than 3% of breast cancers. The typical Paget's cells are believed to develop in subjacent ducts in the nipple. There is an increased frequency of multicentric lesions with a prolonged duration of symptoms before either a breast mass or lymph node enlargement can be distinguished.

Tubular carcinoma, mucinous carcinoma, cystosarcoma phylloides, sarcomas, and pure squamous cell lesions are all quite rare and will not be discussed.

CHOICE OF OPERATION

Countless clinical studies have shown that one out of four breast cancer patients with negative lymph nodes will succumb to their disease within 10 years and that approximately three out of four will not survive a decade if tumor is present in their lymph nodes at the time of operation. These data have led many oncologists to conclude that by the time a clinical diagnosis of breast cancer is established most patients will have potentially disseminated disease. The primary aim of the modern surgical oncologist dealing with breast cancer is directed toward removal of primary regional macroscopic disease, followed by election of an adjuvant program for controlling residual microscopic disease.

During the past 40 years a number of extended radical mastectomy operations have been devised, but none has significantly improved survival statistics and, for the most part, all have been discouraged for future usage. Radical mastectomy continues to be the most commonly employed surgical procedure in this country for the treatment of primary operable carcinoma of the breast. The morbidity associated with radical mastectomy in terms of wound problems, body deformity, and arm complications is quite significant. Thirty years ago Patey and Dyson[11] introduced modified radical mastectomy; at present this operation is being employed with increasing frequency and in many medical centers has almost totally supplanted radical mastectomy. Reported studies indicate that results are quite comparable with the standard radical mastectomy.[7,11] Segmental mastectomy does not offer local control for multicentric lesions, nor does it allow study of the regional lymph nodes. Documentation of disease in lymph nodes is quite important not only for discussion of prognosis with the patient but also for selection of the adjuvant program to be employed. For the most part, noninvasive lesions are made up of lobular carcinoma *in situ*, papillary breast cancers, and intraductal lesions without stromal invasion. As previously stated, these malignancies are relatively uncommon and have a tendency to be multicentric. If, after histopathologic evaluation, invasion is found to have occurred, most physicians would agree that modified radical mastectomy is indicated. If no invasion is evident subcutaneous mastectomies with implants may be adequate. It has been estimated that approximately 10%[12] of women who survive the removal of a primary breast malignancy will develop disease in the opposite breast. Even though numerous authors have reported an excess of 20% positive biopsies from random sites in the opposite breast, overt clinical disease would not support such a high frequency. The biologic significance of disease in the opposite breast remains an unanswered question.

Breast skin involvement with tumor may vary from ulceration to simple dimpling or to the classic inflammatory carcinoma. Histopathologic examination of inflammatory lesions reveals lymphatic extension within the neoplasm, and surgery is to be recommended only as a "toilet mastectomy." Radical mastectomy or reconstructive procedures should not be considered for this type of disease. Simple cutaneous involvement with dimpling is present in approximately 5% of breast cancer cases. This occurs with involvement of lymphatics in either the dermis alone or with the dermis and epidermis. It is more commonly seen with primary lesions of diameter greater than 2 cm. Lymph node involvement is a common feature. Reconstructive efforts should be discouraged if skin dimpling is present at the time of initial examination. Nipple involvement with Paget's disease and nipple retraction have been discussed at length. Relatively little has been written, however, concerning the direct involvement of the nipple with non-Paget's disease. Nipple involvement occurs in less than 15% of all breast cancers; it is most common in primary lesions of ductal origin located beneath the nipple, in medullary carcinomas, and in mucinous carcinomas. If nipple transplantation is to be considered for the reconstructive phase, careful assessment must be made prior to completion of this part of the procedure (see p. 165).

ADJUVANT THERAPY IN PRIMARY BREAST CANCER CONTROL

During the past 50 years the disease-free interval and long-term survival rates in patients being treated for primary breast cancer have not varied a great deal. The different selected surgical procedures, both with and without x-ray therapy, have not greatly altered the statistics. As previously stated, a significant number of patients with primary breast cancer have disseminated disease at the time of the original clinical diagnosis. Improvement in the disease-free interval and long-term survival of such patients will result only when effective systemic adjuvant therapy is used in conjunction with surgery and radiation. A number of study protocols evaluating adjuvant chemotherapy, hormonal therapy, and both nonspecific and specific immunotherapy have produced noteworthy gains relative to both survival and disease-free interval. The effectiveness of adjuvant chemotherapy is determined by the response of micrometastases to the cytotoxic agents employed. Skipper has emphasized the importance of considering different types of chemotherapeutic agents designed to effect the cell metabolic cycle at different points.[13] The studies suggest that tumor cell growth kinetics include proliferating clonogenic cells undergoing active anabolism, nonproliferative cells in a resting phase, and nonclonogenic cells that do not contribute to tumor growth but are important to overall tumor volume.

Chemotherapeutic agents seem to have their greatest efficiency in interfering with cell-cycle activity. The drugs are used in a pulse-type fashion, and as the resting cells become proliferative, they are suppressed or cytolysed by the chemotherapeutic drugs. Constant drug administration may keep tumor cells suppressed and in a resting phase and thus not reflect efficiency for tumor cell death. Early trials utilizing adjuvant chemotherapy usually consisted of single drugs administered for a short period of time. These were given only to patients with the highest likelihood of developing recurrent disease, therefore, the statistics were not very encouraging.

It was not until the 1970s that patients with clinically curable breast cancer were considered for combination therapy consisting of surgery followed by chemotherapy. Little enthusiasm had been generated by the scores of patients treated with different chemotherapeutic regimens for advanced recurrent disease. It became increasingly apparent that nondiscernible micrometastases present at operation could perhaps be destroyed by prolonged administration of pulse-type chemotherapy. The first large cooperative program undertaken by the Breast Task Force was a controlled study using L-phenylalanine mustard administered to patients following conventional or modified radical mastectomy. Patients with potentially curable breast cancer who had one or more axillary nodes that had been proved histologically to contain tumor were considered eligible for inclusion in the evaluation. Patient categories were broken down into two groups consisting of those 49 years or age or younger and those between the ages of 50 and 75 years. Half of the patients were given the drug and half were administered a placebo. Patients were treated with 0.15 mg/kg/day by mouth of L-phenylalanine mustard during the first 5 days of each 6-week period. Treatment was begun no sooner than 2 weeks and not later than 4 weeks postoperatively and was continued until there was documented evidence of treatment failure or for 2 years, whichever occurred first. In premenopausal women the difference with respect to the disease-free interval of treated and control groups was highly significant. Treatment failures occurred in approximately one third of premenopausal patients receiving placebo and in only 3% of those receiving L-phenylalanine mustard. A similar trend was observed in postmenopausal patients, but the difference was not deemed to be statistically significant.[4]

In 1973 Bonadonna and associates initiated an adjuvant regimen consisting of cyclophosphamide (Cytoxan), methotrexate, and 5-fluorouracil. The patients received either twelve cycles of drug or no treatment. A 2-week rest period between drug cycles was observed. Data accumulated from this regimen revealed that approximately one fourth of control patients had recurrent disease at the end of 1 year whereas only 5% of treated patients demonstrated a recurrence.[2]

Since the turn of the century there has been a general appreciation that hormonal manipulation results in a measurable effect for breast cancer patients. A variety of studies have reflected an approximate 35% response rate in patients with recurrent breast cancer who were treated with estrogens and an approximately 20% response rate if the patients were treated with androgens. Oophorectomy, bilateral adrenalectomy, and hypophysectomy have resultant response rates varying from 30% to 50%. Recent studies concerning hormone receptor sites in mammary tumor tissue have provided specific patient selection for hormonal manipulation, and thus the response rates in patients treated empirically has drastically been improved. Normal target tissues contain specific receptors for hormones—cytoplasmic proteins for steroids and surface receptors for polypeptides—and these receptor sites are responsible for the initial interaction between the hormone and the cell.[9] They function to trigger the biochemical chain of events characteristic for the particular hormone. Hormone-dependent tumors also contain receptors, but it now appears that independent or autonomous tumors often may not.[9] If, with malignant transformation, the breast tumor cell retains the hormonal receptor sites, its growth and function, like those of the normal cell, are potentially capable of being regulated by its hormonal environment. If the cell loses the receptors as a consequence of its malignant transformation, it is no longer recognized as a target cell by circulating hormones and endocrine control is abolished. Such data indicate that determination of hormonal receptor sites can indeed identify the 20% to 40% of breast cancer patients who will actually benefit from endocrine therapy. Prolactin, estrogen, and progesterone all appear to have regulatory effects on breast tumor growth. Specific receptor assays for each are now clinically available. The functional role of hormone receptor sites has not been established in the mechanism of tumor regression caused by utilization of antiestrogens, androgens, and progestins. Be that as it may, when estrogen receptors are absent in tumor, prediction can be made with a high degree of accuracy that endocrine therapies will fail. However, when they are present, the likelihood of a successful response to pharmacologic or ablative therapy is high.

Immunotherapy for breast cancer is based on the supposition that the host can be made to respond to this particular tumor type. Tumor-associated antigens have been reported by a number of investigators. The neoantigens expressed on the membrane of breast tumor cells may indeed be differentiation-type antigens, and specific immune surveillance of this class has been questioned. Immunotherapy can be active or passive and nonspecific or specific. Active nonspecific immunotherapy refers to the use of adjuvants such as bacillus Calmette-Guerin, *Corynebacterium parvum,* and vaccinia. These agents usually stimulate the reticuloendothelial system, which, it is hoped, will then activate specific cell killing and macrophage activity directed toward tumor destruction. Active specific immunotherapy refers to specific vaccination with the tumor antigen. This can be accomplished by administering intact tumor cells, partially purified membrane, or purified soluble tumor antigen extract. This is designed to increase specific antitumor immunity. Passive cellular immunotherapy refers to the transfer of lymphocytes or cell products of immune lymphocytes after in vitro or in vivo sensitization. This particular type of immunotherapy utilizes classical adoptive transfer. It has its greatest efficiency if the host lymphocyte is sensitized in vitro to the tumor-specific antigen and then the host immune cell is infused. If a separate donor is utilized, the host will respond to the foreign HL-A antigens present on the cell surface and the cells will thus be destroyed by a host-vs-graft reaction. Passive serotherapy utilizes antitumor antibodies from an immune donor. Only anecdotal experience has been reported using passive immunotherapy for breast cancer. A number of investigators have reported some efficiency with active nonspecific immunotherapy, and more recently active specific immunotherapy has shown a significant prolongation of patient survival to 7 years (61% as compared to 30% not receiving immunotherapy).[1] Clinical experience with transfer factor, immune RNA, lymphokines, and thymosin have not as yet generated enough data to permit adequate interpretation. Studies are being pursued that hopefully will allow interpretation of combining adjuvant chemotherapy, immunotherapy, and hormonal therapy. If we are to have a meaningful impact on this disease, such studies must clearly be advanced.

CONCLUSION

The management of breast carcinoma patients is an enormously complex endeavor requiring a team approach. The endocrinologist, pharmacologist, immunologist, radiologist, pathologist, surgical oncologist, and plastic and reconstructive surgeons all play important roles. Careful assessment of the patient by the endocrinologist is of prime importance. Routine blood chemistries, xeroradiograms, carcinoembryonic antigen assay, routine diagnostic x-ray studies, bone scan, and appropriate skeletal x-ray studies if indicated must be completed prior to planning combined modality therapy. Patients with ulcerated lesions, inflammatory carcinoma, skin dimpling or nipple retraction, primary lesions greater than 2 cm in diameter, or an age of 50 years or more should not be considered for early breast reconstruction. If patients have invasive ductal carcinoma with poor differentiation and a high mitotic index, they also are poor candidates for consideration for this procedure. If patients have more than three positive axillary lymph nodes or if level II and III lymph nodes are involved, there is a high probability of systemic disease, and reconstructive procedures should not generally be attempted.

Lobular carcinoma in situ, noninvasive intraductal carcinoma, and invasive carcinoma either lobular or ductal forming a mass no greater than 0.5 cm in diameter have been defined as minimal breast cancer.[6] These patients are the more favorable candidates for early breast reconstruction. Following modified radical mastectomy, if the primary lesion is favorable and there is no lymph node involvement, early breast reconstruction can be considered. Whether or not these lymph node–negative patients should receive adjuvant therapy remains an open question. But the fact that among those patients followed for 10 years one in four will succumb to breast cancer tends to support the thesis that some type of systemic therapy for nondiscernible disease should be undertaken. At the present time studies are underway evaluating Tamoxifen for patients with estrogen receptor–positive tumors either as a single agent or combined with intermittent single drug chemotherapy. Alternating L-phenylalanine mustard and

Corynebacterium parvum is also being studied in patients in this category. If the patient is premenopausal or perimenopausal, oophorectomy should be considered. Results with specific active immunotherapy for invasive melanoma without documented metastasis would support clinical trials using this regimen in breast cancer patients with invasive lesions but with no documented lymph node involvement.

Following modified radical mastectomy, if the patient has a more aggressive primary lesion with first-order lymph node involvement, early breast reconstruction should not be considered. These patients should receive either pulse-type multiple drug chemotherapy, hormonal therapy, or combination chemohormonal therapy and should be followed for at least 12 months prior to breast reconstruction. The questions and debate concerning the opposite breast will for the most part be resolved by subcutaneous mastectomy and implant completed by the plastic surgeon in the second phase of reconstruction. If breast cancer patients are assessed and managed by a team approach, careful selection for combined modality treatment can not only preserve self-image but may indeed result in a prolonged disease-free interval and significantly improve patient survival.

REFERENCES

1. Anderson, J. M.: Prolonged survival after autograph immunotherapy of mammary cancer, Proc. Am. Assoc. Cancer Res. **17:**186, 1976.
2. Bonadonna, G., and associates: Combination chemotherapy as an adjuvant treatment in operable breast cancer, N. Engl. J. Med. **294:**406-410, 1976.
3. Dockerty, M. B.: The grading and typing of carcinoma of the breast, J. Iowa Med. Soc. **54:**289-294, 1954.
4. Fisher, B., and associates: L-Phenylalanine mustard (1-PAM) in the management of primary breast cancer: a report of early findings, N. Engl. J. Med. **292:**117-122, 1975.
5. Foote, F. W., Jr., and Stewart, F. W.: Lobular carcinoma in situ—rare form of mammary cancer, Am. J. Pathol. **17:**491-496, 1941.
6. Gallaher, H. S., and Martin, J. E.: An orientation to the concept of minimal breast cancer, Cancer **28:**1505-1507, 1971.
7. Handley, R. S.: The technique and results of conservative radical mastectomy (Patey's operation), Prog. Clin. Cancer **1:**462-470, 1955.
8. Kraus, F. T., and Neubecker, R. D.: The differential diagnosis of papillary tumors of the breast, Cancer **15:**444-455, 1962.
9. McGuire, W. L., Chamness, G., and Costlow, M. E.: Progress in endocrinology and metabolism: "hormone dependence and breast cancer," Metabolism **23:**75-100, 1974.
10. Murier, R.: The evolution of carcinoma of the mamma, J. Pathol. **52:**155-172, 1941.
11. Patey, D. H., and Dyson, W. H.: The prognosis of carcinoma of the breast in relation to the type of operation performed, Br. J. Cancer **2:**7-13, 1948.
12. Robbins, G. F., and Berg, J. W.: Bilateral primary breast cancers: a prospective clinical pathological study, Cancer **17:**1501-1527, 1964.
13. Skipper, H. E.: Kinetics of mammary tumor cell growth and indications for therapy, Cancer **28:**1479-1499, 1971.

CHAPTER 8

Reconstruction of the breast: rationale, prognosis, and timing

Donald Serafin

Patients requesting breast reconstruction are motivated by a variety of reasons. In this discussion an attempt will be made to present my criteria for reconstruction of the breast in patients who have undergone mastectomy for breast carcinoma. In as much as breast carcinoma is a spectrum of diseases with varying biologic behavior, I will attempt to define that group of patients with favorable prognosis for whom reconstruction is most clearly indicated. Finally attention will be given to the timing of the reconstructive effort, recognizing its interdependence on both the rationale for reconstruction and the ultimate prognosis of any given patient.

RATIONALE FOR RECONSTRUCTION

Until the last several years, women desiring breast reconstruction following mastectomy sought consultation directly from a plastic and reconstructive surgeon. Referrals from the extirpative surgeon who performed the mastectomy were uncommon. This probably reflected a conservative "wait and see" attitude on the part of the general surgeon with reluctance to refer a patient with an uncertain disease status for reconstruction. It no doubt also reflected a true lack of appreciation for the need for reconstruction in some patients, with emphasis being primarily on cure and survival.

Several things have become apparent during the past 5 years, with a resultant change in the attitudes of both surgeon and patient. Epidemiologic reports[27] from large groups of patients in widespread geographic locations suggest that the incidence of carcinoma of the breast is increasing. With this increase in incidence, mortality rates have not changed (Fig. 8-1).[28] The present 5-year survival for patients with carcinoma of the breast with negative axillary nodes is still 80% to 85%, which has remained the same since Halsted's introduction of the radical mastectomy in 1890.[8] A static mortality rate in the face of an increased incidence of breast cancer raises several questions regarding the etiology and natural history of this disease. More data will be required to evaluate the systemic effects of invasive breast cancer. What influence the early detection and treatment of breast cancer and premalignant breast disease will have on these observations is only speculative at present.

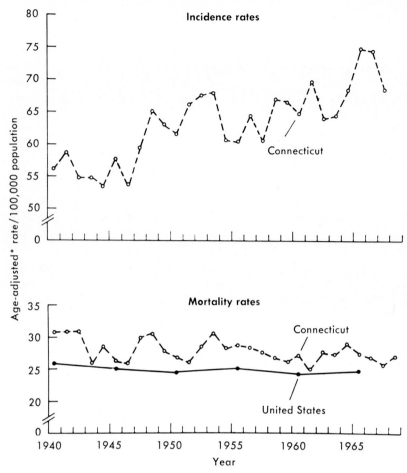

*Age-adjusted to 1950 total U.S. population

Fig. 8-1. Graphs depicting progressive increase in incidence of carcinoma of the breast. Mortality rates are unchanged. (From Cutler, S. J., Christine, B., and Barclay, T. H. C.: Cancer **28**(6):1376-1380, 1971.)

Whereas in the past a unilateral mastectomy was recommended without hesitation for operable carcinoma of the breast, the prospect of an additional mastectomy in those high-risk patients for premalignant disease in the opposite breast was a formidable therapeutic consideration. Consultation was sought from the reconstructive surgeon, and the subcutaneous mastectomy has been increasingly utilized as a diagnostic-therapeutic approach to many of these premalignant conditions. Attention now could also be directed to the previous mastectomy site and reconstruction considered.

Public awareness of the possibility of breast reconstruction paralleled the increased medical interest. Frequent articles appeared in nonmedical magazines and journals. Interest was also heightened by television documentaries. Patients, now aware that future reconstruction was a possibility, began to query their extirpative surgeon preoperatively for additional information.

Most of these patients expressed negative concerns about their altered body contour. Many expressed feelings of self-consciousness, especially when trying to buy or fit clothing. Surprisingly anxiety about their husband's response to an altered contour did not appear to be a dominant factor in those patients seeking reconstruction. The restoration of form and contour to enhance a feeling of diminished femininity rather than sexuality predominated.

The attitudes and anxieties of patients seeking reconstruction as well as their responses preoperatively and postoperatively to an altered body contour and that of their families is discussed in Chapters 1 and 2.

DETERMINATION OF PROGNOSIS

Inherent in the investigation of any tumor is the study of those factors that directly influence survival. Only after a thorough appreciation of those factors can one evaluate various treatment modalities. This is especially relevant when reconstruction is also being considered. The literature is replete with factors thought to influence prognosis in carcinoma of the breast. Alderson and Hamlin[1] selected twenty-one of these prognostic factors and subjected them to a multiple regression analysis to determine their independent effect on survival. Nine of these factors were found to be independently associated with survival (Table 8-1).[7] The multivariate analysis also permitted an estimate to be made of the relative contribution that each of these factors makes toward survival (Table 8-2).[7]

Table 8-1. Correlation coefficient between each of twenty-two prognostic factors and survival for 258 patients with breast cancer*

Clinical stage	−0.41	Immunoblasts in axillary nodes	0.12
Axillary node metastases	0.40	Infiltration around tumor	0.11
Size of primary	−0.35	Laterality	0.09
Stromal reaction	−0.32	Duration of symptoms	0.09
Radiotherapy given	0.28	Plasma cell content in axillary nodes	0.08
Site of primary	0.23	Mast cell infiltration in tumor	0.08
Malignancy grading	−0.21	Germinal centers in axillary nodes	0.07
Year of treatment	0.21	Age	−0.07
Host defense response†	0.16	Sinus histiocytosis in axillary nodes	0.06
Infiltration within tumor	0.15	Edge of tumor	0.04
Menopausal status	0.14	Marital status	−0.02

From Alderson, M. R., Hamlin, I., and Staunton, M. D.: The relative significance of prognostic factors in breast carcinoma, Br. J. Cancer **25**:646-656, 1971, p. 651.
*If correlation coefficient >0.12 or <-0.12 then $p < 0.05$
  >0.16 or <-0.16 then $p < 0.01$.
†Host defense response derived from combined score of five items; lymphocytic and plasmacytic infiltration around and within the tumor; the number, size, and activity of the germinal centers in the axillary nodes; the immunoblast content of the axillary nodes; and the plasma cell content in the axillary nodes.

Table 8-2. Percentage of total variance in survival independently explained by each of twenty-two prognostic factors for 258 patients with breast cancer*

	Per- centage		Per- centage
Axillary node metastases	7.6	Menopausal status	1.1
Clinical stage	7.0	Immunoblasts in axillary nodes	0.6
Size of primary	6.4	Sinus histiocytosis in axillary nodes	0.4
Radiotherapy given	3.6	Duration of symptoms	0.4
Stromal reaction	3.5	Mast cell infiltration in tumor	0.3
Malignancy grading	3.4	Laterability	0.2
Year treatment	3.4	Plasma cell content in axillary nodes	0.2
Site of primary	3.0	Age	0.1
Host defense response†	2.9	Edge of tumor	0.0
Infiltration around tumor	1.4	Marital status	0.0
Infiltration within tumor	1.3	Germinal centers in axillary nodes	0.0

From Alderson, M. R., Hamlin, I., and Staunton, M. D.: The relative significance of prognostic factors in breast carcinoma, Br. J. Cancer 25:646-656, 1971, p. 651.
*If variance explained >1.5% $p < 0.05$
  >2.6% $p < 0.01$.
†Host defense response derived from combined score of five items; lymphocytic and plasmacytic infiltration around, and within the tumor; the number, size, and activity of the germinal centers in the axillary nodes; the immunoblast content of the axillary nodes; and the plasma cell content in the axillary nodes.

Table 8-3. Classification of histologic types (Ackerman)

Type I	Rarely metastasizes (not invasive)
	Intraductal carcinoma
	Lobular carcinoma
	Noninvasive papillary carcinoma
Type II	Rarely metastasizes (always invasive)
	Pure extracellular mucinous or colloid carcinoma
	Medullary carcinomas with lymphocystic infiltration
	Well-differentiated carcinoma
	Invasive papillary carcinoma
Type III	All carcinomas not definitely classified as types I, II, or IV constitute type III
Type IV	Undifferentiated carcinomas
	Also includes all types of tumors invading blood vessels

From del Regato, J. A., and Spjut, H. J.: Ackerman and del Regato's cancer: diagnosis, treatment, and prognosis, ed. 5, St. Louis, 1977, The C. V. Mosby Co.

Histologic type

Histologic type was not included as an independent factor influencing survival in Table 8-1. Rather a greater emphasis was given to malignancy grading. This in part probably reflected the predominance of invasive ductal carcinoma, accounting for at least 80% of the patients under study. Other authors[5] (Table 8-3) believe that the histologic type is of such importance that complete grading systems were devised as an index to prognosis. Schiödt concluded that the histologic classification of breast cancer as an index to prognosis has little value except with colloid and mucinous carcinoma.[11] Undoubtedly a prospective study utilizing techniques described in Table 8-1 with multifactoral analysis is needed to resolve the issue. This study should include among others the separation of histologic type and the grade of malignancy into separate variables for analysis.

Carcinoma of the breast has a variety of histologic types but for simplicity is generally categorized into ductal and lobular carcinoma (Table 8-4). Each of these categories can be further subdivided into noninfiltrating and infiltrating forms, the former representing a more favorable lesion with a better prognosis.

Intraductal epithelial hyperplasia is believed by some authors to have a significant correlation to the eventual development of carcinoma of the breast. Early forms of hyperplasia, for example, papillary, are more frequently seen in premenopausal patients, whereas more hyperplastic lesions, for example, cribriform, are not generally hormonally responsive and are seen more commonly in the postmenopausal patient (see Chapter 9).

The true incidence of noninfiltrative and hyperplastic lesions is difficult to determine since most lesions cannot be palpated and are often incidental findings in biopsy and subcutaneous mastectomy specimens. Studies have demonstrated

---

Table 8-4. Carcinoma of breast classification

I. Carcinoma of mammary ducts
  A. Noninfiltrating
    1. Papillary carcinoma
    2. Comedocarcinoma
  B. Infiltrating
    1. Papillary carcinoma
    2. Comedocarcinoma
    3. Ductal carcinoma
    4. Colloid carcinoma
    5. Medullary carcinoma
II. Carcinoma of mammary lobules
  A. Noninfiltrating
    1. In situ lobular carcinoma
  B. Infiltrating
    1. Lobular carcinoma
III. Sarcoma and other relatively rare carcinomas

Table 8-5. Comparison of special histologic types of infiltrating breast carcinoma with infiltrating duct carcinoma with productive fibrosis

Histologic type	Infiltrating duct carcinoma with productive fibrosis	Infiltrating lobular carcinoma	Infiltrating medullary	Infiltrating colloid	Infiltrating comedocarcinoma	Infiltrating papillary
Percent of total*	78.1%	8.7%	4.3%	2.6%	4.6%	1.2%
Average age (years)	50.7	53.8	49.0	49.7	48.6	51.9
Average size (cm)	3.1	3.5	3.4	3.8	3.9	3.4
Node involvement	60%	60%	44%	32%	32%	17%
Median survival of treatment failures (years)	3.75	3.25	2.25	4.3	2.7	5
Actuarial survival						
5 years	59%	57%	69%	76%	84%	89%
10 years	47%	42%	68%	72%	77%	65%

Modified from McDivitt, R. W., Stewart, F. W., and Berg, J. W.: Tumors of the breast second series fascicle 2, Washington, D.C., 1968, Armed Forces Institute of Pathology, p. 86.

*Eight cancers of miscellaneous type excluded from tabulation.

an increased incidence of epithelial hyperplasia in subcutaneous mastectomy specimens in the contralateral breast in patients who previously underwent a radical mastectomy for carcinoma of the breast (see Chapter 9).

Intraductal carcinoma, papillary variant.[10] This is a rare form of breast carcinoma that is thought to antedate the infiltrating variety (Table 8-5). It is frequently multifocal, arising in large, intermediate, and small ducts. The microscopic appearance is characterized by atypical ingrowths of duct epithelium (Fig. 8-2). Malignant change is reflected in a disturbance of cell polarity. Hyperchromatism is not marked, and cell division is low. As outlined previously (see Chapter 5), there is evidence to suggest that noninfiltrative papillary carcinoma may be antedated by intraductal epithelial hyperplasia.

Intraductal carcinoma, comedocarcinoma variant.[10] This type is characterized by a solid growth within the ducts with marked cellular pleomorphism and is most often accompanied by central necrosis (Table 8-5). This can frequently be expressed from the cut specimen, thus the name comedo. Microscopically the cells evidence greater atypia, hyperchromatism, and loss of polarity (Fig. 8-3). This variety arises in intermediate and small ducts, less often in larger ducts.

Infiltrating ductal carcinoma, papillary variant.[10] This type of tumor is character-

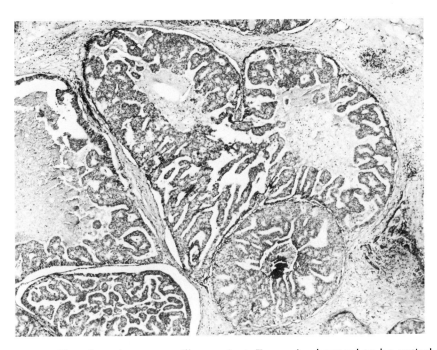

Fig. 8-2. Intraductal carcinoma, papillary variant. Tumor is observed to be entirely in intraductal space with definite basement membrane. Pronounced papillary nature of this tumor is emphasized. Central necrosis is apparent, and papillary character is retained in lower duct. (Courtesy Kenneth S. McCarty, Jr.)

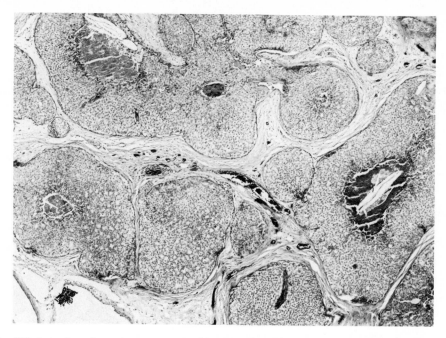

Fig. 8-3. Intraductal carcinoma, comedocarcinoma variant. Tumor is noted to be entirely within borders of basal lamina. There is extensive filling of ducts with pleomorphic cells. Characteristic comedocarcinoma feature of central necrosis is readily apparent. (Courtesy Kenneth S. McCarty, Jr.)

ized by a slow rate of growth and a long delay before metastasizing (Table 8-5). Having once metastasized, there is a slow progression to fatality. The tumor is frequently a bulky one, well circumscribed, and freely movable on palpation. This, in part, reflects its limited invasiveness. It is often confused preoperatively with a cyst or fibroadenoma. The microscopic appearance of this tumor is similar to the noninfiltrating form except that tumor cells extend beyond the duct and into the fibrous stroma.

Infiltrating ductal carcinoma with comedocarcinoma variant.[10] This tumor is also characterized by its large size and its slow rate of metastasis (Table 8-5). The microscopic appearance is similar to that of the noninfiltrative form. Once infiltration has occurred, however, tumor cells in the stroma appear to be indistinguishable from infiltrating ductal carcinoma with productive fibrosis. Because infiltration is often limited, these tumors may be well circumscribed. The biologic behavior of this tumor is related to the extent of the infiltrative portion rather than to total tumor size.

Infiltrating ductal carcinoma.[10] This type of tumor represents the most common of all mammary carcinomas, occurring with a frequency of about 80% (Table 8-5). Nodal metastasis at the time of primary recognition and treatment occurs with a frequency of 60%. The tumor is characterized by its infiltrative, irregular margin. Microscopically a variety of cell types can be seen (Fig. 8-4). In well-

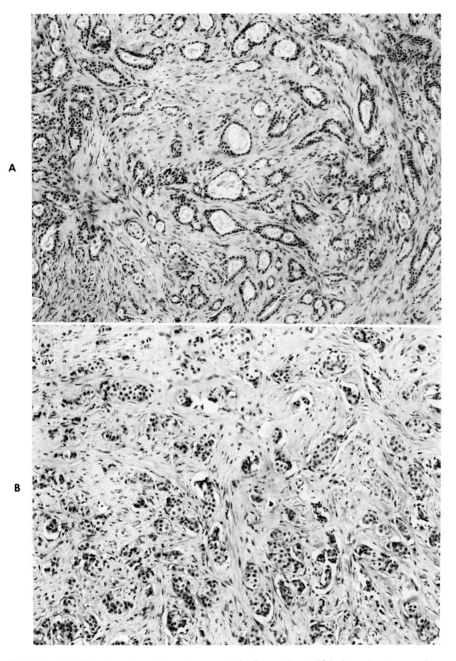

Fig. 8-4. A, Infiltrating ductal carcinoma, tubular variant. This invasive tumor is among the best differentiated of infiltrating ductal carcinomas. Whereas well-defined tubular arrangements are apparent, no basal lamina and free invasion of tumor cells into stroma are present. **B,** Infiltrating ductal carcinoma, not otherwise specified. Infiltrating nature of tumor cells into fibrous stroma is shown. Typically infiltrating ductal carcinomas infiltrate as clusters of pleomorphic invasive cells. Degree of tubule and/or glandular formation is important reflection of degree of differentiation. Tumor demonstrated shows little or no tubule formation. (Courtesy Kenneth S. McCarty, Jr.)

differentiated forms tubule formation is common. When stromal fibrosis is marked and cell compression occurs, the tumor cells may appear spindle shaped and fusiform. Tumor size correlates well with the frequency of regional axillary metastasis and ultimate survival.

Infiltrating ductal carcinoma, colloid variant.[10] This type is characterized by its abundant mucin (Table 8-5). Microscopically the cells appear orderly and mature looking (Fig. 8-5). The greater the differentiation, the greater the amount of mucin produced. This correlates well with the presence of axillary metastases and ultimate survival. Thus a pure gelatinous tumor has a lower incidence of axillary metastasis and a 78% 5-year survival. Tumors with less differentiation have survival figures the same as for unselected breast cancers.

Infiltrating ductal carcinoma, medullary variant.[10] This type of tumor is also characterized by its large size, often measuring 4 to 6 cm in diameter (Table 8-5). A circumscribed border with intense lymphocytic infiltrate is present, perhaps reflecting a low-grade infiltrative potential. Microscopically the tumor is among the most pleomorphic, composed of large oval or rounded cells with abundant cytoplasm and large nuclei (Fig. 8-6). The lymphocytic infiltration that frequently accompanies the tumor cells may represent a positive host response. The size of the lesion does not correlate well with the presence of axillary metastases or with ultimate survival. The configuration of the tumor border, whether circumscribed or irregular, however, is a better determinant of long-term survival.[20] Circumscribed borders have the best prognosis in the entire group. If metastases do occur, fatility occurs early. Interestingly no deaths occur after 5 years.

Invasive lobular carcinoma.[10] This type arises from the intralobular ducts and their terminal ramifications in the lobule (Table 8-5). Lobular hyperplasia is a change frequently observed in premenopausal patients and in patients on estrogenic hormones. No increased incidence of breast cancer in premenopausal patients with lobular hyperplasia has been observed; however, the incidence of malignancy is uncertain in postmenopausal patients (see Chapter 9).

The tumor is frequently bilateral (35% to 59%) and often multicentric (88%). Grossly the tumor has an irregular border and is poorly demarcated. Microscopically atypical lobules are noted (Fig. 8-7).[29] If the infiltrative area is inspected, lobular architecture is usually not present and diagnosis depends on the pattern of infiltration.

It should be apparent from the foregoing discussion that the histologic type of the primary lesion can influence prognosis considerably. Histologic type, however, is only one of many parameters that determine survival, some of which are incompletely understood.

MacDonald,[1] a proponent of "biologic predeterminism," believes that the complex interrelationship between tumor and host determines its responsiveness to therapy. He has stated that one third of breast carcinomas will rarely metastasize but if untreated will continue to grow and destroy tissue locally. Another one third will have already metastasized before the primary tumor is

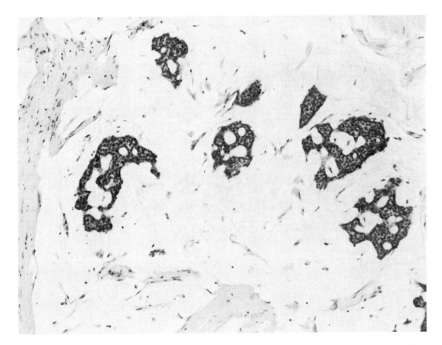

Fig. 8-5. Infiltrating ductal carcinoma, colloid variant. Tumor cells rest in sea of colloid material. With routine hematoxylin-eosin staining, this colloid appears blue. This is typical of the mucin secretory product observed in breast carcinoma cells of infiltrating ductal variant when secretory product is present. Contrast of mucin mixoid pattern with fibrous stroma is noted on left-hand side. (Courtesy Kenneth S. McCarty, Jr.)

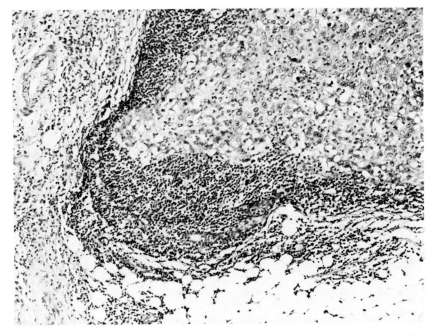

Fig. 8-6. Infiltrating ductal carcinoma, medullary variant. Medullary variant of infiltrating ductal carcinoma is invasive tumor characterized by relatively distinct borders that include profound infiltration of the tumor with lymphocytic elements. This is well demonstrated in the present example. The large bizarre morphology of tumor cells is also apparent. Prominent nucleoli are present in tumor cells. Numerous mitotic figures are seen. (Courtesy Kenneth S. McCarty, Jr.)

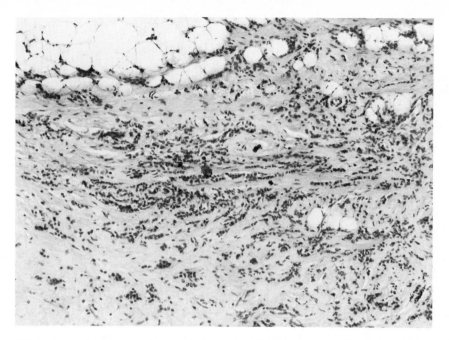

Fig. 8-7. Invasive lobular carcinoma. Lobular carcinoma variant of invasive breast cancer is characterized by presence of lobular orientation of tumor, and in invasive component a characteristic Indian filing is seen. The present example demonstrates this linear array of invasive tumor cells and the characteristic Indian filing. (Courtesy Kenneth S. McCarty, Jr.)

detected. The remaining one third will continue to grow, eventually reaching a size clinically detectable. There is, thus, a latent period during which growth occurs before systemic disease is apparent.

Metastasis in some tumors does not appear to be related to early diagnosis or size but rather to histologic type and host responsiveness. This group includes uncommon variants of breast carcinoma, including papillary, comedo, mucinous, and medullary variants.[2,3,4] It should be emphasized, however, that any of these histologic types, although behaving favorably as a group, can and will in selected hosts metastasize with eventual death (Table 8-3).[5] The likelihood of metastasis is also obviously greater in the infiltrative types.

Histologic grading

Histologic grading of mammary carcinoma has the advantage of indicating the degree of potential malignancy in tumors of varying cell types.[6,9] Epithelial elements in a tumor are evaluated on the basis of (1) tubular and/or adenocystic configuration; (2) nuclear variation; and (3) frequency of hyperchromatic and mitotic figures. Based on these evaluations, the tumor is placed in one of three grades of malignancy: (1) *low* (grade I); (2) *intermediate* (grade II); or (3) *high*

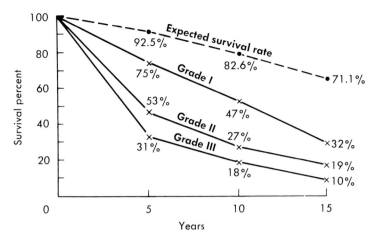

Fig. 8-8. Graph depicting crude survival for mammary carcinoma of different histologic grade. (From Bloom, H. J. G., and Richardson, W. W.: Br. J. Cancer **11:**359, 1957.)

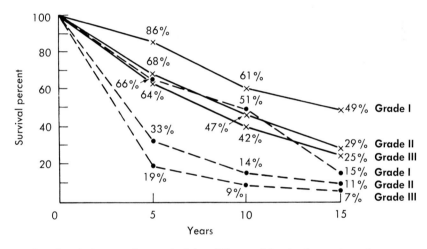

Fig. 8-9. Graph relating crude survival for different histologic grades of mammary carcinoma to presence or absence of axillary metastases. (From Bloom, H. J. G., and Richardson, W. W.: Br. J. Cancer **11:**359, 1957.)

grade (grade III). The crude 5-year survival for grade I was 75% and for grade III, 32% (Fig. 8-8). The crude 10-year survival for grade I was 53% and for grade III, 19%. Thus the number of survivors with low-grade malignancy was two to three times greater than those with high-grade malignancy. If the presence of axillary metastases was related to tumor grade, a more accurate guide to prognosis was obtained (Fig. 8-9). Thus the crude 5- and 10-year survival of patients with tumors of low-grade malignancy and negative axillary nodes was 86% and 61%, respectively. Similarly for high-grade malignancy with positive axillary nodes, crude survival at 5 and 10 years was 19% and 9%, respectively.[9]

Table 8-6. The Columbia Clinical Classification

Stage A	No skin edema, ulceration, or solid fixation of tumor to chest wall. Axillary nodes not clinically involved.
Stage B	No skin edema, ulceration, or solid fixation of tumor to chest wall. Clinically involved nodes, but less than 2.5 cm in transverse diameter and not fixed to overlying skin or deeper structures of axilla.
Stage C	Any one of five grave signs of advanced breast carcinoma: 1. Edema of skin of limited extent (involving less than one third of the skin over the breast). 2. Skin ulceration. 3. Solid fixation of tumor to chest wall. 4. Massive involvement of axillary lymph nodes (measuring 2.5 cm or more in transverse diameter). 5. Fixation of the axillary nodes to overlying skin or deeper structures of axilla.
Stage D	All other patients with more advanced breast carcinoma, including: 1. A combination of any two or more of the five grave signs listed under stage C. 2. Extensive edema of skin (involving more than one third of the skin over the breast). 3. Satellite skin nodules. 4. The inflammatory type of carcinoma. 5. Clinically involved supraclavicular lymph nodes. 6. Internal mammary metastases as evidenced by a parasternal tumor. 7. Edema of the arm. 8. Distant metastases.

From Haagenson, C. D.: Diseases of the breast, ed. 2, Philadelphia, 1971, W. B. Saunders Co., p. 630.

Axillary node metastases

One of the most important indications of long-term survival following the surgical treatment for carcinoma of the breast is the presence or absence of axillary metastases. The presence of regional metastases indicates that the delicate balance between host and tumor has been upset. If the axilla is free from disease, 67.8% of the patients will survive 5 years and 61% will survive 10 years. If axillary nodes are positive, survival rates are 44.4% and 26.6%, respectively.[14]

Haagensen,[15] based on his extensive experience in performing the radical mastectomy and using as an index of operability the Columbia Classification System (Table 8-6), finds axillary metastases to be present 45.5% of the time. This series although extensive was also highly selective. Using this system of classification, occult metastases were found in axillary nodes 33% of the time in clinical stage A.[13]

The presence or absence of axillary metastases as well as the number of involved nodes are important in influencing prognosis (Table 8-7). In clinical stage A, the 10-year survival rate for patients with one to three positive axillary nodes (68%) is almost as good as when there are no positive nodes (76.5%). If four to

Table 8-7. Radical mastectomy for breast carcinoma—extent of axillary metastasis correlated with 10-year survival—personal series of cases, 1935—July, 1963

Columbia Clinical Classification	No. of axillary nodes with metastases	No. of patients	10-year survival	
			Number	Percentage
Stage A	No nodes involved	418	320	76.5
	1-3 nodes involved	131	89	68
	4-7 nodes involved	30	10	33
	8 or more nodes involved	29	6	20
	TOTAL	608	425	70
Stage B	No nodes involved	48	34	70
	1-3 nodes involved	61	27	44
	4-7 nodes involved	37	14	38
	8 or more nodes involved	40	5	12
	TOTAL	186	80	43
Stage C	No nodes involved	17	8	47
	1-3 nodes involved	21	6	29
	4-7 nodes involved	9	4	44
	8 or more nodes involved	29	3	10
	TOTAL	76	21	30
Stage D	No nodes involved	1	0	
	1-3 nodes involved	2	1	
	4-7 nodes involved	1	0	
	8 or more nodes involved	8	1	
	TOTAL	12	2	17
TOTAL		882		

From Haagensen, C. D.: Diseases of the breast, ed. 2, Philadelphia, 1971, W. B. Saunders Co., p. 706.

seven nodes are involved, the 10-year survival rate drops to 33%.[15] These observations are also supported by the findings of the National Surgical Breast Project[12] (Table 8-8). Results of this study failed to demonstrate that the discovery and examination of a greater number of lymph nodes in a surgical specimen were more meaningful in determining prognosis than if a smaller number were found.

Size of primary tumor

The size of the primary tumor has a direct correlation with the presence of axillary metastases and ultimate survival. Statistics relating size of the primary tumor to both 5- and 10-year survival periods should also be reviewed with an understanding of the histologic types. Some tumors, such as infiltrating papillary carcinoma, infiltrating comedocarcinoma, and infiltrating medullary carcinoma, grow slowly and become quite bulky and large before metastasizing. These tu-

Table 8-8. Survival rates according to number of nodes examined

Months after operation	No. of nodes examined								
	1 to 5			6 to 10			11 to 15		
	No.*	S†	Percent‡	No.	S	Percent	No.	S	Percent
Negative nodes									
18§	70	68	97	285	270	95	380	361	95
36§	56	50	89	247	215	87	317	271	85
60‖	35	26	74	161	123	76	211	163	77
Positive nodes									
18	47	40	85	217	179	82	353	297	84
36	44	30	68	188	116	62	293	194	66
60	35	16	46	136	60	44	189	98	52
1 to 3 positive nodes									
18	36	31	86	122	113	93	179	165	92
36	34	24	71	103	76	74	140	112	80
60	27	12	44	74	43	58	99	67	68
4+ positive nodes									
18	11	9	82	95	66	69	174	132	76
36	10	6	60	85	40	47	153	82	54
60	8	4	50	62	17	27	90	31	34
All patients									
18	117	108	92	502	449	89	733	658	90
36	100	80	80	435	331	76	610	465	76
60	70	42	60	297	183	62	400	261	65

From Fisher, B., and Slack, N. H.: Number of lymph nodes examined and the prognosis of breast Gynecology and Obstetrics.
*Number of patients followed up.
†Number of patients surviving.
‡Survival rate.
§Phase 1 patients plus phase 2 patients followed up 18 months or more.
‖Phase 1 patients plus phase 2 patients followed up for 5 years or more.

mors account for only a small percentage of the total, thus explaining the validity of the relationship of tumor size and survival.

Metastasis has already taken place in almost three fourths of the patients with tumors larger than 5 cm when first examined. Studies have shown that a 73% 5-year survival rate existed for those patients whose tumors measured less than 2 cm, 24% for those patients whose lesions measured 3 to 6 cm, and 16% when the lesion measured 7 cm or more.[4,16,17]

Haagensen[14] has noted that only 33% of the patients with a primary tumor size measuring less than 3 cm had axillary metastases. Approximately 50% had axillary metastases if the tumor size was greater than 3 cm. Tumor size was also noted to have a direct relationship to the degree of axillary involvement.

16 to 20			21 to 25			26 to 30			31 or more		
No.	S	Percent	No.	S	Percent	No.	S	Percent	No.	S	Percent
363	346	95	211	203	96	104	100	96	97	94	97
301	271	90	174	155	89	85	74	87	82	73	89
195	154	79	129	104	81	59	45	76	62	50	81
347	295	85	257	222	86	125	99	79	143	117	82
305	192	63	223	143	64	113	65	58	123	75	61
197	86	44	140	67	48	78	44	56	92	44	48
183	174	95	108	99	92	59	53	90	42	41	98
159	121	76	92	71	77	52	39	75	34	29	85
102	56	55	56	38	68	39	26	67	29	22	76
164	121	74	149	123	83	66	46	70	101	76	75
146	71	49	131	72	55	61	26	43	89	46	52
95	30	32	84	29	35	39	18	46	63	22	35
710	641	90	468	425	91	229	199	87	240	211	88
606	463	76	397	298	75	198	139	70	205	148	72
392	240	61	269	171	64	137	89	65	154	94	61

carcinoma, Surg. Gynecol. Obstet. **131**(1): 79-88, July-September, 1970. By permission of Surgery,

Configuration of tumor border

Primary tumors have been classified into groups depending on the macroscopic configuration of their borders. Well-delineated carcinomas are thought to represent a slower, more expansile type of growth, whereas irregular carcinomas are thought to represent a more rapid and malignant growth pattern. Lane concluded, after excluding papillary, comedo, and mucoid carcinomas from the study, that circumscribed lesions were one third larger and that the incidence of axillary metastases was significantly lower than that of the more infiltrative variety.[19,20] Haagensen supports these observations. In the multiple regression analysis of Alderson[5] previously cited, however, the configuration of the tumor border was not a valid factor in determining survival (Tables 8-1 and 8-2).

Host defense response

As outlined earlier, MacDonald[20] in his theory of biologic predeterminism emphasized the importance of the host-tumor interaction in the ultimate survival of the patient. Tumor immunology is a rapidly expanding area of scientific endeavor. A thorough discussion is beyond the scope of this text, however, its importance in understanding the behavior of any malignancy cannot be over-emphasized. There is no question that host defenses influence prognosis directly; however, a direct measurement of this effect is still elusive. Lymphocytic, macrophage, and plasmocytic infiltration both within and around the tumor have been measured as well as the immunoblast and plasma cell content of axillary nodes. When all of these factors were grouped as indices of host defense, the relationship to survival was highly significant.[4]

TIMING OF RECONSTRUCTION

During the past 40 years the surgical treatment of head and neck malignancies has evolved from simple extirpation of the primary tumor to an en bloc wide dissection including the regional nodes. As surgeons became more aggressive in their treatment, the surgical defect similarly increased. Delayed reconstruction often scheduled for an indefinite future date was undertaken earlier both to correct the functional deficit and to improve the appearance of the patient. If a primary tumor did recur locally after surgical treatment, survival was limited, approximately 15%. Because of the many advantages of immediate and early reconstruction and the abysmally poor chance for survival in cases of recurrent tumor, most head and neck surgeons are now skilled in both the extirpative and reconstructive aspects of this surgery. Frequently reconstruction is completed during the initial operative procedure.

Reconstruction of the breast following radical mastectomy is presently being carefully evaluated, especially with regard to its effect on survival. A change in thinking in terms of the timing of reconstruction is also taking place. This evolution of thought from a "wait and see" attitude to early reconstruction has been somewhat retarded because reconstruction to improve the function of the breast is limited. None of the present techniques can restore lactation or nipple sensitivity and erectility. There are functional deficits resulting, however, after mastectomy. Frequently there is a deficiency of healthy, well-vascularized skin, often accentuated by postoperative radiation therapy. Skin atrophy and ulceration occur and lymphedema of the ipsilateral upper extremity can be disabling. Only now are psychologic reasons for restoration of form and contour being appreciated and significance attributed to these valid reasons for early reconstruction. Perhaps as important is the emerging concept that even if a cure is not effected with the primary therapy, why not reconstruct the ablated breast? There is no evidence to suggest that early reconstruction either retards or influences further treatment or adversely affects predicted survival.

During the past 5 years considerable attention has been directed to the contralateral breast of women with a previous mastectomy and to breasts of some women with a significantly higher predicted incidence to develop carcinoma of the breast. Carcinoma of the breast affects 5% to 7% of all women. In women whose mothers, daughters, or sisters have developed a breast cancer, the risk of developing a breast malignancy is two to five times greater than the average incidence.[21,22,23] If a patient develops bilateral breast malignancies, her close female relatives have an even higher risk of developing carcinoma of the breast.

Over the years it has become increasingly apparent that cancer is a systemic, not a local, disease. It is not surprising, therefore, that the incidence of malignancy of the opposite unaffected breast is 6% to 7% greater than in the average female population.[24,26,27]

As the natural history of breast cancer becomes better understood, precancerous mastopathies will be identified (Chapter 5). If untreated, frank malignant change may occur with a predicted frequency.

The subcutaneous mastectomy is being performed with increased frequency and has replaced the more mutilative simple mastectomy and/or multiple biopsy in these high-risk patients. Its role in reconstruction is presently being evaluated (see Chapter 9).

With changing attitudes toward breast reconstruction, the plastic and reconstructive surgeon has had an increasing involvement in the early treatment of these patients. It is not unusual in our present institution for patients to discuss with the general surgeon preoperatively not only the treatment of the contralateral breast but also early reconstruction of the breast with a demonstrated malignancy.

Immediate reconstruction

There is a small group of patients who qualify for immediate reconstruction after radical mastectomy. In these patients malignancy may be suspected by abnormal xeromammograms obtained in a patient in a high-risk category. The lesion may not even be palpable. A small lesion may be encountered on breast biopsy or in a subcutaneous mastectomy specimen.

Candidates considered for immediate reconstruction have: (1) a small lesion (less than 2.0 cm); (2) favorable histologic type and grading, for example, infiltrative papillary carcinoma or comedocarcinoma, infiltrative colloid, mucinous, or infiltrative ductal carcinoma; and (3) negative axillary nodes.

If such a small infiltrative lesion is found, a modified radical mastectomy is done. The nipple is "banked" in the inguinal region if biopsy of the base reveals no involvement and if there is no evidence of the Paget disease. Five days are permitted to elapse until permanent histology of both the primary lesion and the axillary contents are thoroughly evaluated. If these criteria are met and the patient is considered a suitable candidate, a silicone gel prosthesis is inserted at this time. Frequently additional size correction must be done several months later and the problem of the contralateral breast dealt with. Nipple transplantation is usually done at this late date as well.

Early reconstruction

Candidates for early reconstruction (usually within 18 months to 2 years after mastectomy) are those whose primary tumor size, histology, grading, and axillary contents indicate a favorable long-term survival. Criteria for reconstruction include: (1) primary tumor size less than 2.0 cm in diameter (2 to 5 cm in diameter if infiltrating papillary, medullary carcinoma, or comedocarcinoma); (2) favorable histologic type and grading, for example, infiltrating papillary, mucinous, medullary, ductal and lobular carcinoma, or comedocarcinoma with grade I Bloom classification; (3) negative axillary nodes or zero to three positive axillary nodes; (4) no detectable recurrent or metastatic disease.

Delayed reconstruction

Candidates in this group have a less favorable prognosis by the criteria outlined previously. Reconstruction can be considered after 2 years if no recurrent or local disease is evident. Included in this group are less well-differentiated tumors with or without axillary metastases that statistically have a guarded long-term survival. Considerable individual scrutiny must be given to patients in this group, and all parameters that influence prognosis must be carefully assessed. Results from this evaluation must be weighed with all those factors influencing the rationale for reconstruction.

CONCLUSION

In this discussion every attempt has been made to evaluate those multiple factors that influence both the patient and the surgeon to reconstruct an ablated breast for malignancy. Before any decision is made, the malignant potential of the contralateral breast must be carefully considered since both breasts should be included in the total reconstructive effort. The reconstructive surgeon must have a thorough knowledge of the natural history of breast cancer as it relates to prognosis and ultimate survival. Such knowledge will permit wise and careful patient selection.

Once the multiple variables that influence prognosis are understood, the timing of reconstruction can be individualized. Patient satisfaction can thus be achieved through reconstruction that is hopefully accompanied by prolonged survival free from disease.

ACKNOWLEDGMENT

I wish to acknowledge Dr. Kenneth S. McCarty, Jr., for his invaluable critique of the chapter and also for the use of certain illustrations.

REFERENCES

1. Alderson, M. R., Hamlin, I., and Staunton, M. D.: The relative significance of prognostic factors in breast carcinoma, Br. J. Cancer **25:**646, 1971.
2. Anderson, D. E.: Some characteristics of familial breast cancer, Cancer **28:**1500, 1971.
3. Anderson, D. E.: Familial factors in breast cancer and their implications, Hosp. Pract. **7**(6):107, 1972.
4. Bloom, H. J. G., and Richardson, W. W.: Histological grading and prognosis in breast cancer, Br. J. Cancer **11:**359, 1957.
5. Brightmore, T. G., Greening, W. A., and Hamlin, I.: An analysis of clinical and histo-

pathological features in 101 cases of carcinoma of breast in women under 35 years of age, Br. J. Cancer **24:**644, 1970.

6. Cutler, S. J., Christine, B., and Barcley, T. H. C.: Increasing incidence and decreasing mortality rates for breast cancer, Cancer **28**(2):1376-1380, 1971.

7. del Regato, J. A., and Spjut, H. J.: Ackerman and del Regato's Cancer: diagnosis, treatment, and prognosis, ed. 5, St. Louis, 1977, The C. V. Mosby Co.

8. Fisher, B., and Slack, N. H.: Number of lymph nodes examined and the prognosis of breast carcinoma, Surg. Gynecol. Obstet. **131:**79, 1970.

9. Fisher, B., and associates: Cancer of the breast: size of neoplasm and prognosis, Cancer **24:**1071, 1969.

10. Gold, D., and Roth, E. J.: Current operative treatment of carcinoma of the breast and its rationale, Am. J. Surg. **110:**724, 1965.

11. Greenough, R. B.: Varying degrees of malignancy in cancer of the breast, J. Cancer Res. **9:**453-463, 1925.

12. Haagensen, C. D.: Special pathological forms of breast carcinoma. In Haagensen, C. D.: Diseases of the breast, Philadelphia, 1971, W. B. Saunders Co., p. 608.

13. Haagensen, C. D.: The clinical classification of carcinoma of the breast and the choice of treatment. In Haagensen, C. D.: Diseases of the breast, Philadelphia, 1971, W. B. Saunders Co., p. 631.

14. Haagensen, C. D.: The natural history of breast carcinoma. In Haagensen, C. D.: Diseases of the breast, ed. 2, Philadelphia, 1971, W. B. Saunders Co., p. 401.

15. Haagensen, C. D.: The surgical treatment of mammary carcinoma. In Haagensen, C. D.: Diseases of the breast, ed. 2, Philadelphia, 1971, W. B. Saunders Co., p. 706.

16. Lane, N., Goksel, H., and Salerno, R. A.: Clinico-pathologic analysis of the surgical curability of breast cancers: a minimum ten-year study of a personal series, Ann. Surg. **153:**483, 1961.

17. Leis, H. P., Jr., and associates: The second breast, N.Y. State J. Med. **65:**2460, 1965.

18. Lewison, E. F.: Breast cancer and its diagnosis and treatment, Baltimore, 1955, The William & Wilkins Co.

19. Lewison, E. F., and Neto, A. S.: Bilateral breast cancer at Johns Hopkins Hospital, Cancer **28:**1279, 1971.

20. MacDonald, I.: The natural history of mammary carcinoma, Am. J. Surg. **111:**435, 1966.

21. McDivitt, R. W., Stewart, F. W., and Berg, J. W.: Tumors of the breast, Bethesda, Md., 1968, Armed Forces Institute of Pathology.

22. Moore, F. D., and associates: Carcinoma of the breast: a decade of new results with old concepts, N. Engl. J. Med. **277:**293, 1967.

23. Moore, O. S., Jr., and Toote, F. W., Jr.: The relatively favorable prognosis of medullary carcinoma of the breast, Cancer **2:**635, 1949.

24. Norris, H. J., and Taylor, H. B.: Prognosis of mucinous (gelatinous) carcinoma of the breast, Cancer **18:**879, 1965.

25. Robbins, G. F., and Berg, S. W.: Bilateral primary breast cancers: a prospective clinico-pathology study, Cancer **17:**1501, 1964.

26. Rush, B. F., Jr.: Breast. In Schwartz, S. I., editor-in-chief: Principles of surgery, ed. 2, New York, 1974, McGraw-Hill Book Co., p. 540.

27. Schiödt, T.: Breast carcinoma: a histologic and prognostic study of 650 followed-up cases, Copenhagen, 1966, Munksgaard.

28. Spratt, J. S., and Donegan, W. L.: Cancer of the breast: major problems in clinical surgery, Philadelphia, 1967, W. B. Saunders Co., vol. 51.

29. Warner, N. E.: Lobular carcinoma of the breast, Cancer **23:**840, 1969.

CHAPTER 9

Clinical significance of histopathologic lesions observed in the contralateral breast in patients with breast carcinoma

Kenneth S. McCarty, Jr., Gregg H. D. Kesterson, and
Nicholas G. Georgiade

Breast cancer affects one woman in every fifteen in the United States.[8] In properly selected patients the technique of reconstructive breast surgery may provide a means of reducing the physical and emotional stigmata of mastectomy.[6] Patients with the highest probability of long-term survival, as determined by clinical and pathologic staging, are the best candidates for reconstruction.[6,8] With long-term follow-up the likelihood of observing carcinoma in the remaining breast becomes considerable.[20] Carcinoma in this setting occurs at a frequency sixfold to seventeenfold greater than does breast carcinoma in patients with no previous mammary malignancy.[9] Whereas contralateral tumor infrequently occurs synchronously with the first cancer, the likelihood of carcinoma being discovered in the remaining breast increases with each year following the discovery of cancer in the first breast.[20] The techniques of subcutaneous mastectomy with immediate reconstruction[6] may provide a satisfactory approach to the problem of the contralateral breast at high risk for carcinomatous involvement.

The histopathology of the clinically uninvolved breast at a time proximal to mastectomy of the contralateral breast is of considerable interest in view of the eventual frequency of bilaterality of breast cancer (12% to 24%).[9,20,22] The characterization of which epithelial lesions may represent "premalignant" dysplasias would greatly enhance the management of both the breast contralateral to diagnosed carcinoma and the breasts of patients with high clinical risks of developing carcinoma.[2,3,5,19] Explanation of such "premalignant" lesions has been used by Jensen and Wellings to attempt to define these entities.[10] Another approach has been to seek statistical correlation of histopathlogic lesions from uninvolved areas of cancerous breasts[2,13] or to prospectively compare lesions observed in patients who have had a biopsy interpreted as benign, who subsequently develop carcinoma.[4,19] Others have evaluated the remaining breast contralateral to a previous breast carcinoma using autopsy-acquired specimens.[15,23] These approaches have shown certain epithelial proliferative lesions to be closely associated with carcinoma.

As a standard practice in our institution, breasts removed by glandular mastectomy are extensively evaluated by a standardized protocol. The present discussion emphasizes the importance of certain epithelial proliferative lesions observed in breasts contralateral to diagnosed breast cancer. The findings in fifty subcutaneous glandular mastectomy specimens obtained from patients who had previously undergone mastectomy for carcinoma are compared to those in age-, side-, and date-matched breasts from fifty patients who underwent bilateral glandular mastectomies for indications other than the histopathologic diagnosis of malignancy.

MATERIALS AND METHODS

Sixty consecutive subcutaneous mastectomies in patients who had previously undergone mastectomy for carcinoma of the contralateral breast were selected as a study population. Of these, ten were excluded because either: (1) histologic material from the original surgery was unavailable (eight patients) or (2) histologic diagnosis of the original cancer was questionable (two patients). The fifty patients remaining in the study population ranged in age from 28 to 55 years with one patient age 71 years. The patients underwent subcutaneous mastectomy in the period from 1974 to 1977. The mean interval from mastectomy for carcinoma to contralateral subcutaneous mastectomy with reconstruction was 34 months (range <1 to 30 years; Table 9-1). Among the study population were 20 patients who had normally cycling menstrual periods, five patients who had received chemotherapy that interfered with menstrual cycling, and twenty-five patients who were either surgically or naturally menopausal (twenty menstruating; thirty nonmenstruating). The control population consisted of women who were age-matched within 2 years of the study population and who were operated on with bilateral subcutaneous mastectomies in the same period, 1974 to 1977. The control population consisted of twenty-two patients who were apparently normally cycling, with the remainder being naturally or surgically menopausal (twenty-two menstruating; twenty-eight nonmenstruating).

The mammary glands from both the study and control populations were obtained from the operating room in the fresh state, with sutures placed for quadrant orientation and identification of the subareolar region. The breasts were sectioned at 3-mm intervals in the sagittal plane and examined on a stereomicroscope with transillumination and/or epi-illumination at four to fifty magnifications. Areas containing subgrossly apparent lesions were selected in addition to representative sections of the four quadrants to include a minimum of 20 cm^2 from the four quadrants and the subareolar region. The tissue was fixed in 0.1M phosphate buffered 4% formalin pH 7.2 and subsequently dehydrated and embedded in paraffin. Sections were prepared at 6μ to 8μ and stained with hema-

Table 9-1. Study population characteristics

Age at radical or modified radical mastectomy (years)	Histologic type of carcinoma	Nodes (involved/total)	Age at subcutaneous mastectomy (years)	Menstrual status*
27	Infiltrating ductal	0/12	28	C, TL
27	Medullary	0/18	29	hys, oop
30	Infiltrating ductal	0/18	30	**Chemo R_x
29	Infiltrating ductal	0/19	30	C, TL
30	Infiltrating ductal and intraductal	0/28	30	C
29	Infiltrating ductal	-/-	31	C
32	Infiltrating lobular	0/8	32	C
33	Colloid	-/-	33	C
33	Infiltrating ductal and lobular / Lobular carcinoma in situ and intraductal	0/17	33	**Chemo R_x
33	Infiltrating ductal	0/12	34	**Chemo R_x
36	Infiltrating ductal	0/12	36	C
36	Scirrhous	1/18	36	C
35	Infiltrating ductal and intraductal	0/12	36	C
36	Intraductal	0/17	37	C
32	Infiltrating ductal	0/16	38	C, TL
37	Intraductal	0/21	39	*oop
40	Intraductal	0/9	40	C
40	Intraductal	0/25	40	+hys, oop
40	Tubular	0/17	40	hys, C
38	Scirrhous	3/28	40	***Chemo R_x
35	Infiltrating ductal and intraductal	0/14	41	hys, oop
39	Infiltrating ductal	0/19	41	hys, C
39	Infiltrating ductal and intraductal	0/7	42	C, TL
44	Infiltrating ductal	0/23	44	MP
32	Medullary	0/13	44	C, TL
42	Infiltrating ductal	0/23	44	C
44	Intraductal	0/12	44	C
42	Intraductal and lobular carcinoma in situ	0/32	45	MP
41	Infiltrating ductal	0/9	45	hys, oop
38	Infiltrative ductal	-/-	45	*hys, oop

*C, cycling menses; TL, tubal ligation; hys, hysterectomy; oop, oophorectomy; **, Alkeran, 12 months; Chemo r_x, chemotherapy received; *, 3000 rads cobalt; +, L-PAM 6 weeks; ***, see Table 5-3 adjuvant therapy; MP, menopausal; ++, prednisone 15 mg/qd. (asthma); +++, levothyroxine (Synthroid).

Table 9-1. Study population characteristics —cont'd

Age at radical or modified radical mastectomy (years)	Histologic type of carcinoma	Nodes (involved/total)	Age at subcutaneous mastectomy (years)	Menstrual status
39	Infiltrating ductal	0/14	46	C
43	Infiltrative ductal	7/31	46	***Chemo R_x
43	Infiltrating ductal	0/12	47	MP
47	Infiltrating ductal	-/-	47	MP
42	Infiltrating ductal	1/25	47	C
39	Infiltrating ductal	0/18	48	++MP, hys
47	Lobular carcinoma in situ	0/8	48	C
31	Infiltrating ductal	-/-	48	hys
40	Infiltrating ductal	0/7	49	hys
30	Intraductal	0/4	51	hys
27	Intraductal	0/13	51	MP
49	Tubular	0/18	51	oop
48	Intraductal	0/17	51	MP
51	Intraductal	0/0	52	MP
51	Infiltrating ductal	0/6	53	hys
50	Infiltrating lobular	3/14	53	Chemo R_x
53	Scirrhous	0/11	54	MP
51	Medullary	2/16	55	*hys
43	Infiltrating lobular		55	+++hys
41	Infiltrating ductal		71	MP

toxylin and eosin. Following age and date matching of the control population to the ipsilateral matched breast from the bilateral control was utilized), each slide was coded and examined without knowledge as to whether it was from the control or study population.

Table 9-1 shows the histopathologic diagnosis of the initial mastectomy specimen containing carcinoma as well as the nodal status of patients in the study population. The menstrual status is indicated as well as the age of subcutaneous mastectomy and age of initial radical or modified radical mastectomy for cancer of the contralateral breast. Those patients who received medications or other therapies that might have altered the histopathology of their subsequent subcutaneous mastectomy are also noted in Table 9-1. Patients with a family history of breast cancer are indicated in Table 9-2.

Those patients with positive axillary nodes in the original surgical specimen are shown in Table 9-3. The histopathologic diagnosis, nodal status, and interval in months between initial and contralateral breast surgery are noted for these six patients. Three patients as noted received adjuvant chemotherapy. The mean

Table 9-2. Association of family history with proliferative lesions

Family history*	Histologic type of carcinoma	Nodes (involved/ total)	Age at subcutaneous mastectomy (years)	Menstrual status†	Epithelial lesion‡
A, A, GM (P)	Infiltrating ductal	0/12	28	C, TL	P
S, M	Infiltrating ductal (medullary)	0/18	29	hys, oop	
S	Infiltrating ductal	0/18	30	Chemo R$_x$	P
S, M	Infiltrating lob- ular	0/8	32	C	P, C
M	Infiltrating ductal and intraductal	0/12	36	C	P, S
M, GM	Intraductal	0/17	37	C	P/C
M	Intraductal	0/21	39	oop	S, S/C, P/C
S, A, M	Infiltrating ductal and intraductal	0/14	41	hys, oop	
M	Infiltrating ductal	0/19	41	hys, C	
S	Infiltrating ductal	0/23	44	S	P, S
A (P), S	Infiltrating ductal	0/9	45	hys, oop	
S	Infiltrating ductal	-/-	47	MP	P
S	Infiltrating ductal	0/18	48	MP, hys	
S	Infiltrating ductal	0/7	49	hys	C
S	Intraductal	0/0	52	MP	C, P/C
GM	Infiltrating lob- ular	3/14	53	Chemo R$_x$	P, C

*A, Aunt; GM, grandmother; (P), paternal; S, sister; M, mother.
†See Table 5-1 for abbreviations.
‡Moderate or severe lesions. P, papillary intraductal hyperplasia; C, cribriform intraductal hyperplasia; S, solid intraductal hyperplasia.

Table 9-3. Management of patients with positive axillary nodes in original surgical specimen

Tumor histology original mastectomy	Nodes (involved/ total)	Age at subcutaneous mastectomy (years)	Interval between radical or modified radical mastectomy and subcutaneous mastectomy (months)	Adjuvant therapy (duration)*
Scirrhous (right)	3/28	40	24	5FU, MTX, CYT (18 months)
Infiltrating ductal (right)	7/31	46	30	5FU, MTX, CYT (18 months)
Infiltrating lobular (left)	3/14	53	34	L-PAM (12 months)
Medullary (right)	2/16	55	38	
Infiltrating ductal (left)	1/25	47	60	
Scirrhous (right)	1/18	36	22	

*5FU; 5-fluorouracil; MTX; Methotrexate; CYT, cyclophosphamide (Cytoxan); L-PAM, L-phenyl-alanine mustard.

interval between mastectomy for carcinoma and subsequent subcutaneous contralateral mastectomy was 34.7 months for women in this group.

RESULTS

The patient study population included fifty patients of whom sixteen had positive family histories for breast cancer (Table 9-1). Of these sixteen patients, ten were 45 years old or younger (Tables 9-1 and 9-2). Of the breast carcinomas associated with a positive family history, 30% included a significant component of intraductal carcinoma. The intraductal epithelial proliferative lesions are prominent in this subpopulation (Table 9-3).

Moderate or severe epithelial proliferative changes of papillary, solid, and cribriform hyperplasia (Figs. 9-1 to 9-3) as well as combinations of these have a statistically significant (p=0.025 to 0.005) increased incidence in the patients who have had previous contralateral breast carcinoma compared to patients who had no such history. For specific age-matched pairs (cases/controls) the lesions in this group were statistically significant more frequently than that for the control population. Sclerosing adenosis, cystic duct dilation (gross or

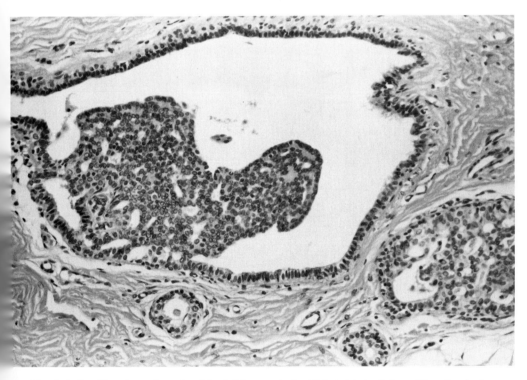

Fig. 9-1. Papillary intraductal epithelial hyperplasia. This intraductal proliferative lesion demonstrates a distinct stalk and a mixed cell population (H & E; 100X).

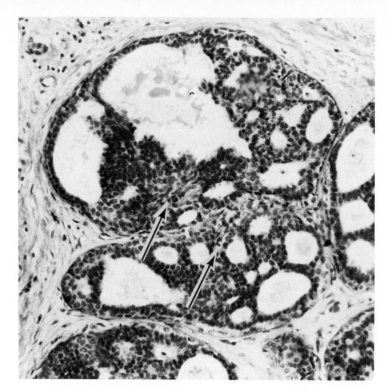

Fig. 9-2. Cribriform intraductal epithelial hyperplasia. This proliferative lesion contains mixed epithelial components arranged in a cribriform pattern, without necrosis and demonstrating some stalk formation *(arrows)* as well as myoepithelial elements. There is marked variation in the cribriform pattern in areas (H & E; 100X).

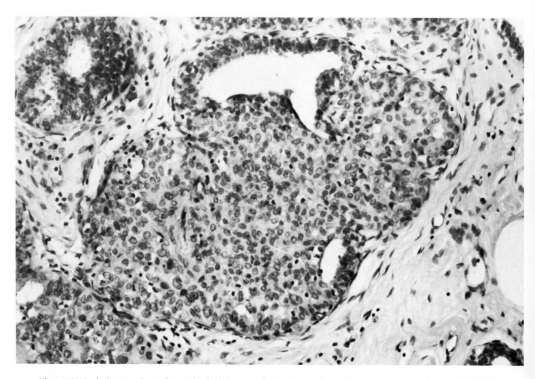

Fig. 9-3. Solid intraductal epithelial hyperplasia. The ductal lumen is nearly occluded by proliferation of the ductal epithelium. Some cellular variation is noted (H & E; 100X).

microcystic), lobular hyperplasia, subepithelial calcification, or any of the other lesions classified (Table 9-4) failed to demonstrate a statistically significant association with carcinoma. The significance of the increased proportions of eipthelial hyperplastic lesions is emphasized when it is realized that the control population contained many patients believed clinically to be at a high risk for the development of breast cancer (family history, ethnic extraction, late parity, multiple previous biopsies, etc.) who displayed severe fibrocystic disease of both breasts (Table 9-4).

In order to segregate the possible contribution of ovarian influence on the relative frequency of the various lesions observed, a comparison of histopathologic characteristics of the study population separated into premenopausal and either naturally or surgically postmenopausal patients is shown in Table 9-5. These data suggest that the papillary proliferative form is more commonly seen in the premenopausal group, whereas the cribriform intraductal proliferation is seen primarily in the postmenopausal group. The mixed patterns and solid proliferative lesion are seen with approximately equal frequency with respect to menstrual status, as is sclerosing adenosis. It is of interest that lobular hyperplasia is of equal frequency in the premenopausal and postmenopausal groups, as is apocrine metaplasia. Blunt duct adenosis, fibroadenoma, and fibroadenomatous changes are lesions of the premenopausal group. Carcinoma in the contra-

Table 9-4. Association of lesions with carcinoma of contralateral breast

	Cases		Controls		Statistical significance*
	Present	Absent	Present	Absent	
Intraductal epithelial hyperplasias					
Papillary	21	29	10	40	$x^2 = 5.66$, p = 0.025
Solid	8	42	0	50	$x^2 = 8.70$, p = 0.005
Cribriform	10	40	1	49	$x^2 = 9.27$, p = 0.005
Papillary/cribriform	8	42	2	48	$x^2 = 5.55$, p = 0.025
Solid/cribriform	2	48	1	49	PSI
Papillary/solid	1	49	2	48	PSI
Apocrine metaplasia	19	31	17	33	$x^2 = 0.17$ NS
Sclerosing adenosis	19	31	12	38	$x^2 = 2.29$ NS
Blunt duct adenosis	23	27	21	29	$x^2 = 0.16$ NS
Cystic duct dilation	20	30	25	25	$x^2 = 1.01$ NS
Subepithelial calcification	6	44	7	43	$x^2 = 0.09$ NS
Fibroadenomatous change	7	43	8	42	$x^2 = 0.08$ NS
Lobular hyperplasia	18	32	11	39	$x^2 = 2.38$ NS

*x^2, CHI-squared; PSI, population size inadequate to assess significance (that is, too few lesions observed); NS, not statistically significant.

Table 9-5. Comparison of cellular lesions in premenopausal and postmenopausal cases*

Lesion (moderate or severe degree)	Premenopausal (twenty cases) (%)	Postmenopausal (twenty-five cases) (%)
Intraductal epithelial hyperplasias		
Papillary	55	20
Solid	30	12
Cribriform	5	28
Papillary/solid	5	
Papillary/cribriform	20	20
Solid/cribriform		8
Other lesions		
Sclerosing adenosis	35	28
Lobular hyperplasia	30	36
Apocrine metaplasia	45	32
Blunt duct adenosis	45	36
Fibroadenoma and fibroadenomatous change	20	8

*Five patients whose menses ceased secondary to chemotherapy are excluded.

lateral breast is exhibited once in each study subgroup—those patients who received chemotherapy, those who were postmenopausal, and the premenopausal subjects. In each case the cancerous subcutaneous mastectomy specimen had been contralateral to a breast containing intraductal carcinoma.

Patients who received chemotherapy were noted to have fewer epithelial proliferative lesions than the patients who did not receive chemotherapy. Remarkably, cellular atypia was uncommon in this group. The patients having received chemotherapy were excluded from the premenopausal and postmenopausal designation. The three study cases exhibiting carcinoma (6%) had 1-, 2-, and 4-year intervals from the time of initial mastectomy to the time of subcutaneous mastectomy.

DISCUSSION

The prognosis of a patient with carcinoma of the breast is directly related to the stage of the disease at the time of mastectomy.[8] The probability of a malignancy being discovered in the contralateral breast becomes increasingly important in the patient in whom prolonged survival or surgical "cure" is likely.[5,9,20,22] In Foote and Stewart's now classical work on the breast contralateral to a diagnosed carcinomatous breast, it was concluded that "the most frequent antecedent of cancer in one breast is the history of cancer in the opposite breast."[5] To approach this problem, Urban proposed generous biopsies of the upper outer quadrant and mirror image site of the contralateral breast at the time of amputation of a carcinomatous breast.[22] Utilizing this technique, Urban observed seven of sixty (11.7%) biopsies demonstrating a second tumor in the opposite breast when no clinical signs were noted in that breast, whereas twenty-four of ninety-nine biopsies (24%) contained tumor when minimal signs were noted.[22]

Such biopsy procedures are effective in optimizing management of the patient when the biopsies obtained contain a clear-cut histologic picture of malignancy.[22] Difficulties arise when there is no tumor seen since the biopsied breast is rendered considerably more difficult to examine and follow clinically by the scarring that inevitably accompanies biopsy of the mammary gland. The proportion of cases in which a simultaneous or subsequent tumor was observed by Urban is higher than that observed by others[9,15,17,20]; however, the problems encountered in the long-term clinical follow-up of the breast after multiple biopsies must be considered.

If reconstruction of the amputated (cancerous) breast is indicated by the patient's clinical and psychologic setting,[6] an effective approach to the problem of the high carcinoma risk in the contralateral breast is to perform a subcutaneous glandular mastectomy on the remaining breast, with immediate or staged reconstruction of both breasts. This approach is optimally applied to those patients in whom staging (pathologic and clinical) provides a prognosis commensurate with prolonged survival (that is, negative adequate nodal examination and primary tumor less than 2 cm in diameter).[6] When the initial mastectomy is associated with one to three lymph nodes containing tumor or the primary tumor is greater than 2 cm in diameter, a minimum of 18 months is allowed to elapse before the patient's request for reconstruction is considered. This 18-month period covers the median interval for tumor recurrence.[8] The potential for the presence or development of metastatic disease must be clearly explained to the patient before the procedure is planned. In the situation of more than three lymph nodes involved by tumor or with large or poorly differentiated lesions, reconstruction is generally not performed unless the patient has major psychologic problems with her deformity and is clearly appraised of the probability of metastatic disease.

When a specimen is removed in the subcutaneous procedure, it must be methodically examined by subgross and histopathologic techniques to evaluate all cellular areas, the four quadrants, and the subareolar region. This allows the determination of the extent of epitheliosis and/or clinically occult neoplasm. This approach in the present study emphasizes several aspects of the significance of various lesions: (1) intraductal epithelial hyperplasias of the solid (Fig. 9-1), cribriform (Fig. 9-2), and papillary (Fig. 9-3) forms are closely associated (statistical significance ($p = 0.005$ to 0.025) with carcinoma; (2) sclerosing adenosis is *not* associated with carcinoma ($p = NS$); (3) cysts, both gross and microscopic, do *not* correlate with carcinoma ($p = NS$); (4) typical lobular hyperplasia is not associated with carcinoma ($p = NS$); and (5) other typical features included in the fibrocystic complex (for example, blunt duct adenosis, fibroadenomatous change, apocrine metaplasia) do *not* correlate with malignancy.

Wellings, Jensen, and Marcum,[23] Foote and Stewart,[5] and Jensen, Rice, and Wellings[11] observed similar associations in autopsy-acquired or cancerous breasts. The findings of the present study provide additional support to the concept of a "premalignant" epitheliosis[1,11,21] that may be observed prior to the development of classical in situ or invasive cancer. To gain wider recognition of the preneoplastic lesions, multiple lines of evidence must converge with observations regarding statistical associations with malignancy.[1]

The management of the patient with fibrocystic disease may be greatly enhanced by the recognition of which lesions are of clinical significance.[14] The risk factors of breast cancer have been found to be sufficiently similar to those of benign breast disease[16] to preclude precise discrimination, by clinical criteria alone, of which patients may benefit from aggressive surgical management. As more is understood of the etiology and natural history of breast cancer[13,14] and the putative "precancerous" mastopathy patterns become more widely recognized,[1] the histologic presence of these mastopathies with their high correlation with the eventual development of invasive breast cancer[12] may then permit the selection of patients in whom glandular mastectomy may be indicated prior to the development of a frankly malignant histologic pattern. Successful reconstruction of the extirpated breast would make this approach more acceptable to the patient who might not otherwise accept breast amputation in the absence of overt malignancy. As progress in reconstructive breast surgery parallels investigations into the natural history of the premalignant mastopathies, wider acceptance of such an approach may possibly provide the potential to improve the outlook for a disease whose mortality remains unchanged in the last 50 years.

ACKNOWLEDGMENTS

We wish to thank Drs. D. Serafin, K. Pickrell, C. Peters, R. Riefkohl, and R. Georgiade for their assistance in the management of the patients in this study and in data acquisition. We also gratefully acknowledge Dr. B. Fetter for his contributions in the evaluation of the histologic material, Ms. L. Cleveland for her technical excellence, and Ms. Brenda Haley for assistance in the typing of the manuscript. The contributions of Phillip Pickett to the preparation of the histologic material are deeply appreciated. Dr. W. Wilkinson of the Department of Biostatistics, Duke University, is gratefully acknowledged for the data-formatting and statistical evaluations. This study supported in part by National Cancer Institute Contracts No 1-CB-84223 and No 1-CB-63996.

REFERENCES

1. Black, M. M.: Structural, antigenic and biological characteristics of precancerous mastopathy, Cancer Res. **36:**2596-2604, 1976.
2. Black, M. M., and associates: Association of atypical characteristics of benign breast lesions with subsequent risk of breast cancer, Cancer **29:**338-343, 1972.
3. Davis, H. H., Simons, M., and Davis, J. B.: Cystic disease of the breast: relationship to carcinoma, Cancer **17:**957-978, 1964.
4. Donnelly, P. K., Baker, K. W., Carney, J. A., and O'Fallon, W. M.: Benign breast

lesions and subsequent breast carcinoma in Rochester, Minnesota, Mayo Clin. Proc. **50:**650-656, 1975.

5. Foote, F. W., and Stewart, S. W.: Comparative studies of cancerous versus noncancerous breasts, Ann. Surg. **121:**197-221, 1945.

6. Georgiade, N. G.: Immediate reconstruction of the breasts following subcutaneous mastectomy. In Georgiade, N. G., editor: Reconstructive breast surgery, St. Louis, 1976, The C. V. Mosby Co., pp. 283-291.

7. Georgiade, N. G.: Reconstruction of the breasts following mastectomy. In Georgiade, N. G., editor: Reconstructive breast surgery, St. Louis, 1976, The C. V. Mosby Co., pp. 292-317.

8. Haagensen, C. D.: The clinical classification of carcinoma of the breast and the choice of treatment. In Haagensen, C. D., editor: Diseases of the breast, ed. 2, Philadelphia, 1971, W. B. Saunders Co., pp. 617-665.

9. Haagensen, C. D.: The natural history of breast carcinoma. In Haagensen, C. D., editor: Diseases of the breast, ed. 2, Philadelphia, 1971, W. B. Saunders Co., pp. 380-458.

10. Jensen, H. M., and Wellings, S. R.: Preneoplastic lesions of the human mammary gland transplanted into the nude athymic mouse, Cancer Res. **36:**2605-2609, 1976.

11. Jensen, H. M., Rice, J. R., and Wellings, S. R.: Preneoplastic lesions in the human breast, Science **191:**295-297, 1976.

12. Kodlin, D., Winger, E. E., Morgenstern, N. L., and Chen, U.: Chronic mastopathy and breast cancer: a follow-up study, Cancer **39:**2603-2607, 1977.

13. MacCarty, W. C.: The histogenesis of cancer (carcinoma) of the breast and its clinical significance, Surg. Gynecol. Obstet. **17:**441-459, 1913.

14. MacMahon, B., Cole, P., and Brown, J.: Etiology of human breast cancer: a review, J. Natl. Cancer Inst. **50:**21-42, 1973.

15. Nizze, H.: Fibrous mastopathy and epitheliosis in the opposite breast of mammary carcinoma patients, Oncology **28:**319-330, 1973.

16. Nomura, A., Comstock, G. W., and Tonascia, J. A.: Epidemiologic characteristics of benign breast disease, Am. J. Epidemiol. **105:**505-512, 1977.

17. Peacock, E. E.: Biological basis for management of benign disease of the breast: the case against subcutaneous mastectomy, Plast. Reconstr. Surg. **55:**14-20, 1975.

18. Pennisi, U. R., and Capozzi, A.: The incidence of obscure carcinoma in subcutaneous mastectomy, Plast. Reconstr. Surg. **56:**9-12, 1975.

19. Potter, J. F., Slimbaugh, W. P., and Woodward, S. C.: Can breast carcinoma be anticipated? A follow-up of benign breast biopsies, Ann. Surg. **167:**829-837, 1968.

20. Robbins, G. F., and Berg, S. W.: Bilateral primary breast cancers—a prospective clinicopathological study, Cancer **17:**1501-1527, 1964.

21. Toker, C., and Goldberg, J. D.: The small-cell lesion of mammary ducts and lobules, Pathol. Ann. **12:**217-249, 1977.

22. Urban, J. A.: Bilaterality of cancer of the breast, biopsy of the opposite breast, Cancer **20:**1867-1870, 1967.

23. Wellings, S. R., Jensen, H. M., and Marcum, R. G.: An atlas of subgross pathology of the human breast with special reference to possible precancerous lesions, J. Natl. Cancer Inst. **55:**231-243, 1975.

CHAPTER 10

Reconstruction of the breast mound after mastectomy

**Nicholas G. Georgiade, Ronald Riefkohl,
and Gregory S. Georgiade**

Although the emphasis until recent years has been solely concerned with cure of carcinoma of the breast with very little thought given to reconstruction of the breast, Czerny[14] as early as 1895 published the first report on extirpation of the breast for fibroadenoma with simultaneous reconstruction utilizing a lipoma taken from the right flank.

As has been discussed in Chapter 6, Bartlett,[3] Lexer,[23] and Rosenauer[33] attempted to reestablish breast contour, utilizing adipose tissue. Berson,[4] Maliniac,[26] Marino,[27] Longacre,[24,25] Letterman and Schurter,[22] and De Cholnoky[9] employed a variety of dermal fat pedicle flaps and dermal-fat-fascia transplants in reconstruction attempts.

Various types of flaps were designed to reconstruct breast contour. Heidenhain[36] rotated a lateral pedicle flap from the upper abdominal wall. Tansini's flap, described by d'Este in 1912,[10] consisted of a thoracic flap composed of skin and the latissimus dorsi, the teres major, and a portion of the infraspinatus muscles. An axillary abdominal flap was utilized by Kleinschmidt.[21] The contralateral breast flap was used by Sauerbruch in 1925.[36] Reinhard[32] as early as 1932 recommended the splitting and sharing of the opposite breast, as did Pontes.[31]

Harris,[16] Holdsworth,[19] and Alexander and Block[1] utilized a portion of the remaining breast to reconstruct the breast mound in multiple stages. Orticochea[30] transferred buttock, skin, and subcutaneous tissue, using the forearm as a carrier to reconstruct the missing breast.

In 1969 Snyderman and Guthrie[34] described the use of a Silastic gel-filled prosthesis to reconstruct the breast mound. This procedure depended on the presence of good quality skin at the site of mastectomy. Hueston and McKenzie[20] reported the first immediate postmastectomy reconstruction with augmentation 2 to 4 days after ablative surgery.

In the last few years numerous reports have appeared in the literature concerning breast reconstruction after ablative surgery for carcinoma.*

A variety of thoracoabdominal flaps have been utilized to transfer sufficient

*See references 5, 12, 13, 15, 17, 28, 29, and 34.

tissue to the postoperative site prior to augmentation with a Silastic prosthesis.*

As discussed in Chapter 11, the latissimus dorsi musculocutaneous flap has been found to be the most versatile of the various flaps and to afford the best possibility of adequately resurfacing the chest wall and axillary defect, especially after radical mastectomy procedures. This method is particularly useful since this is a one-stage flap and muscle transfer procedure. The final aesthetic result utilizing this technique has been most satisfactory.

The reconstruction of the breast mound may be initiated immediately during the first 5 days after ablative surgery or may be delayed for a longer period of time.

IMMEDIATE RECONSTRUCTION

In our experience immediate reconstruction, when feasible, is extremely beneficial for the patient for several reasons. Our psychologic analysis reveals that in the group of women who underwent breast reconstruction immediately following the ablative surgery, none displayed any of the negative psychologic effects displayed by the group of patients who had ablative surgery without the prospect of breast reconstruction. In addition it is easier to achieve a more satisfactory final aesthetic result if the plastic surgeon and general surgeon work cooperatively in the planning and execution of the surgery from its inception.

Patients considered for immediate reconstruction are evaluated by a team that includes the general surgeon, plastic surgeon, radiologist, pathologist, and endocrinologist. Our criteria for the selection of suitable candidates for an immediate reconstruction of the breast have been discussed in detail in Chapter 8. One cannot overemphasize the fact that each case must be assessed as an individual situation.

SURGICAL METHOD OF RECONSTRUCTION

If an immediate reconstruction is planned, the general surgeon and plastic surgeon work together to plan and execute the surgery. A transverse lateral "S" incision is usually utilized by the general surgeon in performing a modified radical mastectomy. In our experience this type of incision allows adequate exposure and still results in the scar placement most suitable for breast mound reconstruction. The wound closure is accomplished by the plastic surgeon utilizing interrupted 4-0 white multifilament nylon sutures for the subcutaneous layer, interrupted 4-0 white Vicryl sutures for the subcuticular layer, and interrupted 5-0 Prolene sutures for the skin closure (Fig. 10-1). A suction drain is inserted at the time of closure.

The nipple-areolar complex is removed from the specimen as a very thick split-thickness graft. The dermal base of the nipple-areolar graft is sent to the pathology department and is evaluated immediately by the pathologist prior to placement on a dermal bed in the inguinal region (Fig. 10-2).

---

*See references 2, 6, 8, 11, 18, and 35.

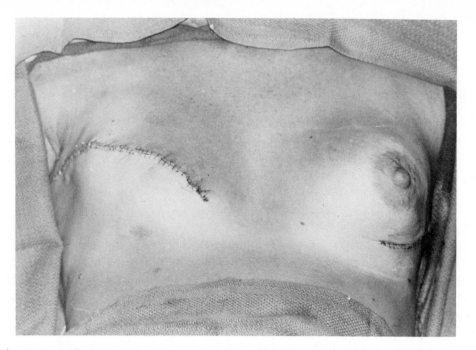

Fig. 10-1. A right modified radical mastectomy has been performed by general surgeon using preferred transverse lateral "S" incision. Wound closure was carried out by plastic surgeon utilizing 4-0 white nylon sutures for subcutaneous layer, interrupted 4-0 white Vicryl sutures for subcuticular layer, and interrupted 5-0 Prolene sutures for skin closure. A left subcutaneous mastectomy with immediate insertion of prosthesis was carried out at same time as ablative surgery.

Fig. 10-2. A, Nipple-areola is removed as thick split-thickness graft before specimen is given to pathologist. Segment of breast tissue at base of nipple and areola is sent to pathologist for immediate evaluation prior to transplantation of nipple-areola to inguinal area. **B,** Nipple-areola has been removed from breast segment as a very thick split-thickness skin graft. Dermal-subdermal bed is sent to the pathology department for immediate evaluation. **C,** Recipient dermal bed in inguinal region has been prepared for nipple-areolar graft by removing split-thickness skin graft. **D,** Nipple-areolar graft is sutured to recipient bed utilizing 5-0 black silk sutures. Scattered "tackers" of 4-0 plain catgut are used to stabilize skin graft in its bed. **E,** The bolus is sutured over nipple-areolar graft. **F,** This 33-year-old patient is shown 2 months after modified mastectomy with transfer of nipple-area graft to left groin. Patient had "immediate" insertion of 165-ml gel-filled prosthesis on the fourth postablative day. **G,** Patient is shown 18 months after a capsulotomy was performed on right breast and prosthesis replaced with a 225-ml gel-filled prosthesis and a subcutaneous mastectomy on left breast with immediate insertion of a 165-ml gel-filled prosthesis and correction of ptosis. Nipple-areolar graft shown was transferred from inguinal region to reconstructed breast mound of right breast. **H,** Lateral view of same patient at same time interval as **G** is shown in final stage 18 months after ablative surgery.

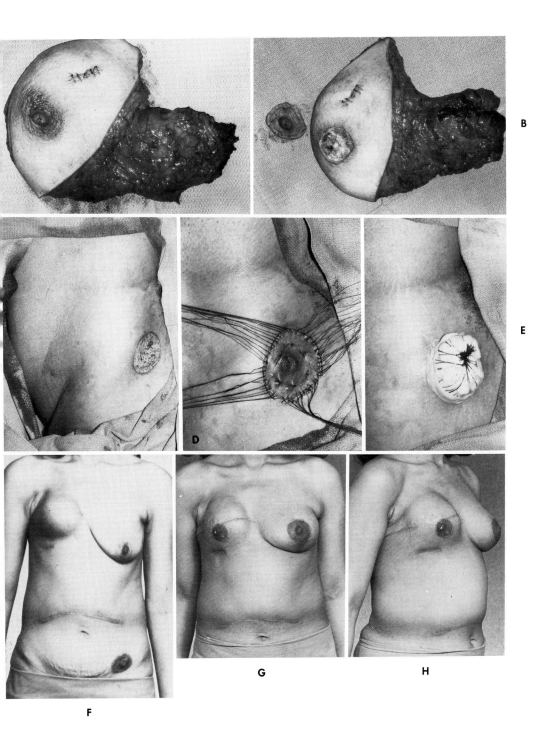

Fig. 10-2. For legend see opposite page.

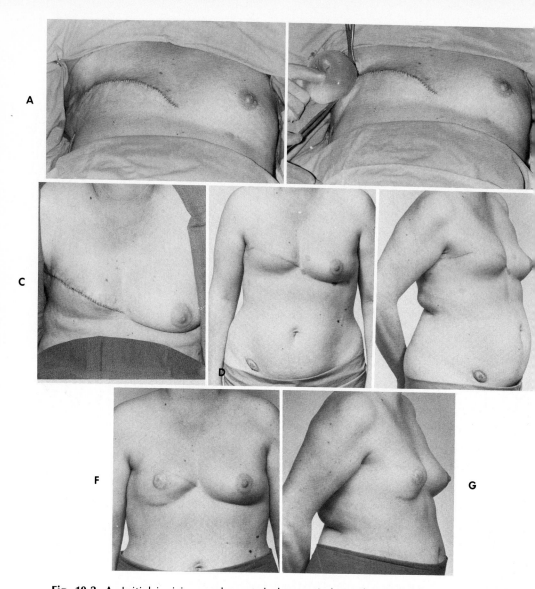

Fig. 10-3. A, Initial incision and wound closure 4 days after a right modified radical mastectomy was performed and the pathology report revealed a small 2-cm intraductal and infiltrating well-differentiated ductal carcinoma in right upper outer quadrant. No tumor was present in nipple bed or in thirty axillary lymph nodes. **B,** A round gel-filled 230-ml prosthesis is inserted through lateral segment of operative area on fourth post-operative day subsequent to final pathology report. **C,** View of same 47-year-old patient 1 day following insertion of preliminary round prosthesis. **D,** Four-month post-operative front view of same patient. Note nipple-areolar graft in right groin. **E,** Four-month postoperative lateral view of same patient. **F,** Front postoperative view of same patient 8 months after a capsulotomy had been performed on right breast and the prosthesis replaced with a 225-ml gel-filled Georgiade contoured Surgitek prosthesis and nipple-areolar graft transferred from inguinal region to right breast. **G,** Lateral view of same patient at same stage of reconstruction as in **F.** Note satisfactory coning of breast mound.

When the final pathologic report has been received, usually on the fourth or fifth postoperative day, a prosthesis approximately two thirds the final desired breast volume is inserted beneath the skin flaps through the lateral segment of the mastectomy closure. The initial prosthesis is round because its orientation is unimportant and it can be inserted with greater facility. Care is taken not to open the mastectomy closure over the dome of the breast mound. The lateral opening is then closed in three layers as before (Fig. 10-3, *A* to *E*). The previously inserted suction drain is allowed to remain or is changed and maintained for an additional 2 days. Sutures are removed on the tenth postoperative day.

By the fourth or fifth month postmastectomy, a capsulotomy is carried out and the prosthesis is replaced with a Georgiade Surgitek contoured prosthesis (usually 185- to 225-ml or similar type prosthesis that has a low profile with a slight axillary projection when properly oriented (Fig. 10-3, *F* and *G*).

The optimum time to transfer the banked nipple-areolar graft depends on the size and shape of the opposite breast as well as on whether a subcutaneous mastectomy is necessary. If possible the subcutaneous mastectomy is accomplished during the initial hospitalization for the ablative surgery after the final pathologic studies from the cancerous breast have been completed. Most often, however, in our patients the subcutaneous mastectomy is carried out during the second stage of reconstruction and the nipple-areolar grafting is carried out during the final or third stage of reconstruction. The subcutaneous mastectomy is performed as discussed in Chapter 6. If a subcutaneous mastectomy is carried out in the contralateral breast along with an immediate reconstruction, the nipple-areolar graft is transferred 6 months later at the time of the completion of a satisfactory breast mound, symmetric with the opposite breast (Fig. 10-4).

If the contralateral breast is hypertrophied, the subcutaneous mastectomy with a simultaneous reduction-ptosis procedure is preferably delayed until the second stage of the reconstructive procedure in order to attain a more satisfactory breast symmetry. The nipple-areolar complex may be transferred anytime after the symmetry is achieved but is usually delayed for 4 to 6 months since capsulotomies are usually indicated and carried out at the same time (Fig. 10-5).

CAPSULOTOMY

To achieve a satisfactory result it is always necessary to release the capsular scar contractures that uniformly occur around the prostheses. The capsulotomy is accomplished through an incision that approximates the eventual inframammary crease and is 6 to 7 cm inferior to the new nipple site. The capsule is incised as previously described in Chapter 6. The prosthesis is removed, and the base of the capsule is visualized and circumferentially incised. Multiple radial incisions are made from the released base over the dome of the capsule. Multiple cross-hatchings are carried out, creating "postage stamp" squares of the capsule. Further undermining of the tissue surrounding the capsule is necessary if enlargement of the breast mound is necessary. Coagulation of all bleeding points

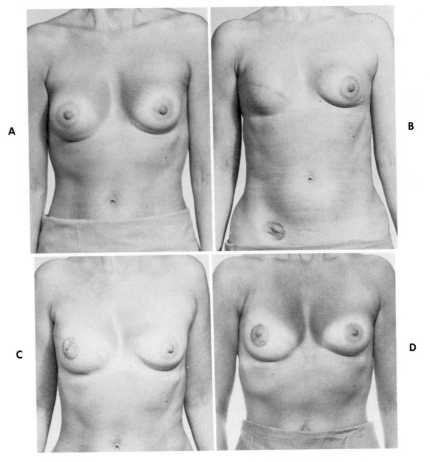

Fig. 10-4. A, Preoperative photograph of 40-year-old patient who had a previous augmentation mammaplasty. She was found to have an early intraductal carcinoma in upper outer quadrant of right breast. **B,** Postoperative view of same patient 5 months after a modified radical mastectomy was performed on right breast. Nipple-areolar complex was removed from right breast and implanted in inguinal area. A 185-ml gel-filled prosthesis was inserted to reconstruct right breast mound 4 days after ablative surgery. At time of ablative surgery a subcutaneous mastectomy was performed on left breast with simultaneous insertion of a 185-ml gel-filled prosthesis. **C,** Front view of same patient 2 months after bilateral capsulotomies were carried out and an 85-ml/165-ml gel-filled Georgiade "piggyback" Surgitek prosthesis was inserted in right breast mound and a 185-ml gel-filled prosthesis in left breast. Nipple-areolar graft was transferred from inguinal area to right breast mound. Depigmentation of reconstructed areola and loss of nipple tissue can be noted. This depigmentation frequently occurs following transfer of areolar grafts. **D,** Front view of same patient 1 year after depigmented area of the areola has been tattooed and a nipple graft transferred from the opposite breast nipple. This photograph was taken 21 months after the initial surgery.

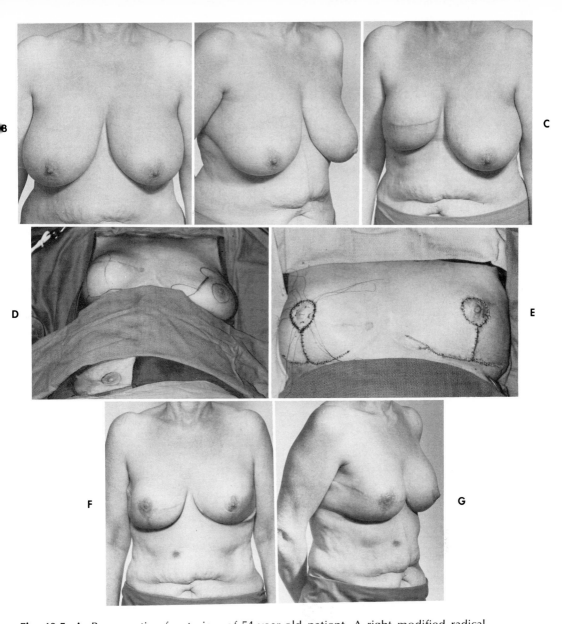

Fig. 10-5. A, Preoperative front view of 54-year-old patient. A right modified radical mastectomy was performed and nipple-areola was transplanted to inguinal area. Lesion was in upper right outer quadrant, and the pathologic diagnosis was infiltrating ductal carcinoma. Base of nipple-areola was free of tumor, and axillary lymph nodes were negative for tumor. A preliminary 230-ml round gel-filled prosthesis was inserted 5 days after ablative surgery. **B,** Preoperative lateral view of same patient. **C,** Seven-month postoperative view of same patient with preliminary 230-ml gel-filled round prosthesis still in place in right breast mound. **D,** Operative view, prior to second stage of reconstruction, 7 months after ablative surgery. The surgical procedures consisted of a capsulotomy of the right breast with replacement of the preliminary prosthesis with a Georgiade bilumen prosthesis, 165-ml gel-filled prosthesis with outer envelope filled with 25 ml of normal saline containing 10 mg of methylprednisolone sodium succinate (Solu-Medrol), and transplantation of nipple-areolar graft from inguinal area to right breast mound. A reduction mammaplasty and subcutaneous mastectomy with simultaneous insertion of a similar Georgiade bilumen prosthesis were carried out on left breast. **E,** Immediate postoperative photograph of procedures illustrated in **D** prior to fixing right nipple-areolar graft with a bolus. **F,** Front view of same patient 7 months after second stage of reconstruction. **G,** Lateral view of same patient 7 months after second stage of reconstruction.

is carefully carried out prior to insertion of a properly oriented prosthesis of a suitable size (usually a 185- to 225-ml gel Georgiade Surgitek) or similar type of prosthesis. The incision is then closed with a deep row of interrupted 4-0 white multifilament nylon sutures followed by 5-0 Vicryl and 6-0 Prolene sutures to approximate the skin edges.

DELAYED RECONSTRUCTION

There are a number of women who have previously undergone a modified radical or radical mastectomy. As more and more of these women have become aware of the available options, there has been an increasing interest in breast reconstructive procedures. Additionally many more general surgeons and gynecologists are referring their patients for reconstructive procedures.

It is necessary to educate the patient regarding what can and cannot be accomplished. It is usually impossible for the plastic surgeon to restore the patient's breast to its exact former status. Obviously the patient must not be allowed to establish unrealistic expectations that cannot be satisfied. The reconstructive surgeon should strive for the best possible result, but the patient must clearly understand the limitations and possible undesirable results. This is particularly important for patients who have had radiation therapy since the results are more likely to be the least satisfactory.

SELECTION OF PROSTHESES

In our experience a variety of sizes and shapes of prostheses are necessary for implantation in order to obtain a final satisfactory aesthetic result in the construction of the breast mound.

Initially a round prosthesis has been found to be easily inserted with the greatest concern being its suitable placement on the chest wall. If the patient has sufficient loose skin, a double-compartment type of prosthesis can be inserted either subcutaneously or subpectorally. This prosthesis can be one that has been custom designed and manufactured. In order to custom design a prosthesis, an impression is obtained of the entire chest, including the opposite breast (Fig. 10-6). From this the manufacturer can make the projected prosthesis in its final size in a stone-type model (Fig. 10-7). This model is placed in a suitable location on the chest, and any necessary adjustments are made by adding plaster to the model or by shaving off some of the model. The final prosthesis is then made in a double- or triple-compartment Silastic prosthesis.

We have been able to eliminate some of this extra time and expense in the fabrication of this type of prosthesis by selecting the projected suitable sized prostheses for the individual patient and cementing together two prostheses one on top of the other ("piggyback"). The top prosthesis is considerably smaller (85 to 100 ml) than the base prosthesis (165 to 265 ml). The top prosthesis gives the needed projection of the breast mound in most of the patients undergoing reconstruction.

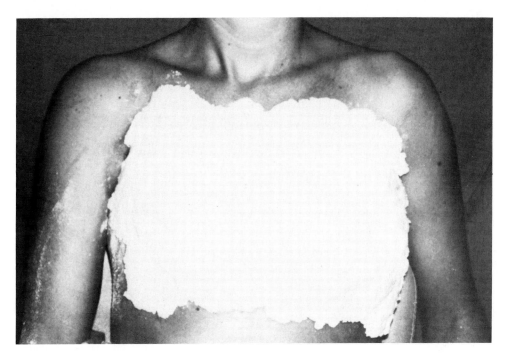

Fig. 10-6. Moulage of patient's entire chest is obtained in order to more accurately create a custom prosthesis.

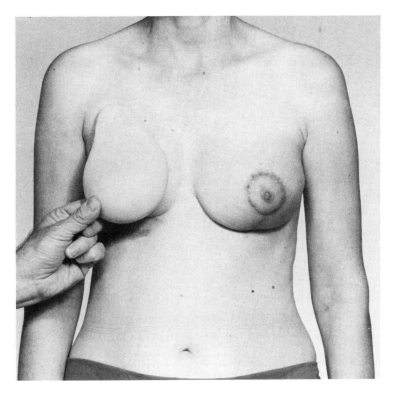

Fig. 10-7. Custom-designed stone model that can be further shaped to fill in the breast defect is placed over the breast defect for final contouring. From this model a double or triple compartment Silastic prosthesis can be manufactured.

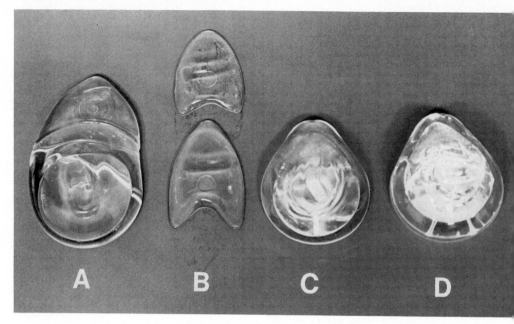

Fig. 10-8. Prostheses. **A,** Custom designed tricompartment prosthesis; **B,** 35- and 50-ml axillary tail prostheses; **C,** Georgiade Surgitek bilumen prosthesis; **D,** Georgiade "piggyback" prosthesis—100-ml gel-filled prosthesis cemented on top of a 185-ml gel-filled prosthesis.

When there is a deficiency of soft tissue in the axillary area, smaller axillary tail prostheses* have been designed in 35- and 50-ml sizes. These prostheses can be inserted at the time the larger prostheses are inserted, or they can be inserted separately via the previous mastectomy scar (Fig. 10-8).

SURGICAL TECHNIQUES
Use of patient's local tissues

If the patient has had a modified radical mastectomy and there is adequate chest wall skin coverage remaining, reconstruction can usually be accomplished by the insertion, either subcutaneously or subpectorally, of a prosthesis of suitable size and shape. The initial prosthesis will be smaller than desired; however, after sufficient stretching of the skin has occurred after a 4- to 6-month interval, a larger prosthesis that approximates the size of the opposite breast may be inserted during the capsulotomy procedure (Figs. 10-9 and 10-10). The use of a multicompartment prosthesis is usually necessary in order to adequately fill the capsulotomy space and still obtain the desired forward projection of the breast mound (Fig. 10-11). Special triangular silicone gel prostheses of 35- to

*Cox-Uphoff, Santa Barbara, Calif.

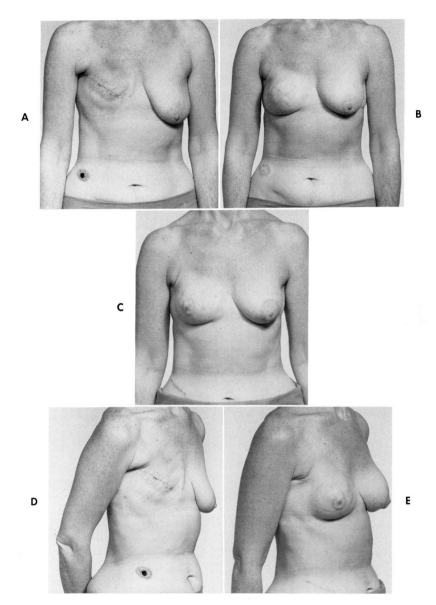

Fig. 10-9. A, Preoperative front view of a 42-year-old patient who had a right modified radical mastectomy with transfer of areola to abdominal area performed at another hospital and was referred 1 month postoperatively. **B,** Four months after ablative surgery a preliminary 225-ml gel-filled prosthesis was inserted in right breast mound and a ptosis procedure and a left subcutaneous mastectomy with immediate insertion of a 185-ml gel-filled prosthesis were performed. This front view was taken 4 months after these procedures. **C,** Four months after initial reconstruction a right capsulotomy was performed and a 225-ml gel-filled prosthesis was reinserted. Nipple-areolar graft was transferred to right breast, and nipple graft obtained from left breast was transferred to right breast. This front view was taken 1 month after these procedures. **D,** Preoperative lateral view of same patient. **E,** Postoperative lateral view taken after second stage of reconstruction 1 year after ablative surgery.

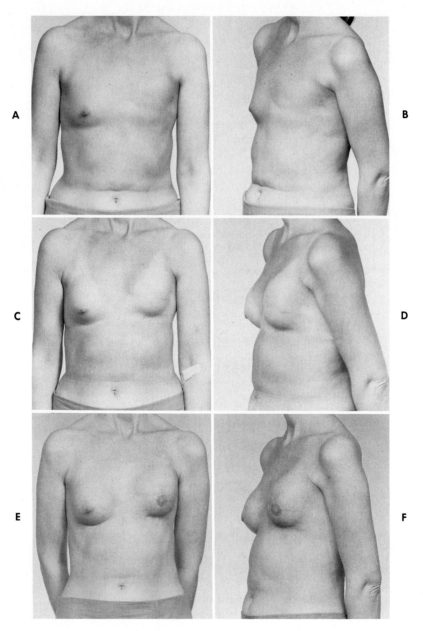

Fig. 10-10. For legend see opposite page.

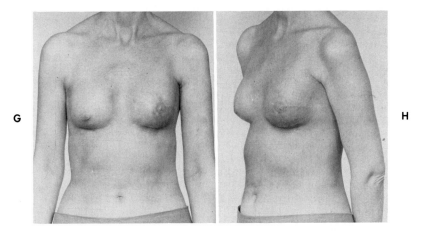

G

H

Fig. 10-10. A, Preoperative front view of 42-year-old patient who had had a left modified radical mastectomy 5 years previously. **B,** Preoperative lateral view of same patient. **C,** Six-month postoperative front view of same patient who had had the left breast augmented with a Georgiade Surgitek "piggyback" 85-ml gel-filled prosthesis cemented to a 245-ml inflatable prosthesis inflated with 100 ml of sterile saline. The right breast was augmented with a 145-ml gel-filled prosthesis. **D,** Six-month postoperative lateral view of same patient. **E,** During second stage of reconstruction 6 months after initial reconstruction, bilateral capsulotomies were performed. A 145-ml gel-filled prosthesis was reinserted on right side and an 85-ml/165-ml gel-filled "piggyback" prosthesis on left side. Nipple-areolar complex was reconstructed utilizing full-thickness postauricular grafts. This is a 5-month postoperative front view of patient. **F,** Lateral view 5 months after second stage of reconstruction. **G,** Five months after second stage of reconstruction, bilateral capsulotomies were again carried out and right prosthesis was replaced with a 165-ml gel-filled Georgiade Surgitek prosthesis and the left with an 85-ml/185-ml gel-filled Georgiade "piggyback" prosthesis. Left prosthesis was repositioned to produce a satisfactory contour. **H,** Lateral view of same patient at stage of reconstruction in **G.**

50-ml capacity have been designed to provide fill for the anterior axillary fold when necessary.

The nipple and areola should be placed and oriented properly with the patient's opposite nipple and areola in the final stage of reconstruction in order to avoid the pitfalls of improperly placed nipple-areolar grafts. Correction of these misplaced grafts is difficult and may necessitate partial excision of the misplaced aveolar graft with resurfacing of the ensuing defect.

The proper placement of the new areola is carried out by marking the new site and proper circumference of the new areola with the patient in an upright position (Fig. 10-12).

Text continued on p. 183.

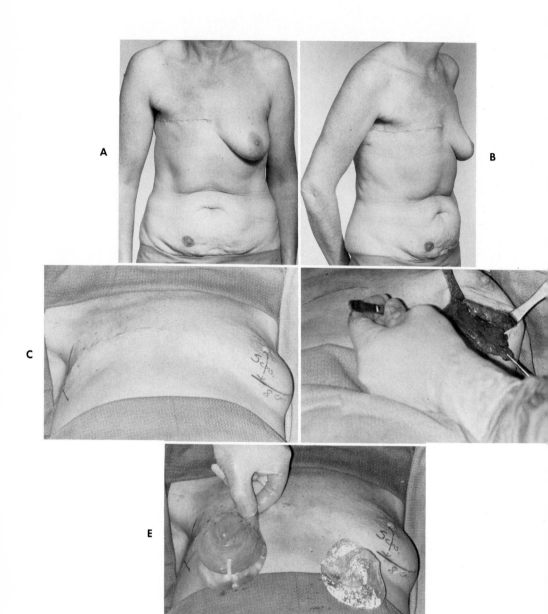

Fig. 10-11. For legend see opposite page.

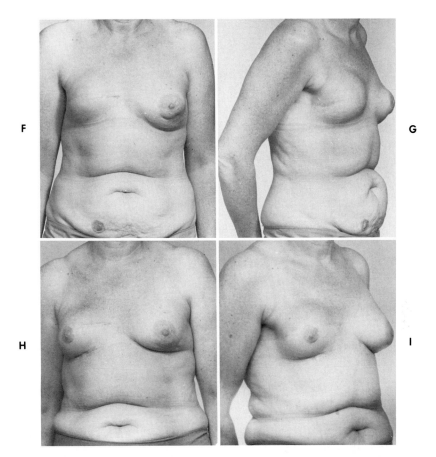

Fig. 10-11. A, Preoperative front view 1 month after extirpative surgery of 40-year-old patient who had had a right modified radical mastectomy with a transplant of nipple-areolar complex to right inguinal area at another hospital. Pathologic diagnosis was early infiltrating ductal adenocarcinoma with negative lymph nodes. Right breast mound was reconstructed by inserting an 85-ml/185-ml gel-filled Georgiade "piggyback" prosthesis through transverse incision of previous right modified radical mastectomy. A subcutaneous mastectomy was performed on left breast with simultaneous insertion of a 190-ml Georgiade Surgitek inflatable prosthesis. **B,** Preoperative lateral view of same patient. **C,** Operative view showing markings for placement of incision for performing subcutaneous mastectomy of left breast. **D,** Operative view illustrating sharp dissection of breast tissue in subcutaneous mastectomy. **E,** Operative view showing prostheses to be inserted. An 85-ml/185-ml gel-filled Georgiade Surgitek "piggyback" prosthesis is shown being held over right breast area and a Georgiade Surgitek inflatable prosthesis on left side. **F,** Six-month postoperative front view of same patient. **G,** Six-month postoperative lateral view of same patient. **H,** Same patient is shown having now had bilateral capsulotomies. A 185-ml gel-filled prosthesis was inserted on left side. On right side an 85-ml/165-ml gel-filled "piggyback" prosthesis was inserted. This front view was taken 4 months after capsulotomies were performed and 15 months after first stage of reconstruction. **I,** Lateral postoperative view taken at same time as **H.**

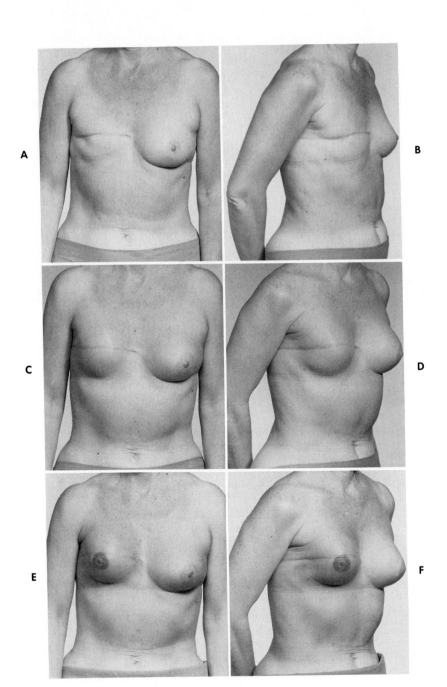

Fig. 10-12. For legend see opposite page.

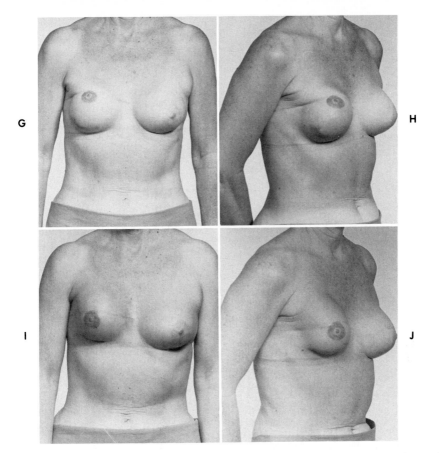

Fig. 10-12. A, Preoperative front view of 54-year-old patient who had had a right modified radical mastectomy 1 year previously. In first stage of reconstruction a 225-ml gel-filled Georgiade Surgitek prosthesis was inserted to reconstruct right breast mound and a subcutaneous mastectomy was performed on left breast with insertion of a 140-ml gel-filled prosthesis. **B,** Preoperative lateral view of same patient. **C,** Postoperative front view taken 4 months after first stage of reconstruction. **D,** Four-month postoperative lateral view of same patient. **E,** Four months after first stage of reconstruction, bilateral capsulotomies were performed. Prosthesis in right breast was replaced with a 100-ml/165-ml gel-filled "piggyback" Georgiade Surgitek prosthesis, and a 145-ml gel-filled prosthesis was inserted in left breast. Areola was tattooed on reconstructed right breast mound and a nipple graft from opposite breast was utilized to place a nipple on reconstructed breast mound. This front view was taken 1 month following second stage of reconstruction. **F,** Lateral view of same patient 1 month after second stage of reconstruction. **G,** Front view 5 months after second stage of reconstruction. Nipple-areolar complex of reconstructed breast mound has shifted upward from normal position because of shifting of prosthesis caused by pressure exerted on prosthesis by intact pectoralis muscle. Bilateral capsulotomies were performed with partial incising of overlying pectoralis muscle of right breast followed by insertion of a smaller 185-ml gel-filled prosthesis. The 145-ml gel-filled prosthesis was reinserted on left side. **H,** Five-month postoperative lateral view of same patient with displacement of prosthesis and nipple-areola. **I,** Front view of same patient 7 months after bilateral capsulotomies were performed and right pectoralis musculature was partially incised along its inferior aspect. **J,** Lateral view of same patient 7 months after replacement procedure.

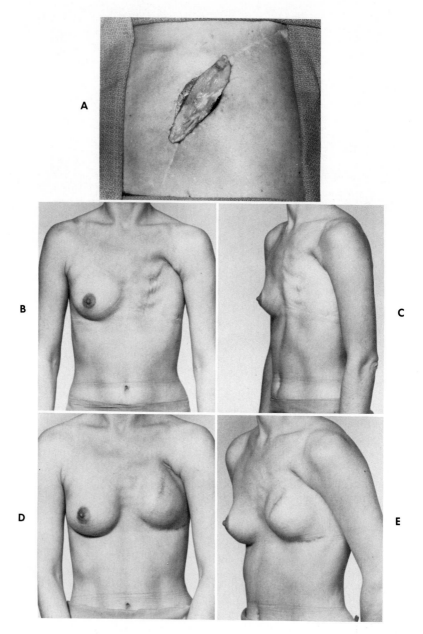

Fig. 10-13. For legend see opposite page.

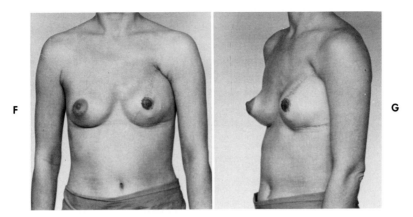

F

G

Fig. 10-13. A, Mastectomy scar has been excised, and a dermal graft that has been obtained from groin is to be inserted beneath skin flaps at site of mastectomy scar to reinforce this area and minimize possibility of breakdown of scar area during reconstructive phase. **B,** Preoperative front view of 29-year-old patient who 2 years previously had had a left radical mastectomy performed for an intraductal carcinoma. Both her mother and sister had carcinoma of the breast. Scar tissue at mastectomy site was of poor quality, necessitating insertion of a dermal graft. Three months after insertion of a dermal graft a 225-ml gel-filled Georgiade Surgitek prosthesis was inserted. A subcutaneous mastectomy with immediate insertion of a 185-ml gel-filled prosthesis was performed on right breast. **C,** Preoperative lateral view of same patient. **D,** Front view of same patient 8 months after insertion of prostheses. At this time bilateral capsulotomies were carried out and a 225-ml inflatable prosthesis was inserted in left breast mound and a 185-ml inflatable prosthesis in right breast. A 35-ml gel-filled axillary prosthesis was inserted into axillary defect. Nipple-areola was reconstructed utilizing a labial graft for areola and a nipple graft from opposite breast for nipple. **E,** Lateral view of same patient. **F,** Front view of patient 27 months after initial reconstruction. **G,** Lateral view of same patient.

Surgical excision of scar and dermal graft

Evaluation of the postmastectomy deformity is very important in order to determine whether reconstruction can be accomplished utilizing a single or multicompartment silicone gel or a combined silicone gel–saline type prosthesis. If the mastectomy scar is wide but the surrounding skin is of good quality and no radiation therapy has been given, local excision of the scar is carried out. A dermal graft obtained from the groin or buttock serves to reinforce the skin closure and is positioned by means of several 4-0 white multifilament nylon sutures to the skin flaps, which are then reapproximated with a deep row of 4-0 white multifilament nylon, a subcuticular row of 5-0 Vicryl sutures, and 5-0 Prolene sutures for the skin closure (Fig. 10-13, A). A pressure type figure eight dressing protects and immobilizes the area for 7 days, at which time the skin

Text continued on p. 188.

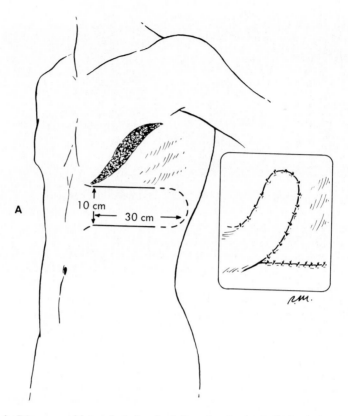

Fig. 10-14. A, Diagram of lateral abdominal flap that is medially based, which is transferred to area of mastectomy scar. Subsequent defect of donor area is closed primarily
leaving a minimal scar. **B,** Preoperative front view of 51-year-old patient who had
a left radical mastectomy 25 years previously with postoperative radiation. A large
left thoracoabdominal flap was elevated to resurface the area of original scar,
which was extremely tight and of poor quality skin. Four months after transfer of
thoracoabdominal flap, a 185-ml gel-filled Georgiade Surgitek prosthesis was inserted
under the flap. A ptosis procedure and subcutaneous mastectomy with simultaneous
insertion of a 145-ml gel-filled prosthesis were performed on right breast. **C,** Lateral
preoperative view of same patient. **D,** Front view of same patient following transfer
of lateral abdominal flap and 6 months after insertion of prostheses. In third stage of
reconstruction bilateral capsulotomies were performed and a 225-ml gel-filled prosthesis and a 35-ml axillary tail prosthesis were inserted in left reconstructed breast.
A 145-ml gel-filled prosthesis was inserted in right breast. Nipple-areolar complex was
reconstructed using a full-thickness skin graft from left groin and nipple sharing from
right breast. **E,** Lateral view of same patient. **F,** Front view of same patient 1 month after
third reconstructive stage and 1 year after initial reconstructive surgery. **G,** Lateral view
of same patient 1 month after third reconstructive stage.

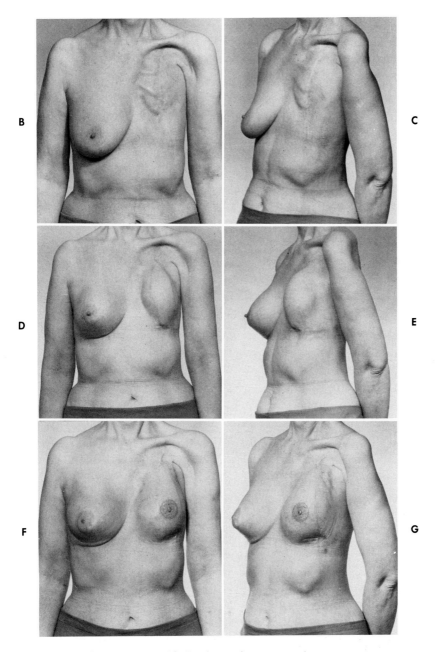

Fig. 10-14, cont'd. For legend see opposite page.

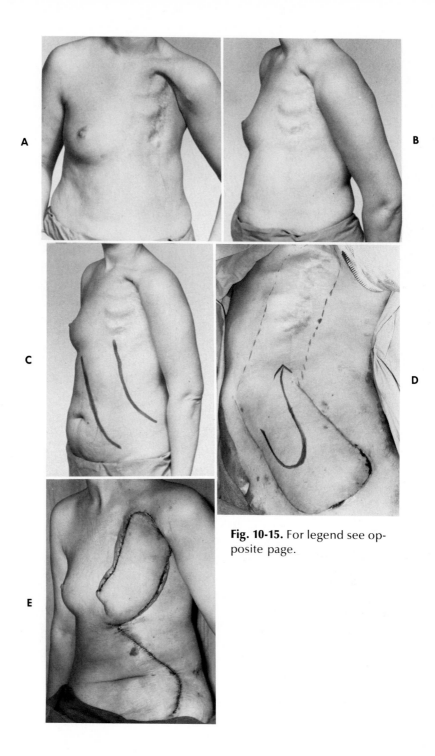

Fig. 10-15. For legend see opposite page.

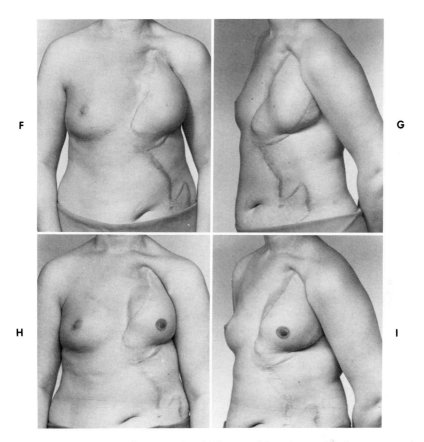

Fig. 10-15. A, Preoperative photograph of 35-year-old patient who 5 years previously had had a left radical mastectomy performed with postoperative irradiation. Because of extensive scar and poor quality of the tissue it was necessary to elevate a large abdominal flap to resurface entire area. **B,** Lateral preoperative photograph of same patient. **C,** Abdominal flap to be elevated is outlined. **D,** Abdominal flap is shown following two delays. **E,** Postoperative view 6 days after transposition and inset of abdominal flap into chest area. **F,** Four months after inset of flap a 225-ml gel-filled prosthesis was inserted beneath newly reconstructed breast flap. This front view was taken 3 months after insertion of prosthesis. **G,** Postoperative lateral view of same patient at same stage of reconstruction as **F. H,** Three months after original prosthesis was inserted, a capsulotomy was performed and the prosthesis was reinserted. Areola was tattooed on reconstructed breast mound and a full-thickness labial graft was sutured in place to provide a nipple. This front view was taken 16 months after final stage of reconstruction and 2 years after initial reconstructive surgery. Note wide abdominal scars inherent with this type of flap. **I,** Lateral view taken 16 months after final reconstruction illustrating excellent reconstruction of breast mound and satisfactory filling of axillary defect with transfer of this large abdominal flap.

sutures are removed. Steri-strips are then applied across the skin edges for an additional 14 days.

Prosthesis insertion can be accomplished approximately 2 months after the dermal grafting procedure. The prosthesis is inserted through an incision approximately 6 cm in length and 6 cm below the contemplated nipple position. Any of the various types of prostheses previously mentioned can be utilized. Usually it will be necessary to replace the initial prothesis and release the capsular contracture 5 to 6 months later. Nipple-areolar reconstruction is also possible during the capsulotomy procedure if there is good bilateral breast symmetry (Fig. 10-13, *B* to *G*). The various methods of nipple-areolar reconstruction are described in Chapter 13.

FLAPS

The mastectomy wound may have required a skin graft, there may have been skin necrosis with delayed healing and a resultant wide scar, or the chest wall may have been irradiated. Each of these situations must be managed by transferring suitable skin flaps to the chest area prior to any attempt to create a breast mound, or else serious complications may result.

A number of flaps are available that transfer an adequate quantity of good quality tissue to the postmastectomy wound. The two most often used are the lateral abdominal flap and the latissimus dorsi musculocutaneous flap.

Lateral abdominal flap

The lateral abdominal flap is particularly useful if the main deficient area involves the lower half of the postmastectomy wound. The flap can be transferred primarily or after one delay procedure, depending on the length and width of the flap design (Fig. 10-14). In many instances the lateral abdominal flap based medially can be transferred successfully, allowing closure of the donor area with a minimal objectionable scar on the abdomen.

Whenever an abdominal flap is utilized to cover the entire postradical mastectomy scarred area from the axillary defect to the inferior chest area, a larger abdominal flap will be needed. The eventual result from transferring this large flap yields a very satisfactory breast mound on which a nipple-areola can be constructed.

The postoperative scar and resultant deformity on the abdomen are objectionable to many patients, particularly since there is a tendency for hypertrophy of the scar (Fig. 10-15).

Latissimus dorsi musculocutaneous flap

The latissimus dorsi musculocutaneous flap has been found to be the most versatile flap to date and because of its importance is described separately in Chapter 11. The use of the latissimus dorsi musculocutaneous flap as an island pedicle is dependent on an intact thoracodorsal artery and vein. When these vessels are absent, a somewhat smaller flap with a shorter arc of rotation may still adequately replace the soft tissue deficiency. Occasionally these limitations may prevent the transfer of sufficient skin necessary to reconstruct a suitable breast mound. In this situation a "free flap" utilizing a latissimus dorsi musculocutaneous flap obtained from the opposite side is quite satisfactory. The use of a free flap is described in Chapter 12.

In summary immediate reconstruction of the breast can usually be carried out in two or three procedures depending on the status of the opposite breast. Delayed reconstruction will of necessity vary, depending on the condition of the chest tissue in the area to be reconstructed, which might initially necessitate the transfer of tissue from the surrounding area. The status of the opposite breast is taken into consideration as to size, shape, and presence of fibrocystic disease. A suitable breast mound is constructed, and the appropriate techniques to obtain symmetry of both breast areas are then carried out. The final stage is the placement of the nipple-areolar complex.

REFERENCES

1. Alexander, J., and Block, T.: Breast reconstruction following radical mastectomy, Plast. Reconstr. Surg. **40:**175, 1967.
2. Baroudi, R., Pinotti, J., and Keppke, E.: A transverse thoracoabdominal flap for closure after radical mastectomy, Plast. Reconstr. Surg. **61:**547, 1978.
3. Bartlett, W.: An anatomic substitute for the female breast, Ann. Surg., **66:**208, 1917.
4. Berson, M. I.: Derma-fat-fascia transplants used in building up the breasts, Surgery **15:**451, 1944.
5. Birnbaum, L., and Olsen, J.: Breast reconstruction following radical mastectomy, using custom designed implants, Plast. Reconstr. Surg. **61:**355, 1978.
6. Bohmert, H. In Georgiade, N. G., editor: Reconstructive breast surgery, St. Louis, 1976. The C. V. Mosby Co., p. 304.
7. Bostwick, J., Vasconez, L., and Jurkiewicz, M. J.: Breast reconstruction after radical mastectomy, Plast. Reconstr. Surg. **61:**682, 1978.
8. Cronin, T. D., Upton, J., and McDonough, J. M.: Reconstruction of the breast after mastectomy, Plast. Reconstr. Surg. **59:**1, 1977.
9. De Cholnoky, T.: Mastectomies with simultaneous reconstruction of breasts, Surgery **44:**649, 1958.
10. d'Este, S.: La technique de l'amputation de la mamelle pour carcinome mammaire par le procede de Tansini et sur une nouvelle application de cette operation; etude anatomoclinique et operatoire, Rev. Chir. **14:**164, 1912.
11. Drever, J. M.: Total breast reconstruction with either of two abdominal flaps, Plast. Reconstr. Surg. **59:**185, 1977.
12. Freeman, B. S.: Experiences in reconstruction of the breast after mastectomy, Clin. Plast. Surg. **3:**277, 1976.
13. Georgiade, N. G.: Reconstruction of the breasts following mastectomy. In Georgiade, N. G., editor: Reconstructive breast surgery, St. Louis, 1976, The C. V. Mosby Co., p. 292.
14. Goldwyn, R. M.: Vincenz Czerny and the beginnings of breast reconstruction, Plast. Reconstr. Surg. **61:**673, 1978.
15. Guthrie, R. H.: Breast reconstruction after radical mastectomy, Plast. Reconstr. Surg. **57:**14, 1976.

16. Harris, H.: Automammaplasty, J. Int. Coll. Surg. **12:**827, 1949.
17. Hartwell, S. W., and associates: Reconstruction of the breast after mastectomy for cancer, Plast. Reconstr. Surg. **57:**152, 1976.
18. Hohler, H.: Reconstruction of the female breast after radical mastectomy. In Converse, J. M., editor: Reconstructive plastic surgery, Philadelphia, 1977, W. B. Saunders Co., vol. 7, p. 3661.
19. Holdsworth, W. G.: A method of reconstructing the breast, Br. J. Plast. Surg. **9:**161, 1956.
20. Hueston, J., and McKenzie, G.: Breast reconstruction after radical mastectomy, Aust. N.Z. J. Surg. **39:**367, 1970.
21. Kleinschmidt, O.: Mammary plastics, Zentralbl. Chir. **51:**653, 1924.
22. Letterman, G. S., and Schurter, M.: Total mammary excision with immediate breast reconstruction, Am. Surg. **21:**835, 1955.
23. Lexer, E.: Die gesamte wiederherstellung, chirurge, Leipzig, 1931, Johann Ambrosius Barth Verlagsbuchhandlung, vol. 2, p. 555.
24. Longacre, J. J.: The use of local pedicle flaps for reconstruction of the breast after subtotal or total extirpation of the mammary gland and for the correction of distortion and atrophy of the breast due to excessive scar, Plast. Reconstr. Surg. **11:**380, 1953.
25. Longacre, J. J.: Correction of hypoplastic breast with special reference to reconstruction of "nipple type breast" with local dermofat pedicle flaps, Plast. Reconstr. Surg. **14:**431, 1954.
26. Maliniac, J. W.: Breast deformities and their repair, New York, 1950, Grune & Stratton, Inc.
27. Marino, H.: Glandular mastectomy: immediate reconstruction, Plast. Reconstr. Surg. **10:**204, 1952.
28. Millard, D. R.: Breast reconstruction after radical mastectomy, Plast. Reconstr. Surg. **58:**283, 1976.
29. Miller, S. H., and Graham, W. P.: Breast reconstruction after radical mastectomy, Am. Family Physician **11:**97, 1975.
30. Orticochea, M.: Use of the buttock to reconstruct the breast, Br. J. Plast. Surg. **26:**304, 1973.
31. Pontes, R.: Single stage reconstruction of the missing breast, Br. J. Plast. Surg. **26:** 377, 1973.
32. Reinhard, W.: Total mastoneoplasty following amputation of breast, Dtsch. Zeitschr. Chir. **236:**309, 1932.
33. Rosenauer, F.: Mammaer satzplastic nach radikaloperation wegen ca, Munch. Med. Wochenschr. **93:**890, 1951.
34. Snyderman, R. K., and Guthrie, R. H.: Reconstruction of the female breast following radical mastectomy, Plast. Reconstr. Surg. **47:**565, 1971.
35. Tai, Y., and Hasegawa, H.: A transverse abdominal flap for reconstruction after radical operations for recurrent breast cancer, Plast. Reconstr. Surg. **53:**52, 1974.
36. Thorek, M.: Plastic surgery of the breast and abdominal wall, Springfield, Ill., 1942, Charles C Thomas, Publisher.

CHAPTER 11

Latissimus dorsi musculocutaneous flap

Ronald Riefkohl and Nicholas G. Georgiade

Breast reconstruction for the majority of women who have been subjected to a radical or modified radical mastectomy may be satisfactorily accomplished by subcutaneous prosthetic augmentation and formation of a nipple-areolar complex.* However, prosthetic augmentation in the presence of poor-quality skin subsequent to chest wall irradiation, thin, tense chest wall skin resulting from wide sacrifice of breast skin and thinly cut mastectomy skin flaps,[12,20] or an atrophic widened mastectomy scar may result in skin erosion and necrosis with ultimate exposure and loss of the prosthesis.[13,31] Even disregarding these complications, the best that can be expected when soft tissue conditions are unfavorable is an immobile and undersized breast relative to its counterpart.

Recognizing obvious soft tissue deficiencies is usually quite easy. However, in most cases the situation is borderline and the decision to transfer additional soft tissue to the breast area prior to augmentation is overruled by the morbidity and generally poor results associated with the various available methods. Thus only a less than optimal breast reconstruction is possible. If there were a simple, reliable, and versatile flap that easily corrected the soft tissue deficiencies, the final result would be considerably better. The latissimus dorsi musculocutaneous island flap appears to be an almost ideal solution to this problem, easily satisfying criteria that other methods dismally fail to achieve.

METHODS OF SOFT TISSUE REPLACEMENT

Bascially there are three approaches to replace skin and subcutaneous tissue in the breast area: local flaps, distant flaps, and breast-sharing procedures.[10,13,17] All require multiple operative procedures for completion; consequently, multiple costly hospitalizations are necessary.

Local flaps should be planned outside the breast area if there has been previous chest wall irradiation. Since most are random flaps, multiple delays are necessary and the size is restricted.[16] It is probable that these flaps are not able to contribute a significant degree of nourishment to the recipient tissues. Since

*See references 7, 10, 11, 13, 24, and 31.

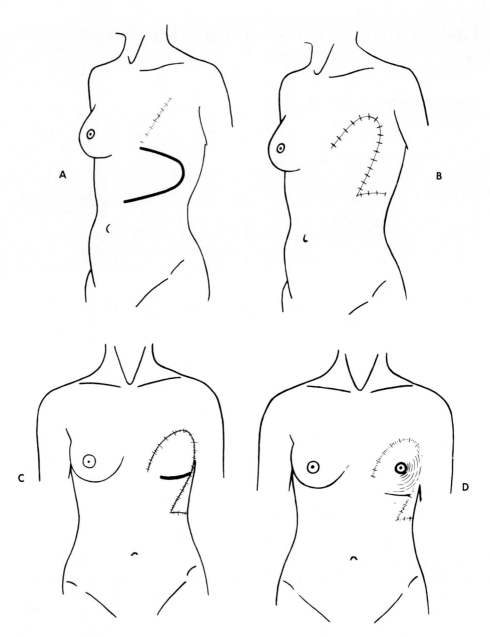

Fig. 11-1. Diagram of the method of breast reconstruction. **A,** Replacement of the missing skin by a rotation flap from the lateral thoracic and abdominal wall, based medially. **B,** Rotation flap in position. **C,** Replacement of the breast volume by a Silastic prosthesis through an incision in the submammary fold. **D,** Reconstruction of the areola and nipple. (Courtesy Dr. H. Bohmert.)

the local blood supply is already compromised after a radical mastectomy and possibly further reduced consequent to irradiation, the flap and adjacent skin may not tolerate the tension generated by an underlying prosthesis and will eventually necrose.

The thoracoabdominal flap[10,13] may be horizontal with a medial base (Fig. 11-1) or vertical with a superior-medial base (Fig. 11-2). An abdominal transposition flap is more reliable when based laterally and superiorly than from the upper midline (Fig. 11-3).

Breast-sharing procedures may be considered if the intact breast is of an adequate size (Figs. 11-4 and 11-5). These procedures are objectionable primarily because they involve the use of tissue at risk for the development of a malignancy.[10] Other criticisms are the limited amount of available tissue for transfer, the parasitic effect of random flaps, and aesthetic considerations.

Distant flaps transported on wrist carriers[10] are inadvisable since prolonged periods of joint immobilization are likely to result in stiffness. Instead tubed flaps may be stepped to the breasts in several stages[18]; however, multiple sites of scarring will result. The segment of tissue destined for the breast area will be entirely dependent on the local tissues for nourishment, this being undesirable for reasons emphasized previously.

Free transfer of dermis-fat-muscle flaps[8,9] or skin-fat flaps[26] to the breast area are quite feasible with recent refinements in microsurgical techniques. Several excellent donor flaps have been defined. Since a free flap transfer re-

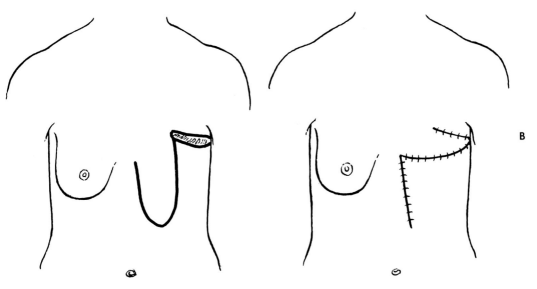

Fig. 11-2. A, Thoracoabdominal flap with superior-medial base. **B,** Mastectomy scar has been excised and flap has been rotated into resultant defect. Donor wound may be closed primarily after appropriate undermining.

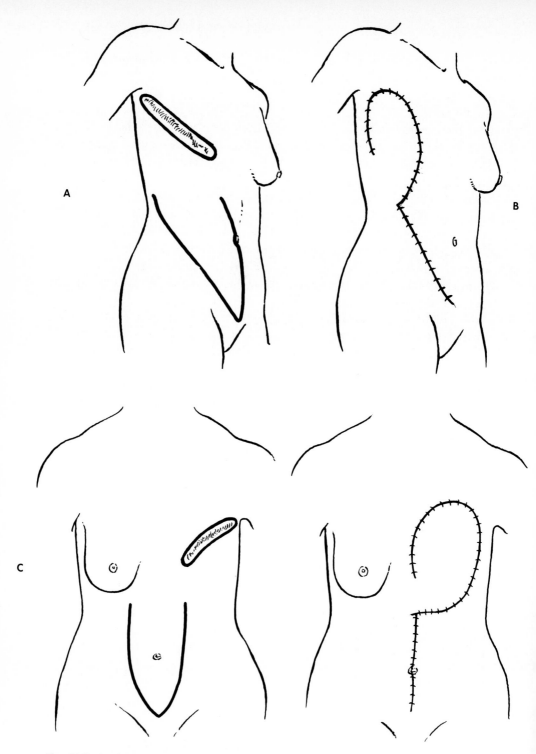

Fig. 11-3. A, Thoracoabdominal transposition flap with superior-lateral base. This is an axial pattern flap receiving its blood supply from the lateral cutaneous branches of the posterior intercostal arteries. **B,** Mastectomy scar has been excised and flap has been rotated into resultant defect. Donor wound may be closed primarily after appropriate undermining. **C,** Superiorly based midabdominal flap. Umbilicus may be incorporated in nipple-areolar complex reconstruction. **D,** Mastectomy scar has been excised and flap rotated into resultant defect. Donor wound is then closed primarily.

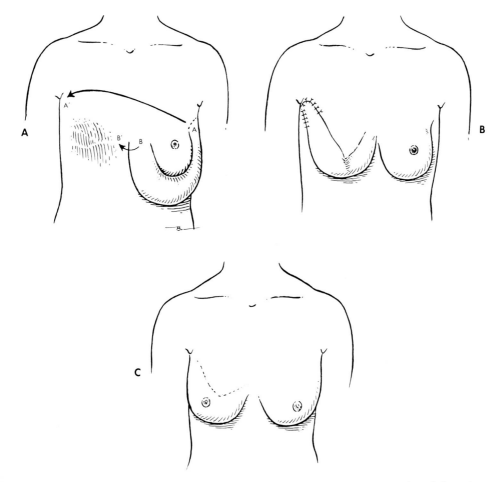

Fig. 11-4. A, Construction of a tube from the remaining breast. **B,** Transfer of the tube to the deficient breast. **C,** Tube inset completed and both right and left breasts newly contoured with areola and nipple on the left simulated with free grafts. (Diagrams modified from the method of Dr. W. G. Holdsworth.)

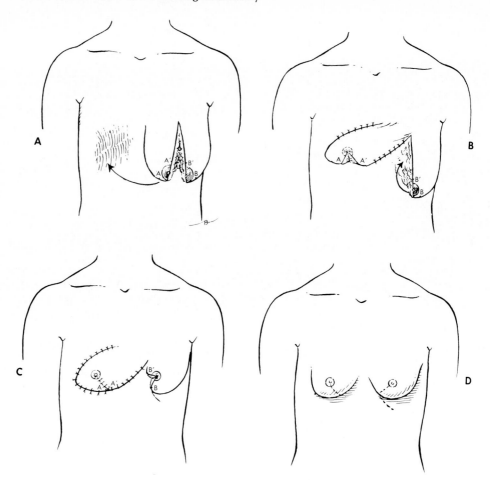

Fig. 11-5. A, An incision of the normal breast bisects the breast into equal parts, each containing half of the breast, areola, and nipple. **B,** The medial portion of the breast is repositioned onto the side of the deficient breast. The lateral portion of the breast is moved superiorly to form a smaller new breast. **C,** The new breasts are then contoured with the areola and nipples placed in the proper position. **D,** The newly contoured breasts with nipples in proper position. (Diagrams modified from the method of Dr. R. Pontes.)

quires a highly skilled, experienced microsurgeon and many hours to accomplish, we reserve this method for those patients found to have ligated thoracodorsal vessels during axillary exploration.

In comparison the latissimus dorsi musculocutaneous island flap is a relatively simple operation, transferring in one procedure a large composite flap of skin, fat, and muscle that has an independent and vigorous blood supply. Consequently the prosthesis is covered by a thick, healthy, and durable layer of tissue. The free sweep of the pectoralis major muscle is restored and the infraclavicular hollow filled in. If the thoracodorsal vessels are intact, the flap is extremely reliable, and its versatility is demonstrated by its ability to replace virtually any type of mastectomy scar. The donor site scar, lying just inside the posterior axillary fold, is readily concealed by the arm. The functional loss of an absent latissimus dorsi muscle is quite minimal, the remaining shoulder girdle muscles substituting for the latissimus dorsi muscle.

EVOLUTION OF LATISSIMUS DORSI MUSCULOCUTANEOUS FLAP

The latissimus dorsi musculocutaneous island flap transfer should be considered a new concept only by virtue of recent clarifications in flap circulatory dynamics.

In a rather detailed report, d'Este[5] in 1912 described a "dorsal flap" used to cover the wound resulting from amputation of the breast. d'Este termed this flap "the technique of Tansini," who apparently conceived it and first reported it in 1896. The method of Tansini is depicted in Thorek's textbook, *Plastic Surgery of the Breasts and Abdominal Wall*[30]; however, the anatomic description of the flap is inaccurate. The Tansini flap, according to d'Este, consisted of the upper portion of the latissimus dorsi and the entire teres major, teres minor, and infraspinatus muscles. The flap was paddle shaped with a base 6 to 7 cm wide that included the thoracodorsal and scapular circumflex vessels, the importance of which is strongly emphasized (Fig. 11-6). The donor wound was closed primarily by the transposition principle.

Davis[3] in 1949 reported using a superiorly based flap of latissimus dorsi muscle to close a 30 × 14 cm anterior chest wall defect. The following year Campbell[2] reported seven cases of chest wall defects reconstructed by latissimus dorsi muscle flaps. Split-thickness skin grafts were applied over the transposed muscle flaps.

Several other reports describe compound flaps of skin, fat, and muscle[4,23]; however, the term "musculocutaneous flap" appears to have been coined by Orticochea in 1972.[22] A musculocutaneous, or "myocutaneous," flap is an axial pattern composite flap[16,19] consisting of skin and underlying muscle. The skin of the flap is vascularized by a system of perpendicular muscle perforating vessels that arise from small segmental muscular arteries, each perforator vessel supplying a limited area of skin and muscle.[29] Segmental muscular arteries in turn originate from one or more relatively independent arteries, one having a dominant vascular territory.[14] This anatomic arrangement permits the elevation and transfer of a major portion of muscle and overlying skin based on a single vascular pedicle. This pedicle becomes the axis of rotation of the flap and its only attachment to the body.[15]

The skin dimensions of a musculocutaneous flap are limited by the length of muscle supplied by the dominant vascular pedicle[15] plus 3 to 5 cm beyond the length and width of this muscle segment.[15,19] These dimensions may be

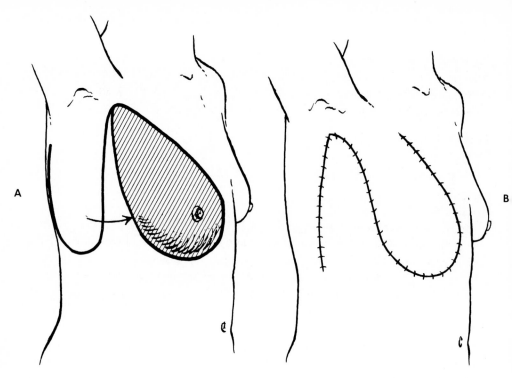

Fig. 11-6. A, Tansini flap. Shaded area represents extent of skin sacrifice included with mastectomy. The flap, as designed, was a musculocutaneous unit incorporating thoracodorsal and scapular circumflex vessels. **B,** Tansini flap has been transposed into mastectomy wound. Donor site is then closed primarily.

extended only by delay procedures intended to extend the vascular territory of the perforator vessels, since muscle arteries are apparently end arteries.[14]

In 1976 Olivari[21] reported using a latissimus dorsi musculocutaneous flap for anterior chest wall reconstruction in two patients. The base of the pedicle included both skin and muscle attachments.

In 1977 Mendelson and Masson[17] reported using latissimus dorsi musculo-cutaneous flaps for radiation injuries about the shoulder region in three cases. They mentioned that the skin bridge at the base of the flap may be very narrow or completely divided. That same year Mühlbauer and Olbrisch[19] reported their experience with twenty-two latissimus dorsi musculocutaneous flaps used for various reconstructive purposes. They recognized that the flap could be isolated on its vascular pedicle, which in their opinion did not offer any particular advantage. Recently Schneider, Hill, and Brown[25] reported reconstructing a single breast with a latissimus dorsi musculocutaneous flap combined with simultaneous insertion of a prosthesis and creation of a nipple-areolar complex. Their flap design differed from ours in that the muscle area was three to four times greater

than the skin area and the skin portion was situated more posteriorly and inferiorly.

The latissimus dorsi musculocutaneous flap has been transferred as a free
flap with microvascular anastomosis.[1,27] It is possible to obtain a rather lengthy
vascular pedicle with vessel diameters ranging from 2 to 3 mm. These features
contribute to reducing the chance of anastomotic thrombosis and flap failure.

ANATOMY

The latissimus dorsi muscle[32] is a broad, triangular muscle inserting as a
band-like tendon in the floor of the intertubercular groove of the humerus and
originating from the lower thoracic, lumbar, and sacral spinous processes in
addition to the posterior crest of the ileum. It pulls the arm down and back and
rotates it medially. It is innervated by the thoracodorsal nerve from the posterior
cord of the brachial plexus and derives its blood supply from the thoracodorsal
artery, the terminal branch of the subscapular artery. Occasionally there is a
branch from the thoracodorsal artery to the serratus anterior muscle as a substitute for the lateral thoracic artery.

TECHNIQUE OF FLAP TRANSFER

Several folded sheets are placed beneath the ipsilateral buttock and scapula,
rotating the lateral thoracic region upward from the operating table. The arm,
abducted 90 degrees with the elbow flexed, is secured to a well-padded malleable
ether screen positioned across the patient's face.

The superior extent of the skin ellipse is marked medial to the posterior
axillary fold 2 cm inferior to the arm. The mastectomy scar is measured, and
this distance is transferred to a point slightly anterior to the palpable anterior
border of the latissimus dorsi muscle inferiorly. These two points are joined
anteriorly by a gentle curving line. The maximum available width of flap is determined by pinching the skin together, and a point is selected that appears to
permit closure of the donor wound without excessive skin tension. The posterior
border is outlined as a curved line several centimeters longer than the anterior
line (Fig. 11-7).

This design will result in a fairly inconspicuous vertical scar since it will lie
high on the medial aspect of the posterior axillary fold. Thus the scar is well
concealed when the relaxed arm is held by the trunk. Any redundant skin encountered during wound closure should be excised toward the axillary hollow
instead of posteriorly around the shoulder or down the inner aspect of the arm.

The upper 5 to 6 cm of the anterior margin of the flap is incised down to
the latissimus dorsi muscle. The axillary fascia is opened along the anterior
border of the muscle, and the thoracodorsal neurovascular bundle is identified
as it traverses the space between the latissimus dorsi muscle and the chest
wall. The neurovascular bundle is mobilized sufficiently to determine the integrity of the artery and vein (Fig. 11-8). If one or both vessels are ligated or of

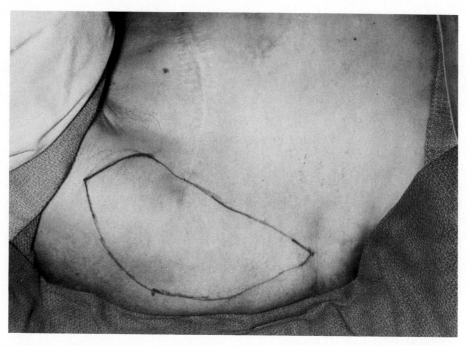

Fig. 11-7. The flap is outlined with brilliant green as described in the text. In this patient a right radical mastectomy had been performed. Patient's head and neck are to left side of photograph.

inadequate caliber to ensure flap viability, transfer of an island flap is not feasible. In this situation several alternatives are available. If there are intact communicating channels between the distal thoracodorsal artery and vein and the serratus anterior vessels, these will adequately nourish a flap of smaller dimensions. Maintaining the integrity of the muscle insertion probably provides additional vascularity (Figs. 11-9 to 11-10). To further ensure an adequate circulation, a deepithelialized skin pedicle may be included (Fig. 11-11). The deepithelialized component will ultimately lie within the tunnel formed between the donor and recipient wounds (Fig. 11-12). However, in the presence of heavily irradiated skin or when a large flap is necessary, it may be safer to transfer a free groin flap or free latissimus dorsi musculocutaneous flap from the opposite side, either immediately or at a future date. When the vessels are suitable, the remainder of the anterior skin incision is completed. The latissimus fascia is incised, and the free anterior border of the latissimus dorsi muscle is sutured at 5-cm intervals to the subcutaneous tissue of the flap.

The delicate loose areolar tissue between the latissimus dorsi muscle and the chest wall is divided, exposing the undersurface of the portion of muscle intended for inclusion with the composite flap. The posterior incision through skin, subcutaneous tissue, and latissimus dorsi muscle is carried out sequentially

Text continued on p. 205.

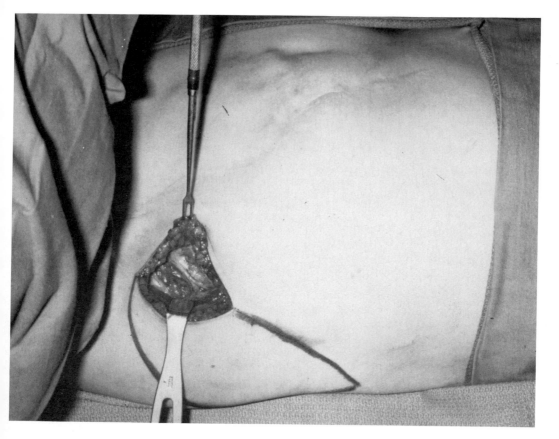

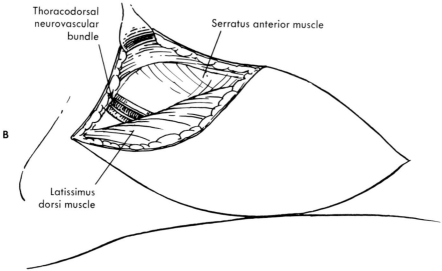

Fig. 11-8. A, Short exploratory incision has been made along upper portion of flap and extended beneath latissimus dorsi muscle. Thoracodorsal vessels and nerve are identified and their integrity established. **B,** Diagrammatic representation of exploratory incision. Vessels and nerve are readily identified once the loose areolar plane is entered between latissimus dorsi muscle and serratus anterior muscle.

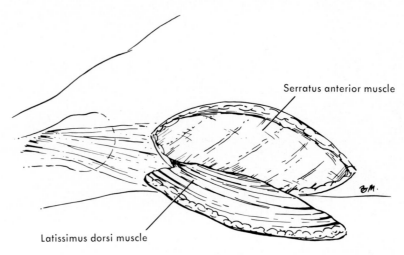

Serratus anterior muscle

Latissimus dorsi muscle

Fig. 11-9. When the thoracodorsal vessels are damaged, it is possible to utilize a smaller flap that receives its blood supply from vascular communications with chest wall and possibly tendinous insertion.

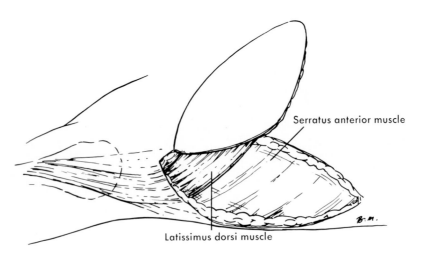

Serratus anterior muscle

Latissimus dorsi muscle

Fig. 11-10. Flap diagrammed in Fig. 11-9 has been transposed. The point of rotation is further inferiorly and laterally than when the flap is rotated as an island pedicle.

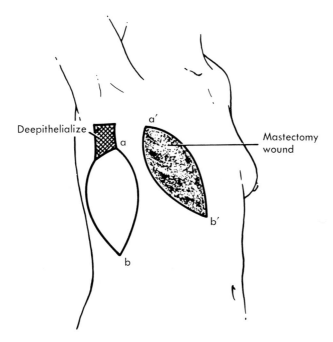

Fig. 11-11. Occasionally a paddle-shaped flap with the base deepithelialized is utilized. Note similarity to flap originally described by Tansini.

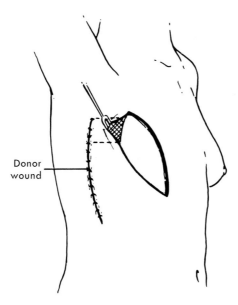

Fig. 11-12. Flap has been tunneled to mastectomy wound and donor site closed. Deepithelialized component lies beneath skin bridge separating the two wounds.

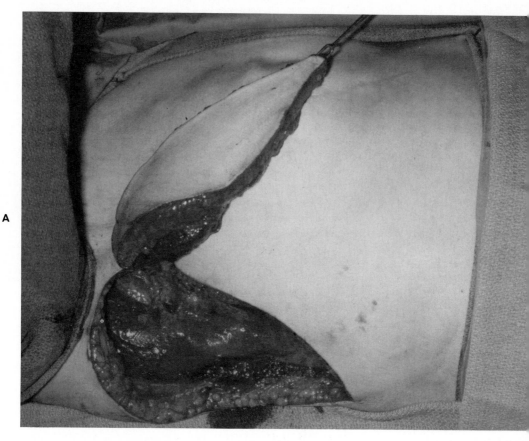

A

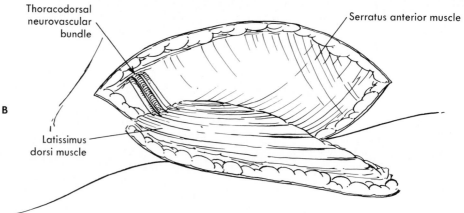

B

Thoracodorsal
neurovascular
bundle

Serratus anterior muscle

Latissimus
dorsi muscle

Fig. 11-13. A, Musculocutaneous unit has been completely freed except for its neurovascular attachments. Further mobilization of the neurovascular bundle is possible if needed. **B,** Diagrammatic representation of completely elevated island flap with its neurovascular attachments.

as the cut edge of the muscle is sutured to the subcutaneous tissue at 5-cm intervals. This maneuver avoids the possibility of injuring those perforator vessels near the margin of the flap by maintaining alignment of the skin with the underlying muscle.

The index finger is passed beneath the narrow tendinous insertion at a level 4 to 5 cm superior to the junction of the neurovascular bundle with the muscle thus protecting the vessels from injury as the insertion is transected. The flap is now completely free except for its neurovascular attachment (Fig. 11-13).

The mastectomy scar is excised and the mastectomy skin flaps are elevated from the chest wall, thus recreating the original mastectomy defect. A tunnel is formed beneath the intact skin bridge separating the two wounds, and the island composite flap is tunneled through (Fig. 11-14).

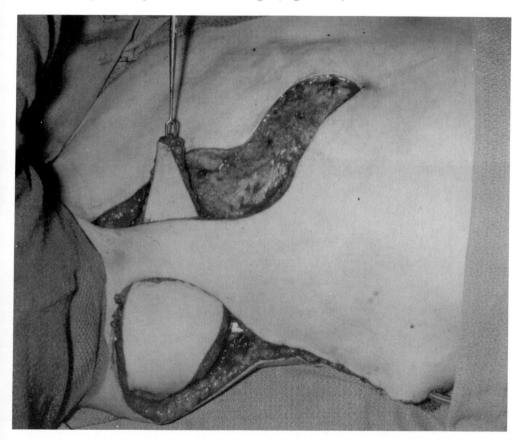

Fig. 11-14. Mastectomy scar has been completely excised and mastectomy skin flaps elevated from chest wall, thus allowing them to retract and reform the original mastectomy defect. It is important to design the flap so that an adequate width of skin bridge separates the two wounds. A tunnel is then formed and flap is brought through into mastectomy wound.

The tension on the vessels is now determined; if they are stretched, further posterior axillary dissection is essential in order to mobilize additional vessel lengths. It may be necessary to divide the branches to the serratus anterior muscle if there is tethering at this point. The subcutaneous tunnel may also require superior enlargement if this will result in a shorter route for the vessels from the axilla to the flap in its transposed position. With a low transverse mastectomy defect, neither of these maneuvers will completely reduce the tension on the vessels, particularly the vein. In this situation the flap should be allowed to retract under the skin bridge until the tension on the vessels is eliminated. The area of the flap skin retracted beneath the skin bridge is then deepithelialized. This modification reduces the skin surface area of the flap a negligible amount and is preferable to designing the skin ellipse at a more inferior-lateral location because of donor scar considerations.

When the flap is not transferred as an island because of damaged thoraco-

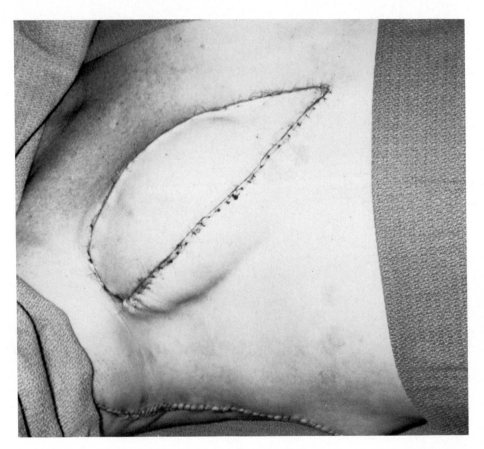

Fig. 11-15. Musculocutaneous flap has been sutured in place with several deep layers of Dexon sutures and three-fourth mattress sutures for the skin. Donor wound has been closed primarily.

dorsal vessels, its mobility will be considerably reduced because of shorter and more inferior attachments to the chest wall, an intact tendinous insertion, and possibly a deepithelialized skin pedicle. Adjustments will be necessary during a later operation to improve the position and contour of the flap.

The flap is sutured within the mastectomy defect and the donor wound closed over a single suction catheter (Fig. 11-15). A bulky occlusive dressing with an inspection window over the distal portion of the flap is applied after the appropriate procedure has been completed on the opposite breast.

Technique of latissimus dorsi muscle flap

When muscle exclusive of skin is intended for transfer, the patient is positioned and the axilla explored in the same fashion as described previously. The undersurface of the muscle is thoroughly exposed, and the latissimus fascia at the free anterior border of the muscle is incised. The subcutaneous layer is

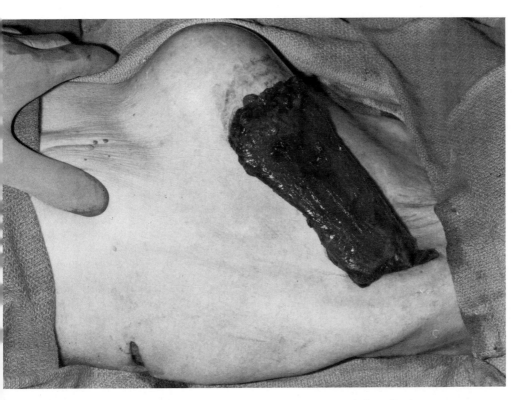

Fig. 11-16. This 70-year-old woman, who had undergone a left radical mastectomy, had completed the left breast reconstruction. However, there was a severe deficiency of soft tissue in the infraclavicular and anterior axillary fold areas. A latissimus dorsi muscle flap was formed through two short incisions, one along the upper posterior axillary fold and a second posterior lateral transverse incision. The muscle flap was then sutured to the chest wall to simulate a pectoralis major muscle.

elevated from the surface of the latissimus fascia, and the perforator vessels are electrocoagulated. Through a short transverse incision located 20 to 25 cm inferior to the junction of the neurovascular bundle with the muscle and 4 to 6 cm posterior to the free edge of the muscle, the mobilization of the muscle flap is completed. While the muscle is still attached above and below, long Metzenbaum scissors with the blades held apart are pushed from above downward in a posterior direction, thus forming a muscle bipedicle shaped like a fan. The muscle bipedicle is then cut across at its inferior attachment and pulled upward through the axillary incision (Fig. 11-16).

The mastectomy skin flaps are elevated through the axillary incision and, if necessary, through an additional short transverse incision placed in the future inframammary crease. The muscle is tunneled beneath the skin and sutured to the chest wall in a splayed configuration. Finally the incisions are closed and a dry sterile occlusive dressing applied.

This procedure is considerably more difficult than that for the musculocutaneous flap. Long instruments, Deaver retractors, and a fiberoptic head lamp are essential to secure complete hemostasis and to properly suture the flap into place.

Clinical experience

As previously discussed, we select patients for a latissimus dorsi musculocutaneous flap who have thin, tight chest wall skin with or without a wide, atrophied mastectomy scar or when there is a moderate deficiency of chest wall skin that has been irradiated (Fig. 11-17). Ordinarily the muscle is easily palpated when voluntarily tensed, but this only establishes continuity of the thoracodorsal nerve. We do not advise arteriography, since it will not visualize the thoracodorsal vein and may be misleading; instead we prefer to explore the axilla. We have encountered three patients with identifiable ligatures on both artery and vein and a fourth patient with only the vein ligated. These four patients subsequently underwent free flap transfers successfully; thus the limited axillary exploration will not jeopardize the suitability of recipient vessels for microvascular anastomoses.[26]

Our experience consists of thirty-eight latissimus dorsi musculocutaneous flaps, of which thirty were island flaps, six were not island flaps, and two were muscle flaps. Among the six musculocutaneous flaps without intact thoracodorsal vessels, three included a deepithelialized skin pedicle. One patient, who had a bilateral subcutaneous mastectomy complicated by extensive skin necrosis, underwent bilateral flaps as one procedure. Because of soft tissue deficiencies, all patients were unsuitable for simple prosthetic augmentation.

At the time of evaluation for breast reconstruction, no patient demonstrated clinical evidence of recurrent or metastatic disease.[28]

The dimensions of the thirty island flaps ranged from 7 to 20 cm in width to 15 to 30 cm in length. Excluding the patient with the extensive chest wall

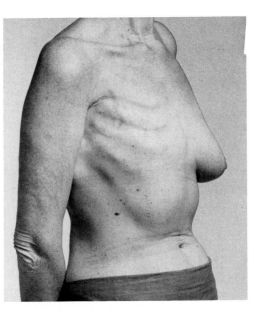

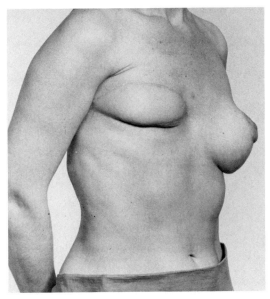

Fig. 11-17. Typical deformity resulting from a radical mastectomy. There is a severe deficiency of chest wall skin and subcutaneous tissue combined with an atrophic mastectomy scar.

Fig. 11-18. Composite island flap oriented transversely.

ulcer subsequent to irradiation, we have not found it necessary to enlarge these dimensions, and in the majority of patients the flap has been larger than the recreated mastectomy defect. In the patient with the radiation ulcer, a 20 × 30 cm flap was transferred after one delay procedure. Though the distal 3 cm of this large flap necrosed we hesitate to define the maximum flap dimensions based on this isolated case.

When the thoracodorsal vessels are absent, the flap circulation is diminished. Two of the six flaps in this category were complicated by skin blistering and skin necrosis of the distal 1 to 2 cm.

Among the island flaps there was only one minor complication of distal flap blistering occurring in a patient with an unusually low, transverse mastectomy scar. In a transverse configuration the flap rotates through an arc of approximately 120 degrees without difficulty (Fig. 11-18); however, if the transverse plane of the wound is lower than the transverse plane of the rotated flap, there will be tension on the vessels when the flap is tunneled to the defect, resulting in impaired venous return. This can be avoided by deepithelializing a small area of skin proximally and allowing the flap to retract beneath the skin bridge until stretching of the vascular pedicle is relieved.

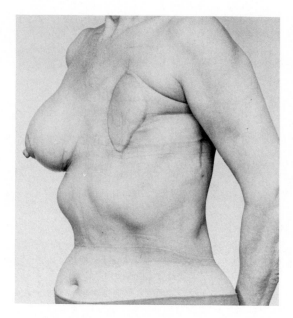

Fig. 11-19. Composite island flap oriented vertically.

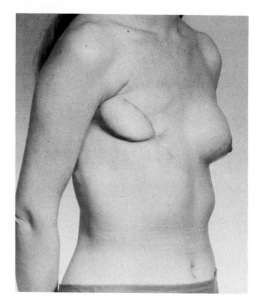

Fig. 11-20. Composite island flap oriented obliquely.

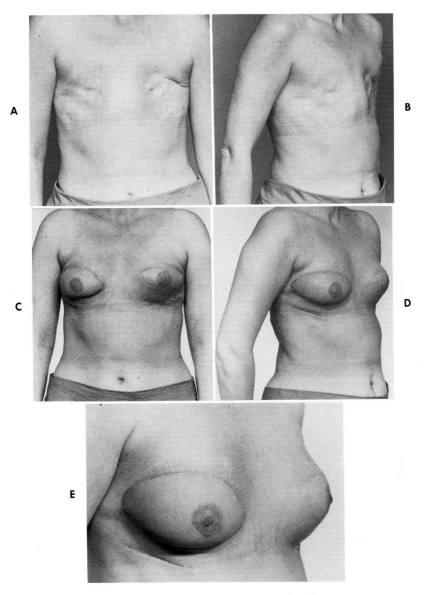

Fig. 11-21. This 32-year-old woman underwent a bilateral subcutaneous mastectomy complicated by an extensive loss of breast skin including the nipple-areolar complexes. Additionally on the left side there is a significant loss of pectoralis major muscle. **A,** Preoperative photograph as seen from front. **B,** Preoperative photograph as seen from right oblique view. **C,** Patient had bilateral latissimus dorsi musculocutaneous flaps followed by reconstruction of both breasts; frontal view. **D,** Right oblique view. **E,** Close-up of breast from oblique view.

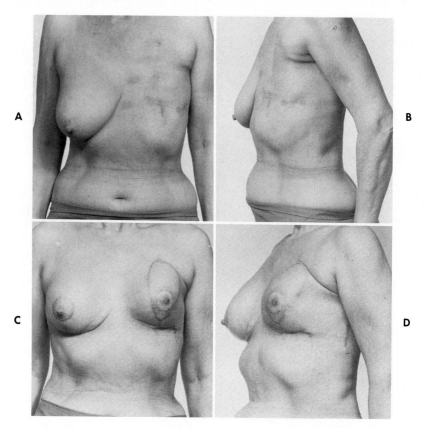

Fig. 11-22. This 59-year-old woman underwent a left radical mastectomy. **A,** As seen from frontal view there is an atrophic and tight mastectomy skin scar and thin mastectomy skin flaps. **B,** Left lateral view. **C,** Breast reconstruction has been completed following a latissimus dorsi musculocutaneous flap. A subcutaneous mastectomy with simultaneous augmentation mammopexy has been performed on right side. **D,** Left oblique view.

Two patients with the vertical flap configuration (Fig. 11-19) required complete mobilization of the thoracodorsal vessels, a tedious dissection in a scarred axilla, to permit tunneling of the flap without tension on the pedicle. The flap in an oblique configuration (Fig. 11-20) presents the least difficulty since the greatest movement occurs at the distal end.

It usually requires 1 to 2 hours to elevate the flap and suture it in place within the recreated mastectomy defect. While the donor wound is closed by an assistant, the opposite breast may be surgically approached.

We do not insert a prosthesis beneath the flap nor attempt to reconstruct the nipple-areolar complex during this procedure. Instead we prefer to accomplish this at least 3 months afterward since there will be some shrinkage of the flap.

About half of the patients have had the breast reconstruction completed

(Figs. 11-21 and 11-22). After critical evaluation we believe that the final results are more acceptable with fewer procedures needed compared to our experience, and that of others, with various other available flaps.

REFERENCES

1. Baudet, J., Garbe, J. F., Guimberteau, J. C., and Lemaine, J. M.: The axillary flap. In Serafin, D., and Buncke, H. J., Jr., editors: Microsurgical composite tissue transplantation, St. Louis, 1978, The C. V. Mosby Co.
2. Campbell, D. A.: Reconstruction of the anterior thoracic wall, J. Thorac. Cardiovasc. Surg. **19:**456, 1950.
3. Davis, H. H., Tollman, P., and Brush, J. H.: Huge chrondrosarcoma of rib—report of a case, Surgery **26:**699, 1949.
4. Desprez, J. D., Kiehn, C. L., and Eckstein, W.: Closure of large meningomyelocele defects by composite skin-muscle flaps, Plast. Reconstr. Surg. **47:**234, 1971.
5. d'Este, S.: La technique de l'amputation de la mammelle pour carcinome mammairre, Rev. Chir. **45:**164, 1912.
6. Drever, J. M.: Total breast reconstruction with either of two abdominal flaps, Plast. Reconstr. Surg. **59:**185, 1977.
7. Freeman, B. S.: Experiences in reconstruction of the breast after mastectomy, Clin. Plast. Surg. **3:**277, 1976.
8. Fujino, T., Harashina, T., and Aoyagi, F.: Reconstruction for aplasia of the breast and pectoral region by microvascular transfer of a free flap from the buttock, Plast. Reconstr. Surg. **56:**178, 1975.
9. Fujino, T., Harashina, T., and Enamoto, K.: Primary breast reconstruction after a standard radical mastectomy by a free flap transfer-case report, Plast. Reconstr. Surg. **58:**371, 1976.
10. Georgiade, N. G.: Reconstruction of the breast following mastectomy. In Georgiade, N. G., editor: Reconstructive breast surgery, St. Louis, 1977, The C. V. Mosby Co., p. 292.
11. Gibson, E. W.: Reconstruction of the breast after mastectomy for carcinoma, Clin. Plast. Surg., vol. 3, 1976.
12. Haagensen, C. D.: Surgical treatment of mammary carcinoma. In Haagensen, C. D.: Disease of the breast, ed. 2, Philadelphia, 1971, W. B. Saunders Co., pp. 559-734.
13. Hohler, H.: Reconstruction of the female breast after radical mastectomy. In Converse, J. M., editor: Reconstructive plastic surgery, Philadelphia, 1977, W. B. Saunders Co., vol. 7, p. 3661.
14. McCraw, J. B., and Dibbell, D.: Experimental definition of independent myocutaneous vascular territories, Plast. Reconstr. Surg. **60:**212, 1977.
15. McCraw, J. B., Dibbell, D., and Carraway, J. H.: Clinical definition of independent myocutaneous vascular territories, Plast. Reconstr. Surg. **60:**341, 1971.
16. McGregor, I. A., and Morgan, G.: Axial and random pattern flaps, Br. J. Plast. Surg. **26:**202, 1973.
17. Mendelson, B. C., and Masson, J. K.: Treatment of chronic radiation injury over the shoulder with a latissimus dorsi myocutaneous flap, Plast. Reconstr. Surg. **60:**681, 1971.
18. Millard, D. R.: Breast reconstruction after a radical mastectomy, Plast. Reconstr. Surg. **58:**283, 1976.
19. Mühlbauer, W., and Olbrisch, R.: The latissimus dorsi myocutaneous flap for breast reconstruction, Chir. Plastica **4:**27, 1977.

20. Nora, R. F.: Operative surgery principles and techniques, Philadelphia, 1974, Lea & Febiger. pp. 188-198.
21. Olivari, N.: The latissimus flap, Br. J. Plast. Surg. **29:**127, 1977.
22. Orticochea, M.: The musculo-cutaneous flap method: an immediate and heroic substitute for the method of delay, Br. J. Plast. Surg. **25:**106, 1972.
23. Owens, N.: A compound neck pedicle designed for the repair of massive facial defects: formation, development, and application, Plast. Reconstr. Surg. **15:**369, 1955.
24. Perras, C.: The creation of a twin breast following radical mastectomy—a report of 50 consecutive cases, 1959-1975, Clin. Plast. Surg. **3:**265, 1976.
25. Schneider, W. J., Hill, H. L., Jr., and Brown, R. G.: Latissimus dorsi myocutaneous flap for breast reconstruction, Br. J. Plast. Surg. **30:**277, 1977.
26. Serafin, D.: Personal communication, February 1978.
27. Serafin, D.: Reconstruction of the thorax and breast following radical mastectomy. In Serafin, D., and Buncke, H. J., Jr., editors: Microsurgical composite tissue transplantation, St. Louis, 1978, The C. V. Mosby Co.
28. Sugarbaker, E. V., Ketcham, A. S., and Zubrod, G. F.: Interdisciplinary cancer therapy: adjuvant therapy, Curr. Probl. Surg. **14:**1, June 1977.
29. Taylor, I. G., and Daniel, R. K.: The anatomy of several free flap donor sites, Plast. Reconstr. Surg. **56:**243, 1975.
30. Thorek, M.: Plastic surgery of the breast and abdominal wall: amastia, hypomastia, and inequality of the breasts, Springfield, Ill., 1932, Charles C Thomas, Publisher, pp. 369-387.
31. Watts, J. T.: Restorative prosthetic mammaplasty in mastectomy for cancer and benign lesions, Clin. Plast. Surg., vol. 3, 1976.
32. Woodburne, R. T.: Essentials of human anatomy, ed. 3, New York, 1965, Oxford University Press, p. 54.

CHAPTER 12

Microsurgical composite tissue transplantation: reconstruction of the breast

Donald Serafin

Mortality statistics for patients with carcinoma of the breast have not changed appreciably during the past four decades.[4] Although treatment modalities may differ, the modified radical mastectomy continues to be the surgical procedure most frequently employed for invasive lesions of the breast. This operative procedure, first introduced 30 years ago, has largely supplanted other, more radical procedures.

Radiation therapy in most major medical centers is still viewed by therapists as adjunctive. It is most often employed with larger, aggressive primary lesions, frequently with positive axillary metastases. Although not an invasive procedure, long-term deleterious effects of this treatment modality may be cumulative and quite destructive.

With increasing public awareness in the early detection of carcinoma of the breast, attention has also been directed to earlier reconstruction. Now it is not unusual to discuss further reconstruction with the patient prior to the proposed extirpative surgery.

Difficulty in reconstruction is inversely related to the amount of well-vascularized tissue remaining at the mastectomy site. This deficiency can be further increased by adjunctive radiation therapy. General principles governing reconstruction in other anatomic regions are also applicable to the breast. The surgical procedure more easily performed with the lowest incidence of tissue morbidity should be considered first.[7] Because the reconstructive effort is frequently initiated to restore form and contour, with emphasis on the aesthetic quality of the final result, donor deformity should be minimal. This frequently influences the procedure selected.

Microsurgical composite tissue transplantation for reconstruction of the breast does not have universal applicability. It should only be performed when existing methods cannot fulfill the proposed requirements. It is in this relatively small population when there is an extreme deficiency of healthy, well-vascularized skin, or when more conventional methods have failed, that this new

215

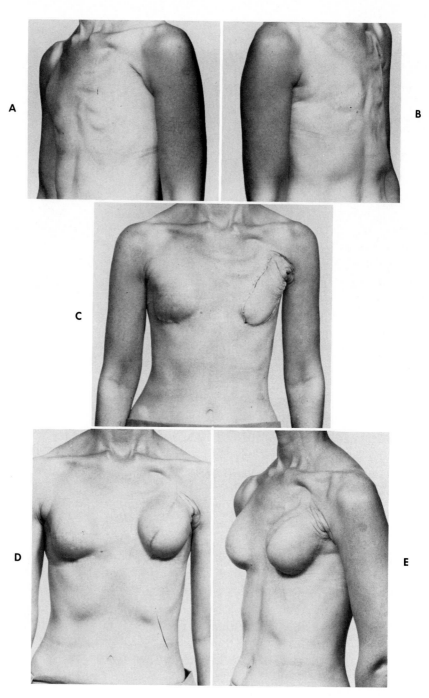

Fig. 12-1. For legend see opposite page.

procedure has its greatest usefulness.[8] The donor deformity resulting from this procedure, especially when the vascularized groin flap is employed, is minimal.

INDICATIONS (PRESENT SERIES)

Twelve patients were selected for breast reconstruction by this new technique (Table 12-1). All patients had previously undergone a standard radical mastectomy for carcinoma of the breast. One patient initially had a left radical mastectomy and then a modified right radical mastectomy for invasive lobular carcinoma of the breast (Fig. 12-1). After mastectomy most of the patients had a

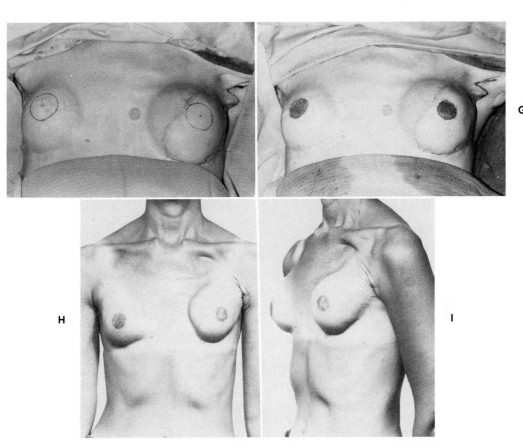

Fig. 12-1. A and **B,** Preoperative photograph demonstrating left radical mastectomy and right modified radical mastectomy for invasive lobular carcinoma of the breast. **C,** Postoperative photograph demonstrating vascularized groin flap to augment deficiency of left breast and reconstruction of right breast with silicone implant. **D** and **E,** Postoperative photograph demonstrating bilateral augmentation to achieve breast mound symmetry. **F** and **G,** Intraoperative photograph demonstrating third stage of reconstruction of nipple-areolar complex with labial grafts. **H** and **I,** Postoperative result. (**A, E, G,** and **I** from Serafin, D., and Georgiade, N. G.: Microsurgical composite tissue transplantation, Ann. Surg. **187**(6):620-628, June 1978.)

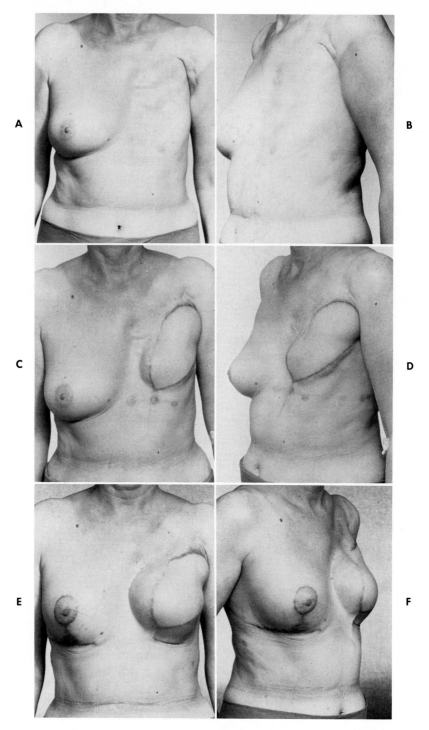

A

B

C

D

E

F

Fig. 12-2. For legend see opposite page.

vertical incision extending from the axilla to the umbilicus (Fig. 12-2). In this series of patients four had primary wound closure effected with a split-thickness graft (Tables 12-1 and 12-2) (Fig. 12-3). Two of these patients had a chronic, recurrent ulceration in the grafted site.

Six patients in the present series also received an average of 4500 R to the chest wall, axilla, and supraclavicular region (Tables 12-1 and 12-2). Most of these patients received adjunctive radiotherapy because of an unfavorable primary lesion or the presence of axillary metastases (Table 12-3). Interestingly two patients in this group had radiographic changes consistent with radiation osteitis. One patient had such extensive changes (that is, multiple rib fractures) that radiation therapy records were obtained and dosages recalculated. Recalculated radiation to the involved areas revealed dosages in excess of 14,000 R (Fig. 12-4, A). A third patient (not included in this series) sought reconstruction of the left breast after mastectomy and postoperative radiation therapy. An upper motor neuron brachial plexus injury was noted on careful neurologic examination. Because of this, breast reconstruction was deferred. Most of the patients who had received postoperative radiation had characteristic skin changes of radiation

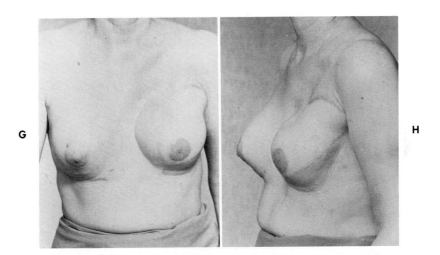

Fig. 12-2. A and **B,** Preoperative photograph demonstrating defect resulting from left radical mastectomy. Note vertical scar. **C** and **D,** Postoperative photograph demonstrating result following completion of first stage of reconstruction with vascularized groin flap. **E** and **F,** Postoperative photograph demonstrating result following completion of second stage of breast reconstruction—right subcutaneous mastectomy with correction of ptosis and immediate insertion of implant, and augmentation vascularized groin flap, left breast. **G** and **H,** Postoperative result. (**A, B, G,** and **H** from Serafin, D., Georgiade, N. G., and Given, K. S.: Transfer of free flaps to provide well vascularized, thick cover for breast reconstructions after radical mastectomy, Plast. Reconstr. Surg. **62**(4):527-536, October 1978.)

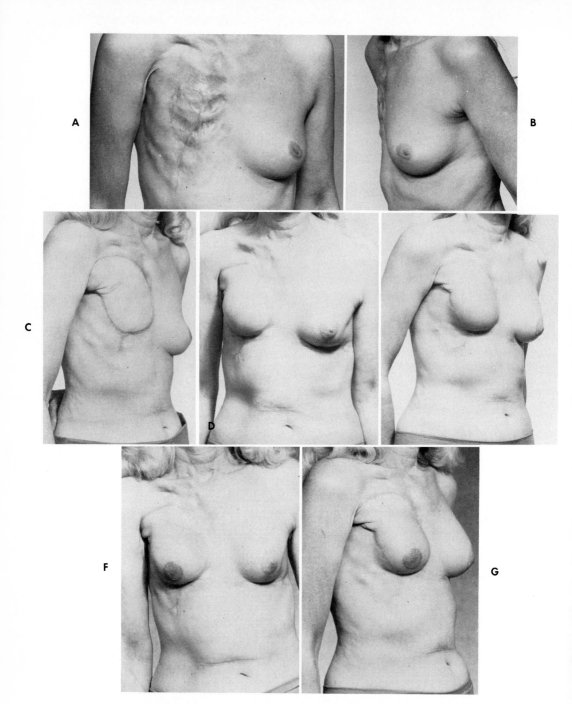

Fig. 12-3. A and **B,** Preoperative photograph demonstrating marked deficiency of healthy, well-vascularized skin with split-thickness skin graft to right chest wall. **C,** Postoperative photograph following completion of first stage with a vascularized groin flap. **D** and **E,** Postoperative photograph following completion of second stage of breast reconstruction—left subcutaneous mastectomy, correction of ptosis and insertion of implant, and right augmentation vascularized groin flap. **F** and **G,** Postoperative result. (**A, C, F,** and **G** from Serafin, D., Georgiade, N. G., and Given, K. S.: Transfer of free flaps to provide well vascularized, thick cover for breast reconstructions after radical mastectomy, Plast. Reconstr. Surg. **62**(4):527-536, October 1978.)

Table 12-1. Factors complicating reconstruction

Case	Extirpative surgery	Skin graft	Cobalt irradiation	Chemotherapy	Ligation subscapular artery and vein
1	Right radical mastecomy	Yes	Yes	No	No
2	Left radical mastectomy	No	No	No	No
	Right modified radical mastectomy	No	No	No	No
3	Right radical mastectomy	Yes	No	No	No
4	Right radical mastectomy	Yes	No	Bil-Salpingo oophorectomy	No
5	Right radical mastectomy	No	No	No	No
6	Left radical mastectomy	No	Yes	No	Yes
7	Left radical mastectomy	No	Yes	Yes	No
8	Right radical mastectomy	Yes	No	No	No
9	Left radical mastectomy	No	Yes	No	No
10	Right radical mastectomy	No	Yes	No	Yes
11	Right radical mastectomy	No	Yes	No	Yes
12	Left radical mastectomy	No	No	No	Yes

From Serafin, D., Georgiade, N. G., and Given, K. S.: Transfer of free flaps to provide well vascularized thick cover for breast reconstruction after radical mastectomy, Plast. Reconstr. Surg. **62**(4): 527-536, October, 1978.

Table 12-2. Factors complicating reconstruction (summary)

Split-thickness graft	4
Radiation	6
Chemotherapy	1
Ligation subscapular vascular pedicle	4
Split-thickness graft and radiation	1
Radiation and ligation of subscapular vascular pedicle	3
TOTAL	19

dermatitis. Telangiectases were common, as were indurated brawney edema, dermal fibrosis, and cutaneous scarring (Fig. 12-4, *B*).

Approximately one third of the patients had mild to moderate edema of the ipsilateral arm. Many patients had limitation in the range of motion of the affected shoulder. This appeared to be more common in the surgery plus radiation group.

Four patients were originally scheduled to undergo breast reconstruction by an island pedicle latissimus dorsi musculocutaneous flap. Axillary exploration revealed a ligated subscapular artery and vein (Fig. 12-5). Reconstruction attempts were abandoned temporarily on the ipsilateral side. All four patients had preoperative mammographic findings consistent with proliferative fibrocystic

Table 12-3. Comparison of gross and microscopic pathology

Case	Microscopic pathology	Size of primary lesion (cm)	Positive axillary nodes	Distant metastases	Local recurrence
1	Poorly differentiated adenocarcinoma	2	0 of 14	0	None
2	Bilateral invasive lobular carcinoma	1-1.5 (left)	0 of 14	0	None
3	Papillary carcinoma	?	0 of 15	0	None
4	Poorly differentiated adenocarcinoma (predominantly intraductal)	2-3?	0	0	None
5	Intraductal carcinoma	2-3	0 of 14	0	None
6	Infiltrating ductal carcinoma	1-2	1 of 12	0	None
7	Poorly differentiated adenocarcinoma (predominantly intraductal)	1-2	0	0	Incisional, 1 cm
8	Moderately well differentiated adenocarcinoma	2-3	0	0	None
9	Poorly differentiated adenocarcinoma	1-2	4 of 9	0	None
10	Poorly differentiated adenocarcinoma	4.0	5 of 31	0	None
11	Moderately well-differentiated carcinoma	2-3	0 of 17	0	None
12	Well-differentiated adenocarcinoma	2-3	0 of 19	0	None

Adapted from Serafin, D., and Given, K. S.: Reconstruction of the thorax and breast following radical mastectomy. In Serafin, D., and Buncke, H. J., Jr., editors: Microsurgical composite tissue transplantation, St. Louis, 1978, The C. V. Mosby Co.

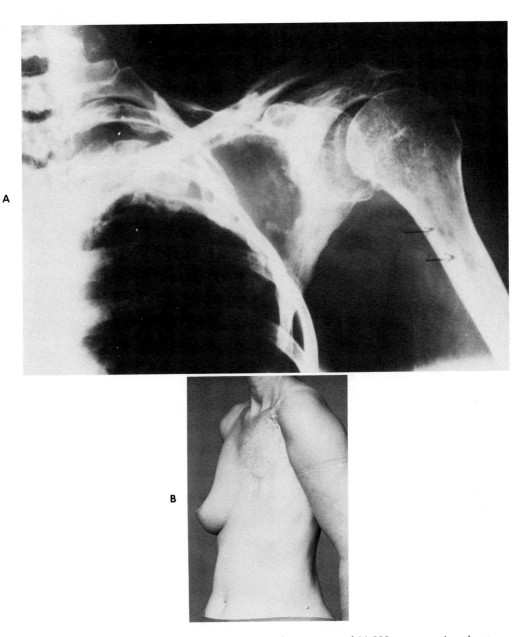

Fig. 12-4. A, Radiograph of patient who received an excess of 14,000 r to anterior chest axilla and left supraclavicular region following left radical mastectomy. Note fractured ribs and radiation osteitis *(arrows).* **B,** Preoperative photograph of same patient demonstrating edema in left upper extremity and cutaneous changes of radiation dermatitis.

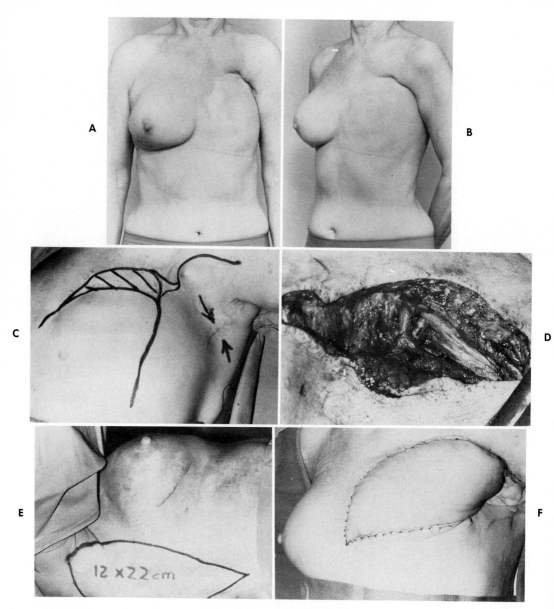

Fig. 12-5. A and **B,** Preoperative photograph demonstrating patient with left radical mastectomy. Split-thickness skin graft and postoperative radiation. **C,** Intraoperative photograph demonstrating unstable scar and skin graft *(stippled area).* Note previous lateral incision *(arrows)* at site of unsuccessful subscapular vascular pedicle exploration. **D,** Intraoperative photograph demonstrating axillary artery and vein. Note subscapular artery and ligature approximately 2 cm distal from origin *(arrow).* **E,** Intraoperative photograph demonstrating outline of vascularized latissimus dorsi musculocutaneous flap from contralateral side. **F,** Early postoperative photograph demonstrating vascularized latissimus dorsi musculocutaneous flap in place. (**A, C,** and **E** from Serafin, D., Georgiade, N. G., and Given, K. S.: Transfer of free flaps to provide well vascularized, thick cover for breast reconstructions after radical mastectomy, Plast. Reconstr. Surg. **62**(4):527-536, October 1978.)

disease. A contralateral subcutaneous mastectomy and immediate insertion of a silicone gel prosthesis was done at this time.[3] These patients all underwent reconstruction with vascularized composite tissue at a second operative procedure (Tables 12-1 and 12-2).

RECONSTRUCTION (FIRST-STAGE) MICROVASCULAR FLAP TECHNIQUE

In all of the patients in the present series, vascularized composite tissue was employed to replace deficient or radiation-damaged tissue. This was accomplished during a single operative procedure with an average duration of 6 hours.

Vascularized groin flap

The vascularized groin flap was used in ten patients (Table 12-4). Using this technique, large segments of well-vascularized tissue, measuring 11 × 27 cm, were available for reconstruction[9] (Fig. 12-6). The suitability of the donor vasculature was first ascertained by direct visualization through a small medial exploratory incision (Table 12-4). If the vasculature was deemed inadequate for transfer, the incision was closed and the opposite groin was explored. Five patients underwent bilateral groin explorations (Fig. 12-6, *F*). A successful groin flap transfer was carried out in two patients. In one, the reconstruction attempt was abandoned. In two additional patients a contralateral latissimus dorsi musculocutaneous flap was successfully transferred.

Once the donor vasculature appears to be suitable for transfer by direct visualization, dissection is begun laterally, joining the medial incision. At the completion of the donor dissection, (45 minutes to 1 hour), flap viability is ensured by careful observation of the composite tissue. Perfusion is totally restricted to the island vasculature, usually the superficial circumflex iliac artery and a single drainage vein (Fig. 12-6, *E*).

Dissection of the axilla is concurrently carried out by the primary operating team (Fig. 12-7). In those patients who received postoperative radiation, dissection is often complicated and may be extremely difficult. Usually a vena comitans of the axillary vein can be identified, however, with a diameter similar to the donor drainage vein, and an end-to-end anastomosis can then be performed (Table 12-4).

Interpositional vein grafts

One patient in the present series had extensive radiation fibrosis involving the axillary artery and vein. Dissection was prolonged and tedious. It was necessary to employ two interpositional vein grafts to bypass the irradiated tissue. One was anastomosed more proximally to a suitable vein in an end-to-end fashion. The other was reversed and then anastomosed end-to-side to the axillary artery (Table 12-3). The problem of finding a suitable branch of the axillary artery with satisfactory flow is circumvented by the use of a reversed segment of an interpositional vein graft anastomosed end-to-side to the axillary artery[6] (Fig. 12-8).

Table 12-4. Composite tissue employed in reconstruction

Case	Composite tissue	Donor vessels	Recipient vessels	Arterial interpositional vein graft	Venous interpositional vein graft
1	Vascularized groin	SCIA* and V	AA† AVC‡	Yes	No
2	Vascularized groin	SCIA and V	AA AVC	Yes	No
3	Vascularized groin	SCIA and V	AA AVC	Yes	No
4	Vascularized groin	SCIA and V	AA AVC	Yes	No
5	Vascularized groin	SCIA and V	AA AVC	Yes	No
6	Vascularized groin	SCIA and V	(Proximal) SA§ AVC	Yes	No
7	Vascularized groin	SCIA and V	AA AVC	Yes	No
8	Vascularized groin	SCIA and V	AA AVC	Yes	No
9	Vascularized groin	SCIA and V	AA AVC	Yes	Yes
10	Vascularized latissimus dorsi musculocutaneous	SA SV	(Proximal) SA AVC	No	No
11	Vascularized groin	SCIA and V	(Proximal) SA AVC	Yes	No
12	Vascularized latissimus dorsi musculocutaneous	SA SV	(Proximal) SA and SV	No	No

Adapted from Serafin, D., Georgiade, N. G., and Given, K. S.: Transfer of free flaps to provide well vascularized thick cover for breast reconstruction after radical mastectomy, Plast. Reconstr. Surg. **62**(4):527-536, October, 1978.
*SCIA, superficial circumflex iliac artery or vein.
†AA, axillary artery.
‡AVC, axillary vena comitans.
§SA, subscapular artery or vein.

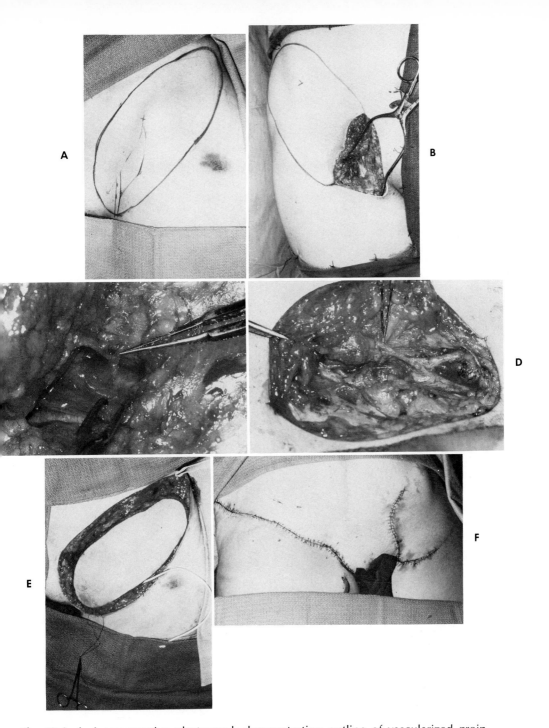

Fig. 12-6. A, Intraoperative photograph demonstrating outline of vascularized groin flap. **B,** Intraoperative photograph demonstrating medial exploratory incision to assess quality of donor vasculature. **C,** Intraoperative photograph demonstrating donor superficial circumflex iliac artery *(instrument)* as seen through medial exploratory incision. **D,** Intraoperative photograph demonstrating drainage vein of vascularized groin flap *(instrument on left)* as visualized through medial exploratory incision. **E,** Vascularized groin flap isolated on island vascular pedicle. **F,** Bilateral groin exploration with vascularized groin flap taken from right inguinal region. Note left medial exploratory incision, which revealed vasculature unsuitable for transfer. (**A** and **E** from Serafin, D., Georgiade, N. G., and Given, K. S.: Transfer of free flaps to provide well vascularized, thick cover for breast reconstructions after radical mastectomy, Plast. Reconstr. Surg. **62**(4):527-536, October 1978.)

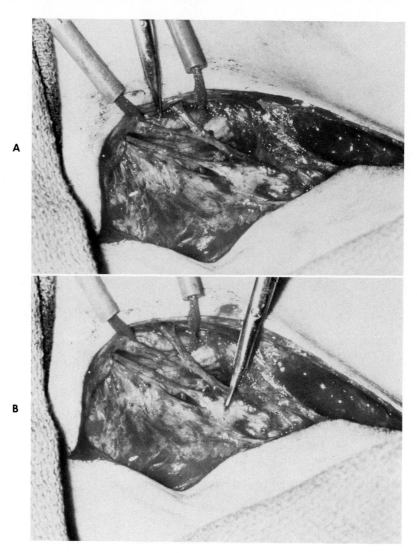

Fig. 12-7. A, Intraoperative photograph demonstrating axillary artery *(instrument).* End-to-side anastomosis will be performed at this location with a reversed segment of an interpositional vein graft. **B,** Intraoperative photograph demonstrating axillary vena comitans to be employed later in end-to-end anastomosis to drainage vein of donor flap. (From Serafin, D., Georgiade, N. G., and Given, K. S.: Transfer of free flaps to provide well vascularized, thick cover for breast reconstructions after radical mastectomy, Plast. Reconstr. Surg. **62**(4):527-536, October 1978.)

If a ligated subscapular artery is identified it can often be transected proximal to the ligature and then anastomosed end-to-end to the reversed interpositional vein graft. Anastomosis to the subscapular arterial stump can usually be accomplished more rapidly than direct end-to-side anastomosis to the axillary artery (Table 12-3).

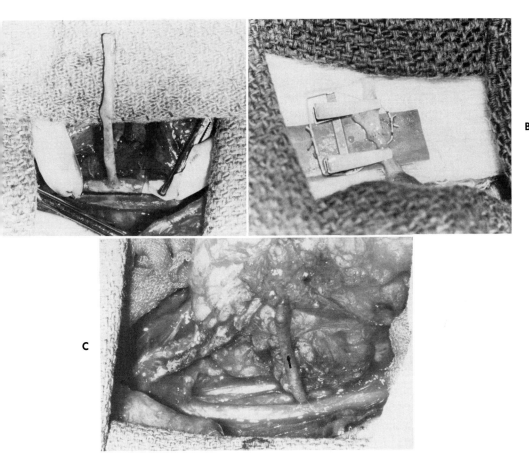

Fig. 12-8. A, Reversed segment of interpositional vein graft with end-to-side anastomosis to donor axillary artery. **B,** End-to-end anastomosis between interpositional vein graft and donor flap artery. **C,** Intraoperative photograph demonstrating interpositional vein graft on right *(arrow)* and end-to-end venous anastomosis on left. (**A** from Serafin, D., Georgiade, N. G., and Smith, D. H.: Comparison of free flaps with pedicled flaps for coverage of defects of the leg or foot, Plast. Reconstr. Surg. **59**(4):492-499, April 1977; **B** from Serafin, D., and Given, K. S.: Reconstruction of the thorax and breast following radical mastectomy. In Serafin, D., and Buncke, H. J., Jr., editors: Microsurgical composite tissue transplantation, St. Louis, 1979, The C. V. Mosby Co.)

The vein graft is frequently selected from the dorsum of the foot or from the distal saphenous system. Lower extremity veins frequently have thick walls with a well-developed media, probably related to higher intraluminal pressures. Suitable veins should be selected and marked preoperatively with the extremity in a dependent position. The extremity should be prepped in the surgical field with a tourniquet available to facilitate rapid, bloodless dissection. Proximal and distal orientation should be maintained with marking solution. Obviously the segment of vein should be reversed when employed as an arterial interpositional graft (Table 12-4). The well-developed media noted in lower extremity grafts also appears better able to withstand arterial pressure for a protracted period of time. Great care should be exercised in graft selection in order to obtain one with a suitable external diameter. During dissection severe vasospasm occurs, obscuring the true diameter. Thus a decision in selection should be made prior to dissection. The distal venous tree is often of smaller diameter, especially when branching occurs. In a reversed segment, the end with the small external diameter (distal) is employed in the end-to-side arterial anastomosis. There should not be an external size discrepancy between the larger (proximal) vein graft and the donor flap artery for a successful end-to-end anastomosis. If the diameter of the vein graft exceeds by one third the diameter of the donor artery, turbulent flow is likely, with later thrombosis.[1]

An interpositional vein graft can be used successfully to provide additional length to existing flap veins or to connect several donor veins to a single recipient vein (Table 12-4). Lower pressure in the venous effluent does not adversely affect anastomotic patency. Following retrieval the lumen of the vein is carefully perfused with a buffered heparinized solution, inspected for leaks, and then kept moist in a similar solution. Atraumatic dissection is essential to minimize endothelial sloughing.

In summary the interpositional vein graft offers many advantages to the reconstructive surgeon: (1) a damaged segment of recipient vasculature can be easily bypassed; (2) mobility of flap placement is enhanced; (3) discrepancies in donor and recipient vascular diameter can be accommodated; (4) the search for recipient vascular branches of suitable external diameter for anastomosis is obviated by an end-to-side anastomosis; and (5) patency is enhanced because exposure is facilitated.

It is apparent that for these reasons the vein graft is frequently indicated in breast reconstruction, especially when postoperative radiation is employed as adjunctive therapy following a radical mastectomy.

Vascularized latissimus dorsi musculocutaneous flap

A contralateral latissimus dorsi musculocutaneous flap was employed for breast reconstruction in two patients (Table 12-4). Large segments of composite tissue can be obtained measuring 10 × 20 cm. The cutaneous portion of the flap is outlined preoperatively and is centralized on the anterior border of the muscle. Skin mobility is measured and proper width is selected to facilitate primary closure of the donor site.

Dissection is begun anteriorly between the border of the latissimus dorsi muscle and the underlying serratus anterior muscle. The neurovascular pedicle is readily identified by a nerve stimulator and is isolated. The thoracodorsal artery and vein are then carefully dissected proximally, ligating communications between the lateral thoracic system. Similarly the circumflex scapular artery and

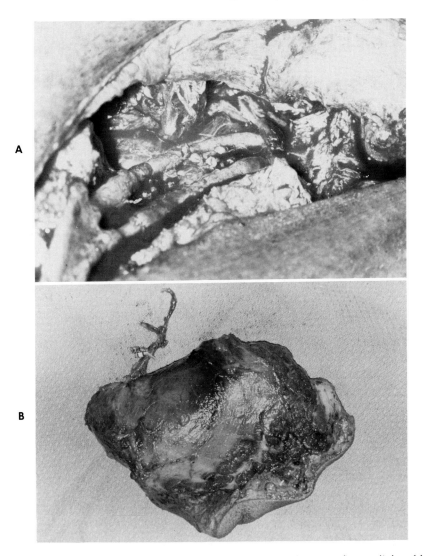

Fig. 12-9. A, Intraoperative dissection demonstrating lengthy vascular pedicle of latissimus dorsi musculocutaneous flap. **B,** Latissimus dorsi musculocutaneous flap with lengthy vascular pedicle (cutaneous portion posterior). (**B** from Serafin, D., and Given, K. S.: Reconstruction of the thorax and breast following radical mastectomy. In Serafin, D., and Buncke, H. J., Jr., editors: Microsurgical composite tissue transplantation, St. Louis, 1979, The C. V. Mosby Co.

vein are dissected to the axillary artery and vein. The external diameter at this location is 3 to 4 mm and is most suitable for anastomosis to the contralateral axillary artery and vena comitans (Fig. 12-9). The vascular pedicle obtained (13 to 15 cm) is quite lengthy and obviates the need for an interpositional vein graft. In breast reconstruction the nerve to the latissimus dorsi muscle is sacrificed. A neural anastomosis, however, may be performed at the recipient site if motor function is required during reconstruction (that is, restoration of flexion to the upper extremity).

The latissimus dorsi musculocutaneous flap is quite suitable for breast reconstruction. It is a bulky flap, however, and recipient site closure, especially in the lower extremity, may require a split-thickness graft.

RECONSTRUCTION (SECOND-STAGE) BREAST MOUND SYMMETRY

After healthy, well-vascularized tissue is transplanted to the deficient recipient area in the first stage, 2 to 3 months are permitted to lapse before the second stage is initiated. Breast mound symmetry is achieved during this procedure (Fig. 12-10).

In the present series the average delay from mastectomy to reconstruction was 6 years (Table 12-5). All of these patients underwent a thorough and complete evaluation prior to reconstruction for recurrent or metastatic disease. A mammogram of the contralateral breast was always obtained as well as a radioactive bone scan. In those patients with fibrocystic disease special attention was given to a mammogram interpretation of P2 and D-Y configuration in Wolfe's classification.[11]

Most of the patients in the present series were over 40 years of age, many with varying degrees of breast atrophy and ptosis.

In order to achieve breast mound symmetry, a subcutaneous mastectomy, often with correction of ptosis, was frequently carried out on the contralateral breast[3] (Fig. 12-11) (Table 12-5). Careful attention was also directed to correction of the infraclavicular depression of the ipsilateral defect and restoration of the anterior axillary fold.

The superior-medial aspect of the previously inserted vascularized flap was deepithelialized and rotated beneath the thin infraclavicular skin.

During the initial procedure of vascularized flap placement, lateral positioning of the tissue along a longitudinal axis accentuated the anterior axillary fold. Following superior-medial rotation during the second stage, this fold achieved a more aesthetic contour, especially following placement of a silicone implant. This result was achieved even though the pectoralis major muscle was no longer present.

Final symmetry is achieved with a silicone double-lumen gel-saline prosthesis placed bilaterally. Size differences are adjusted by altering the volume of saline in each prosthesis.

RECONSTRUCTION (THIRD-STAGE) NIPPLE-AREOLAR RECONSTRUCTION

During the third and final stage, usually 2 to 3 months later, the nipple-areolar complex is reconstructed (Figs. 12-1 and 12-11). Every attempt is made to obtain a suitable color match with the contralateral side. A full-thickness graft is taken from the superior medial thigh, the postauricular region, or the labia if the opposite areola is deeply pigmented. Nipple projection can be obtained by a free

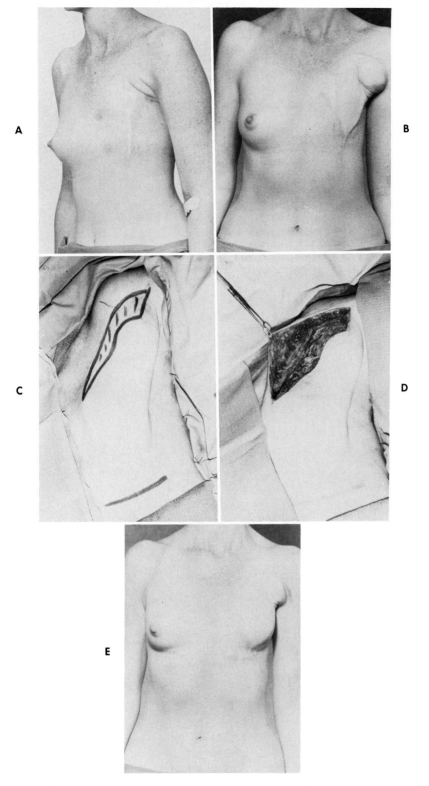

Fig. 12-10. A, Preoperative photograph of patient with left radical mastectomy and post-operative radiation. Note telangiectasis and brawny edema. **B,** Postoperative photograph following first stage of reconstruction with vascularized groin flap. **C** and **D,** Intra-operative photograph demonstrating area to be de-epithelialized to augment infra-clavicular depression. **E,** Postoperative photograph following completion of second stage of breast reconstruction.

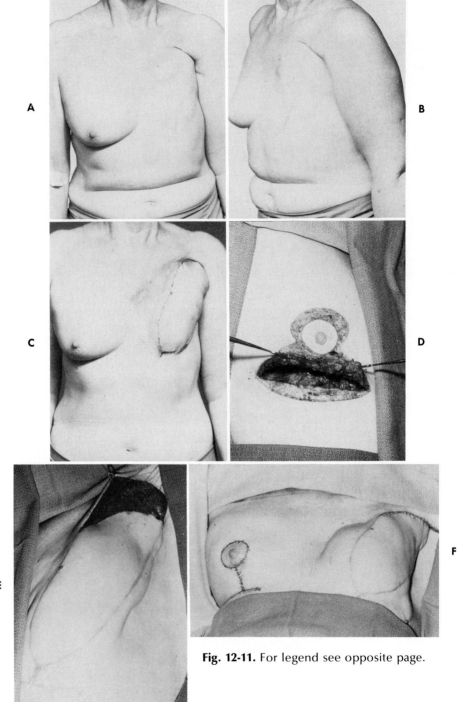

Fig. 12-11. For legend see opposite page.

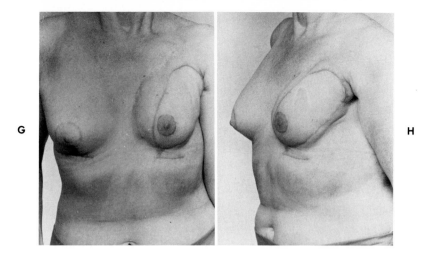

G   H

Fig. 12-11. A and **B,** Preoperative photograph of patient with left radical mastectomy. **C,** Postoperative photograph following completion of first stage of left breast reconstruction with vascularized groin flap. **D,** Intraoperative photograph demonstrating subcutaneous mastectomy of right breast with correction of ptosis and immediate insertion of Silastic implant. **E,** Intraoperative photograph demonstrating deepithelialization of superior aspect of flap to augment infraclavicular depression. **F,** Intraoperative photograph demonstrating completion of second stage of breast reconstruction. **G** and **H,** Postoperative result. (From Serafin, D., and Given, K. S.: Reconstruction of the thorax and breast following radical mastectomy. In Serafin, D., and Buncke, H. J., Jr., editors: Microsurgical composite tissue transplantation, St. Louis, 1979, The C. V. Mosby Co.)

Table 12-5. Reconstruction of contralateral breast

Case	Stage II	Time interval from stages I to II (approximate)	Stage III	Time interval from stages II to III (months) (approximate)
1	Augmentation mammoplasty	3 months	FTG* labial graft	3
2	Augmentation mammoplasty	1 week	FTG labial graft	6
3	Subcutaneous mastectomy	6 weeks prior to stage I	FTG medial thigh	6
4	Subcutaneous mastectomy, correction of ptosis	3 months	FTG medial thigh	3
5	Subcutaneous mastectomy, correction of ptosis	3 months	FTG medial thigh	3
6	Subcutaneous mastectomy, correction of ptosis	3 months	FTG medial thigh	3
7	Subcutaneous mastectomy, correction of ptosis	3 months	FTG medial thigh	3
8	Subcutaneous mastectomy, correction of ptosis	3 months	FTG medial thigh	3
9	None		None	
10	Subcutaneous mastectomy	6 weeks prior to stage I	FTG medial thigh	6
11	Subcutaneous mastectomy	6 weeks prior to stage I	Awaiting stage III	
12	Subcutaneous mastectomy	6 weeks prior to stage I	Awaiting stage III	

*FTG, Full-thickness graft.

graft from the contralateral nipple. If a nipple was previously "banked" during the initial mastectomy, it can now be conveniently transposed to its former location. Discrepancies in size and position related to capsular contracture and tissue shifting can best be appreciated at this time and the new nipple-areolar site positioned correctly.

Thus total breast reconstruction, consisting of three stages, separated by 2 to 3 months, can be completed within 1 year.

DISCUSSION

Microsurgical composite tissue transplantation offers a satisfactory solution for breast reconstruction in those patients with an excessive deficiency of well-vascularized skin. This technique is especially useful in irradiated tissue in which deficient cutaneous and osseous blood supply can be augmented by vascularized tissue. Existing methods of reconstruction employing flaps with a random blood supply are less likely to be successful.

This method is offered as an alternative surgical solution when other procedures cannot be employed. The procedure may be a lengthy one, the average duration lasting approximately 6 hours. A two-team surgical approach is also required, with all surgeons being skilled in microsurgical technique. In addition an operative microscope as well as microsurgical instruments are required. If vascular insufficiency to the transferred tissue occurs, exploration should be undertaken before necrosis supervenes. Dissection of the recipient vasculature may be difficult especially if the patient received postoperative radiation. The only failure in this series occurred with a patient who had an extensively irradiated recipient site. Axillary dissection was made difficult by severe fibrosis. Isolation of a suitable recipient vein was difficult. In retrospect an immediate interpositional vein graft should have been done early in the procedure, rather than a prolonged search for an axillary vena comitans with a diameter equal to that of the drainage vein of the flap. An end-to-side anastomosis to this larger proximal vein could have been done more rapidly and safely.

The amount of tissue transferred with this new technique may be considerable. The vascularized groin flap provides the greatest amount of tissue, 11 × 27 cm; the latissimus dorsi musculocutaneous flap, 10 × 20 cm, provides somewhat less if the donor site is to be closed primarily. This permits the subsequent dissection of a large subcutaneous pocket and the insertion of a suitable silicone implant. A tight skin envelope with restrictive band scars is not seen when vascularized composite tissue of this magnitude is transferred.

In addition, as previously outlined, the anterior axillary fold is easily recreated and the infraclavicular depression augmented by deepithelization and rotation of the large flap.

Four patients in the present series underwent an unsuccessful exploration of the subscapular vascular pedicle for contemplated breast reconstruction with an island latissimus dorsi musculocutaneous flap (Fig. 12-5). The vascular pedicle was apparently ligated during the original radical mastectomy. An ipsilateral

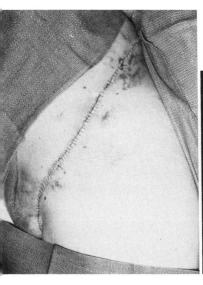
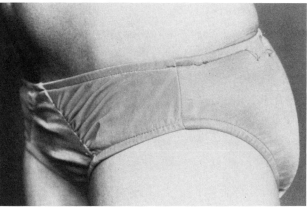

B

Fig. 12-12. A, Intraoperative photograph demonstrating minimal donor defect resulting from vascularized groin flap transfer. **B,** Incision concealed by bikini bathing suit. (**A** from Serafin, D., and Given, K. S.: Reconstruction of the thorax and breast following radical mastectomy. In Serafin, D., and Buncke, H. J., Jr., editors: Microsurgical composite tissue transplantation, St. Louis, 1979, The C. V. Mosby Co.; **B** from Serafin, D., Georgiade, N. G., and Given, K. S.: Transfer of free flaps to provide well vascularized, thick cover for breast reconstructions after radical mastectomy, Plast. Reconstr. Surg. **62**(4):527-536, October 1978.)

island musculocutaneous flap was believed to be contraindicated in this group of patients. Two patients eventually underwent breast reconstruction with a vascularized latissimus dorsi musculocutaneous flap from the contralateral side. Recent experience indicates that even though an island flap cannot be transferred following subscapular pedicle ligation, sufficient cutaneous tissue can be transposed by leaving the musculocutaneous pedicle intact.

Although more difficult to dissect than the latissimus dorsi musculocutaneous flap, the donor deformity of the groin flap is minimal. The incision can be carefully concealed even by a brief bikini (Fig. 12-12). No thoracic or abdominal scars are evident. The donor deformity of the latissimus dorsi musculocutaneous flap is more obvious, but this definitely improves with time. The depression that results from the excised muscle becomes less conspicuous as the remaining muscle atrophies.

Not only is the groin flap more difficult to dissect, but vascular anomalies are encountered more frequently.[2,10] This requires more experience for successful tissue transfer. The use of the interpositional vein graft has permitted the use of the axillary artery and vein as suitable recipient vasculature. This lengthens the operative procedure, however, in comparison to the lengthy vascular pedicle afforded by the latissimus dorsi musculocutaneous flap.

In contrast to many existing methods of breast reconstruction, the first stage is completed in a single operative procedure during a short hospital admission. This shortens the total time of reconstruction.

SUMMARY

A new method of breast reconstruction following radical mastectomy is presented. Eleven cases (92%) were totally successful without any flap morbidity or loss. One vascularized groin flap failed and reconstruction was abandoned. Patients who demonstrate a marked deficiency of healthy, well-vascularized skin following radical mastectomy are suitable candidates for this new operative procedure. When the vascularized groin flap is employed, the donor defect is minimal.

REFERENCES

1. Büchler, U., and Buncke, H. J., Jr.: Experimental microvascular autografts. In Serafin, D., and Buncke, H. J., Jr., editors: Microsurgical composite tissue transplantation, St. Louis, 1978, The C. V. Mosby Co.
2. Harii, K., and Ohmori, K.: Free skin flap transfer, Clin. Plast. Surg. **31:**111, 1976.
3. McCarty, K. S., Jr., Kesterson, G. H., and Georgiade, N. G.: Clinical significance of histopathologic lesions observed in the contralateral breast in patients with breast carcinoma. In Georgiade, N. G.: Breast reconstruction following mastectomy, St. Louis, 1979, The C. V. Mosby Co.
4. Schnotten, D.: Epidemiology of breast cancer, Clin. Bull. **5:**135-143, 1975.
5. Seidran, H. L.: Statistical and epidemiological data on cancer of the breast, New York, 1972, American Cancer Society.
6. Serafin, D., and Georgiade, N. G.: Microsurgical composite tissue transplantation: a new method of immediate reconstruction of extensive defects, Am. J. Surg. **133:**752, 1977.
7. Serafin, D., and Given, K. S.: Reconstruction of the thorax and breast following radical mastectomy. In Serafin, D., and Buncke, H. J., Jr., editors: Microsurgical composite tissue transplantation, St. Louis, 1978, The C. V. Mosby Co., pp. 541-572.
8. Serafin, D., Georgiade, N. G., and Given, K. S.: Transfer of free flaps to provide well vascularized thick cover for breast reconstruction after radical mastectomy, Plast. Reconstr. Surg. **62:**541, 1978.
9. Serafin, D., Georgiade, N. G., and Smith, D. H.: Comparison of free flaps with pedicle flaps for coverage of defects of the leg or foot, Plast. Reconstr. Surg. **59:**492, 1977.
10. Taylor, G. I., and Daniel, R. K.: The anatomy of several free flap donor sites, Plast. Reconstr. Surg. **56:**243, 1975.
11. Wolfe, J. N.: Breast patterns as an index of risk for developing breast cancer, Am. J. Roentgenol. Radium Ther. Nucl. Med. **126:**1130, 1976.

CHAPTER 13

Management of the nipple-areolar complex in reconstruction

Nicholas G. Georgiade

For a variety of reasons, some patients are satisfied with the reconstruction of just the breast mound, which enables them to have freedom of movement without fear of dislodging an external prosthesis. In addition they can once again comfortably wear bathing suits and form-fitting clothing. However, many patients will not accept an incomplete breast and request the additional reconstruction of the nipple-areolar complex.

Each patient presents a unique challenge for the plastic surgeon, who must determine a technique, or combination of techniques, that best creates a nipple-areolar complex. The reconstruction of the nipple and areola should be the last step of the breast reconstruction after a mastectomy. The exact time interval between this step and the breast mound reconstruction varies considerably because one must wait until the best possible result has been obtained by the initial reconstructive procedures. The surgeon must be aware that frequently it is necessary to make adjustments in the size, configuration, or position of the prosthesis and that capsular contractures must be released several times before the final desired breast form is attained. If the nipple-areolar reconstruction is carried out prior to the expected shifting or settling of the prosthesis, the displacement will result in loss of the optimum position of the nipple-areolar complex on the breast mound, as has been shown in Chapter 10.

NIPPLE-AREOLAR POSITION IN RECONSTRUCTION

The best location for the areola, as determined while the patient is in an upright position, is a compromise between its relationship with the nipple-areolar complex on the normal breast and its relationship to the breast mound. When the two breasts are fairly symmetric, direct measurements from the sternal notch and xyphoid process define the exact location for the new areola. However, in most cases there will be slight discrepancies in the size, configuration, and position of the breast; accordingly the placement of the new areola depends more on the aesthetic sense of the surgeon than on direct measurements.

The diameter of the opposite areola is measured. A suitable metal ring slightly

239

smaller than the opposite areola is selected and the circumference of the new areola is outlined with a permanent ink-type pen or brilliant green dye. The recipient site is then prepared by removal of a split-thickness layer of skin (leaving a satisfactory dermal bed) from within the outlined circle.

The following various types of nipple-areolar grafts can be utilized.

Stored nipple-areolar graft

The most satisfactory method of nipple-areolar reconstruction is utilization of the nipple-areolar graft, which was transferred to the groin, or elsewhere, during the ablative surgery.[11] With certain types of malignancies in the absence of lymphatic invasion, it seems reasonable to transfer the nipple-areolar complex to the groin despite the remote possibility of tumor cell transfer to the groin. Adherence to strict criteria would have avoided this unfortunate sequela in the few reported occurrences.[2,3] Close proximity of the primary carcinoma to the nipple-areolar area precludes the transfer of the nipple-areola as a free graft.

At the time of ablative surgery, frozen sections of the breast tissue at the base of the nipple-areolar complex must be meticulously examined by the pathologist prior to transfer of the nipple-areolar graft to the groin. If, in the judgment of the pathologist, the base of the nipple-areolar complex is free of carcinoma and the carcinoma is less than 2 cm in diameter and is a safe distance of at least 4 cm from the nipple and areola, then it seems reasonable to bank the nipple-areolar complex in the groin just lateral to the pubic area. It may be more acceptable in some instances to remove only the areola, leaving the nipple attached to the specimen.

The banked nipple-areolar graft is transferred from the groin to the recipient site on the reconstructed breast mound approximately 6 months after the ablative surgery, provided a suitably sized prosthesis has been inserted previously. A capsulotomy is invariably necessary at this time. The nipple-areolar graft is secured in place with multiple 5-0 silk sutures around the periphery of the graft and several 3-0 plain catgut sutures through the center and the underlying dermal bed. A layer of nitrofurazone (Furacin) or povidone-iodine (Betadine) gauze is applied over the graft followed by slightly moistened mechanic's waste gauze. The 5-0 silk sutures are tied over a bolus in order to immobilize the graft. The stent dressing is maintained for 1 week and then removed along with all sutures except for the catgut. A light Telfa dressing is worn for 2 to 3 weeks to protect the graft, and the patient is fitted with a suitable brassiere that is worn constantly for 2 to 3 weeks except for bathing purposes.

It should be noted that an undesirable depigmentation of the areola may occur. In these instances light tatooing of the depigmented area will yield the desirable result. Occasionally insufficient nipple substance is present following transfer of the nipple-area graft. Quite often a portion of the patient's opposite nipple may be used in a nipple-sharing procedure (Fig. 13-1).

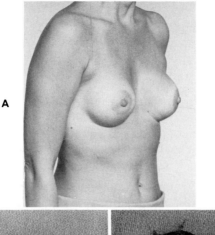

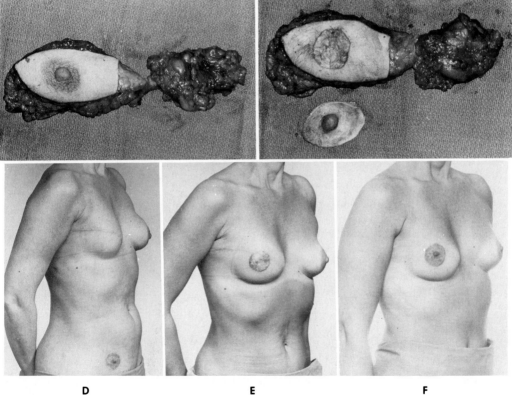

Fig. 13-1. A, Preoperative lateral view of 40-year-old patient who had had a previous augmentation mammaplasty and was found to have an early intraductal carcinoma in the upper outer quadrant of the breast. **B,** Segment of breast tissue removed with nipple-areola. **C,** Nipple-areola is removed as a split-thickness skin graft, and dermal-subdermal breast specimen is sent to pathology for histologic evaluation. **D,** Five-month lateral postoperative view of same patient illustrating initial reconstruction of breast mound and nipple-areolar graft implanted in groin area. **E,** Postoperative lateral view of same patient 2 months after a capsulotomy had been performed, initial prosthesis was replaced with an 85-ml/165-ml gel-filled Georgiade ''piggyback'' Surgitek prosthesis, and nipple-areola was transferred from inguinal area to right breast mound. Depigmentation of areola and loss of nipple tissue are noted. **F,** Postoperative lateral view of same patient 1 year after areola has been tattooed to match pigmentation of areola to that of opposite breast and nipple graft from opposite breast has been utilized to restore nipple tissue.

If a stored nipple-areolar graft is not available, the following alternatives are available.

Split-thickness areolar grafts

In 1950 Kiskadden[8] reported the necessity of using split-thickness skin grafts from the chest area including the nipple and areola to resurface areas of a severely burned patient. Since the nipple-areolar graft was visible on the grafted arm, it was suggested that this technique could be applicable to areolar reconstruction.

Klein,[9] in 1952 used a split-thickness areolar graft 0.010 inch thick that was removed with a dermatome to reconstruct the missing nipple and areola in a male patient.

Millard[10] in 1972 further modified this method by removing an areolar graft as a medium split-thickness graft with either a #10 BP blade or a Reese dermatome shimmed at 0.012 inch. The upper 3 to 5 mm of the nipple is then amputated with a scalpel. This provides two grafts, which as Millard suggested resemble "a doughnut (areola) and a plug for the hole (nipple)." However, the surgeon must be careful to remove only a thin split-thickness graft from the areola to avoid the possibility of depigmentation of the donor areola, particularly if the areola is a light shade. If cut too thin, the areolar graft will not contain sufficient pigmentation. By varying the thickness of the areolar graft, a good color match can usually be obtained. A variant of this scheme is a split-thickness graft from the lower half of the areola transferred to the superior half of the new site, after which the lower half of the new areola can be tattooed.

Areolar sharing from opposite breast

If the areola of the opposite breast is sufficiently large, it may serve as donor tissue to form a new areola. Since the patient with the large areola will usually have some degree of breast hypertrophy and ptosis necessitating correction in order to obtain breast symmetry, the outer portion of this large areola is removed as a thick split-thickness skin graft the width necessary to result in two areolae roughly equal in size may be calculated.[14] On the reconstructed breast mound, a split-thickness graft is removed from the marked recipient site for the new areola. The areolar graft from the opposite breast is rotated in concentric circles and sutured into position with multiple 5-0 Vicryl interrupted sutures. At this time consideration for reconstructing a nipple is also made (see p. 249). A number of long 5-0 silk sutures are placed around the periphery after a suitable nipple, obtained from either the opposite nipple or the labia majora–labia minora area has been sutured in place with 3-0 plain catgut sutures. A stent dressing is constructed and secured with the 5-0 silk sutures. The dressing and silk sutures are removed 1 week later (Fig. 13-2, *A*). Areas of depigmentation may occur in the areas of approximation of the concentric areolar grafts. Tattooing of these depigmented areas will make the newly constructed area aesthetically satisfactory (Fig. 13-3).

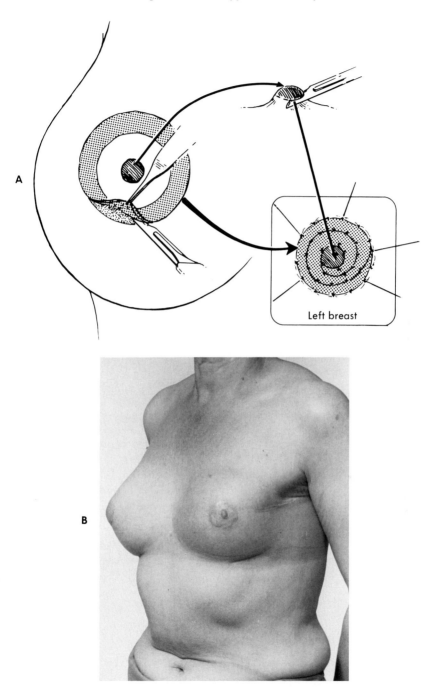

Fig. 13-2. A, Split-thickness graft from outer perimeter of opposite areola is sutured in a spiral fashion to deepithelialized area of reconstructed breast mound. Portion of opposite nipple is utilized to reconstruct nipple. **B,** Six-month postoperative view of nipple-areolar complex that was reconstructed utilizing a split graft of a portion of the areola from the opposite breast. Areolar split graft was sutured in place in a spiral fashion on the deepithelialized area of reconstructed breast mound. Nipple was reconstructed by utilizing half of nipple from opposite breast (as shown in **A**).

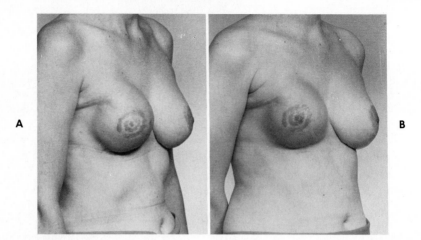

Fig. 13-3. A, Areola has been reconstructed utilizing split-thickness graft from opposite areola and sutured in place in a spiral fashion on deepithelialized area of reconstructed breast mound. Nipple was reconstructed by utilizing half of nipple from opposite breast. Note areas of depigmentation, a characteristic finding along the approximating margins of areolar graft and following the concentric circle. **B,** Same reconstructed nipple-areolar complex after depigmented areas have been tattooed. Additional nipple size was achieved by obtaining a further portion of nipple from opposite nipple.

Full-thickness labial grafts

A full-thickness graft of labia minora was used by Adams[1] in 1949 to reconstruct an areola that had necrosed subsequent to a reduction mammaplasty.

The use of thick split-thickness skin grafts from either the labia minora or labia majora usually produces a satisfactory esthetic result, particularly in bilateral reconstruction, since this skin has the desired roughness and pigmentation. In unilateral reconstruction the color match is not usually as satisfactory because labial grafts either have a darker brown tone than the normal areola or, in some instances, may even be pinker, depending on the location of the donor area (Fig. 13-4).

Buccal mucosal grafts

Since some patients object to the use of labial grafts, other areas have been suggested from which to obtain grafts. Buccal mucosal split-thickness grafts would appear to have the desired texture and pigmentation necessary to reproduce the areola; however, the color match is usually quite poor because of the pinkness of the buccal mucosa. The amount of donor buccal grafts is limited and often precludes the use of this source.

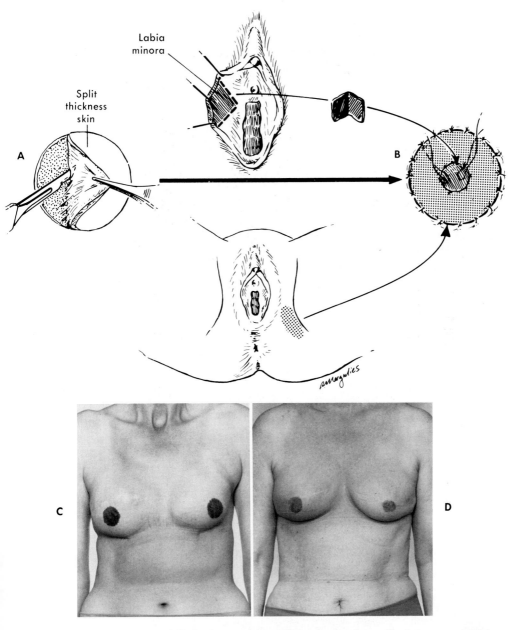

Fig. 13-4. A, Very thick or full-thickness skin graft is obtained usually from para labial area (inner aspect of thigh) after deciding appropriate size and transferred to dermal bed on breast mound. **B,** Nipple is obtained as full-thickness labia minora graft, opened by sharp dissection and sutured in place to construct nipple. Location from which these grafts are taken from the labia minora or majora will vary depending on desired degree of pigmentation. **C,** Bilateral reconstruction of the breast with labial grafts. Note darkness of reconstructed areola. **D,** Bilateral reconstruction of the breast with labial grafts in which the pigmentation is much lighter.

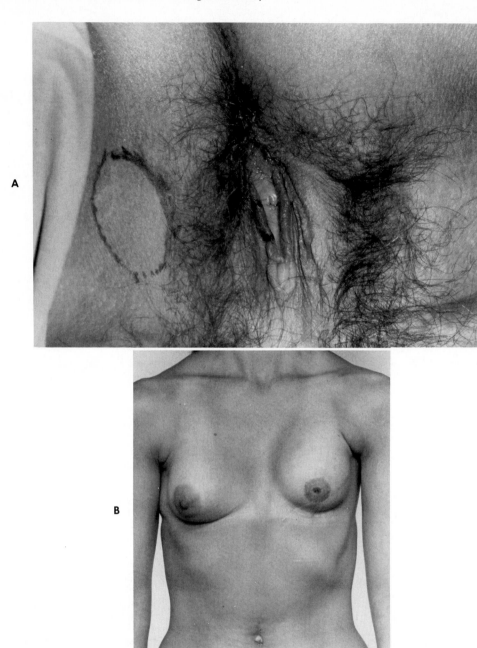

Fig. 13-5. A, Area of inner thigh from which full-thickness skin graft is removed to be used in reconstruction of the areola. This area appears to give best color tones characteristic of normal-appearing areola. **B,** Left areola has been reconstructed utilizing full-thickness graft from inner thigh area. Nipple was reconstructed utilizing split-thickness graft from labia minora. Note good color match with existing nipple-areola.

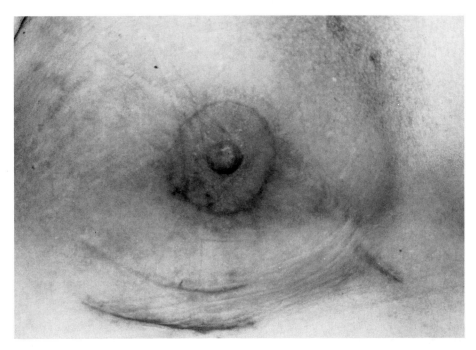

Fig. 13-6. Nipple-areolar complex was reconstructed utilizing full-thickness graft from groin area (see Fig. 13-5, *A*) for areola, and nipple was reconstructed utilizing a portion of opposite nipple.

Full-thickness skin grafts from lower abdomen, groin, and inner thigh area

The skin color of the lower abdomen, groin, and upper thigh area is darker because of a greater degree of melanin pigmentation.[7] Full-thickness skin grafts removed from these areas are suitable for use in the reconstruction of the areola.[5] The upper inner thigh area is hairless, and the scar will be relatively inconspicuous following removal of the graft, which may be either a thick split-thickness or full-thickness skin graft. There is considerable variability regarding the degree of pigmentation in these areas, allowing a wide choice of potential donor sites. The use of thick to full-thickness skin grafts obtained from these areas, which more closely resemble the color tones of the opposite areola, are used as the areas of choice routinely. Grafts obtained lateral to the pubic area will be the most pigmented (Figs. 13-5 and 13-6).

Retroauricular skin

If an areola of a lighter pink tone is required, full-thickness skin grafts obtained from the retroauricular area are quite satisfactory. The grafts must

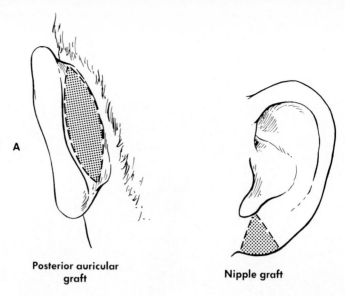

A

Posterior auricular
graft

Nipple graft

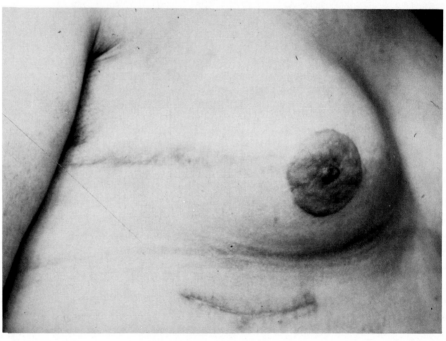

B

Fig. 13-7. A, Diagram of areas from which retroauricular full-thickness skin grafts are removed to reconstruct areola. Grafts must be removed from both ears to obtain sufficient skin to reconstruct suitably sized areola. Nipple may be constructed using composite graft of skin and fat from stippled area of ear lobe. Areolar reconstruction utilizing posterior auricular full-thickness skin grafts will invariably yield a pinker-appearing area. **B,** This nipple was reconstructed in stages utilizing a combination of methods. Areola was originally reconstructed utilizing bilateral posterior auricular grafts. Six months later full-thickness left groin graft was transferred to areola. Nipple was reconstructed using a portion of opposite nipple and a labial graft to complete nipple reconstruction.

be removed from both ears to obtain sufficient size for a suitable areola and still permit primary closure of the donor sites (Fig. 13-7).

Alternative methods of simulating the areola and nipple include tatooing and nipple reconstruction.

TATTOOING

In bilateral reconstruction tattooing the skin can produce a very satisfactory appearing nipple-areolar complex.[13] This is a relatively simple procedure in the hands of an experienced surgeon. Many patients who refuse other methods of nipple-areolar reconstruction will accept tattooing quite readily. Tattooing is also valuable for adding additional pigment to areola-sharing grafts or nipple-areolar grafts transferred from the groin. These grafts have a tendency to develop small areas of depigmentation that may be tattooed with various shades of brown pigment to obtain a homogeneously colored areola (Figs. 13-8 and 13-9).

NIPPLE RECONSTRUCTION

If a suitably sized nipple is present on the opposite breast, approximately half can be excised with a V-type incision that allows the donor nipple to be closed without a deformity. If carefully trimmed to conform to the dermal bed, a graft up to 5 mm in thickness will survive. Ordinarily the areola is re-

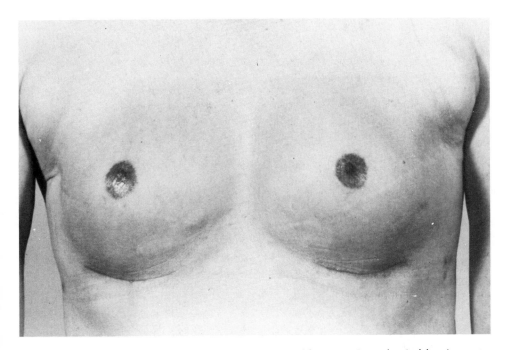

Fig. 13-8. Nipple-areolar complex was reconstructed by tattooing of suitable pigments with darker pigments utilized for nipple area.

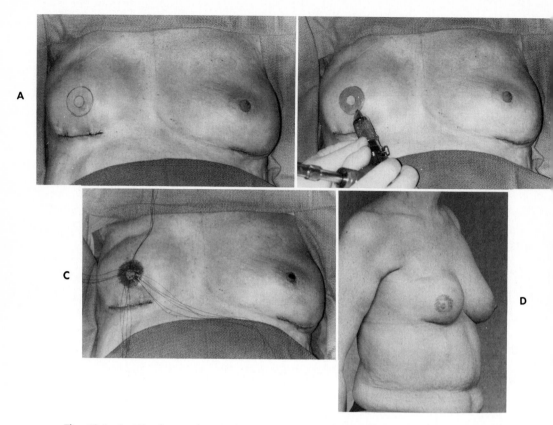

Fig. 13-9. A, Nipple-areolar reconstruction is outlined slightly smaller than opposite areola on reconstructed breast mound. **B,** Areola is tattooed with desired color blended pigment. **C,** Nipple graft is obtained from opposite breast and sutured in center of reconstructed tattooed areola. **D,** Simulated nipple-areolar complex 1 year postoperatively.

constructed simultaneously and the entire nipple-areolar complex is dressed with a tie-over stent. The nipple-sharing technique produces the best aesthetic result[6] (Fig. 13-10).

However, if the normal nipple is inadequate for sharing, several other procedures may be used to produce a nipple prominence.

Labial grafts

The labial majora gives a suitably thick graft that is deeply pigmented and can be used quite readily for construction of the nipple in most patients. The labial graft is attached to a dermal bed utilizing techniques previously described (Figs. 13-4 and 13-11).

Cartilage implantation

The ultimate in nipple-areolar reconstruction, which unfortunately is difficult to obtain since most patients do not wish to undergo the additional surgical

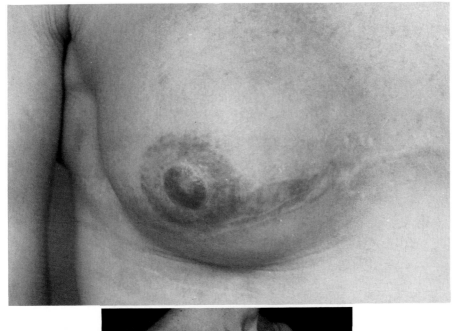

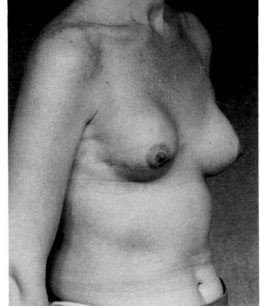

Fig. 13-10. A, Nipple-areolar complex was reconstructed by tattooing of areola and nipple sharing from opposite breast. B, Lateral view of same patient. Notice satisfactory breast mound and accurate location of reconstructed nipple-areola.

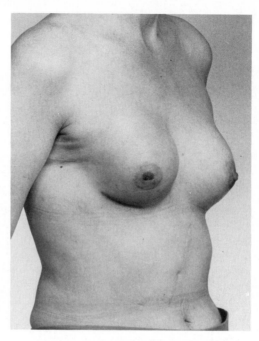

Fig. 13-11. Six-month postoperative view of nipple-areolar complex in which areola was reconstructed utilizing full-thickness posterior auricular grafts and a thick split-thickness labial majora graft for reconstruction of nipple.

intervention and expense, is implantation of small segments of conchal cartilage (Brent) to simulate nipple projection. The cartilage graft is shaped and then inserted within a pocket formed beneath the nipple site of a previously reconstructed nipple-areolar complex. Additionally minute pieces of cartilage dispersed under the skin grafts in order to simulate Montgomery glands result in an even more realistic appearing areola. Care must be exercised in inserting larger portions of cartilage, and there is a tendency for these pieces of cartilage to erode through the thin skin graft.

Dermal flaps

Provided the soft tissue overlying the prosthesis is sufficiently thick, dermal-fat flaps of a variety of designs may be sutured in such a manner that a prominence results that may be covered with a labial graft.[12] I have found this procedure to be of only limited usefulness because of the usual close proximity to the underlying prostheses.

Composite grafts

A circular composite graft of skin and fat may be obtained from the earlobe and reportably attains adequate nipple projection.[4] The color match of the earlobe does not usually correspond to the opposite nipple; however, tattooing of the nipple at a later date is of value. Further nipple projection is attained by Brent and Bostwich[4] by the insertion of two 6- to 8-mm conchal cartilage grafts obtained by means of a corneal-type punch under the previously constructed nipple graft (Fig. 13-7).

SUMMARY

The surgeon must determine which procedure or combination of procedures is the most desirable in reconstructing the nipple-areolar complex in each patient. Consideration of the availability of tissue for transfer, the color match required, and the patient's ultimate goals are all contributing factors in the final outcome.

REFERENCES

1. Adams, W. M.: Labial transplant for loss of nipple, Plast. Reconstr. Surg. **4:**295, 1949.
2. Allison, A. B., and Howorth, M. B., Jr.: Carcinoma in a nipple preserved by heterotopic auto-implantation, N. Engl. J. Med. **298:**1132, 1978.
3. Bouvier, B.: Problems in breast reconstruction, Med. J. Aust. **1:**937, 1977.
4. Brent, B., and Bostwick, J.: Nipple areola reconstruction with auricular tissues, Plast. Reconstr. Surg. **60:**353, 1977.
5. Broadbent, T. R., Woolf, R. M., and Metz, P. S.: Restoring the mammary areola by a skin graft from the upper inner thigh, Br. J. Plast. Surg. **30:**220, 1977.
6. Cronin, T. D., Upton, J., and McDonough, J. M.: Reconstruction of the breast after mastectomy, Plast. Reconstr. Surg. **59:**1, 1977.
7. Edwards, E. W., and Duntley, S. W.: The pigments and color of living human skin, Am. J. Anat. **65:**1, 1939.
8. Kiskadden, W. S.: Case report on skin grafting of nipple, Plast. Reconstr. Surg. **5:**184, 1950.
9. Klein, D.: Correction of loss of the areola mammae, Plast. Reconstr. Surg. **10:**469, 1952.
10. Millard, D. R., Jr.: Nipple and areola reconstruction by split-thickness skin graft from the normal side, Plast. Reconstr. Surg. **50:**350, 1972.
11. Millard, D. R., Devine, J., and Warren, W. D.: Breast reconstruction: a plea for saving the uninvolved nipple, Am. J. Surg. **122:**763, 1971.
12. Muruci, A., Dantas, J., and Nogueira, L. R.: Reconstruction of the nipple-areola complex, Plast. Reconstr. Surg. **61:**558, 1978.
13. Rees, T. D.: Reconstruction of breast areola by intradermal tattooing and transfer, Plast. Reconstr. Surg. **55:**620, 1975.
14. Schwartz, A. W.: Reconstruction of the nipple and areola, Br. J. Plast. Surg. **29:**230, 1976.

Index

A

A cells, superficial (luminal), 38
Abdomen, lower, full-thickness skin grafts from, 247
Abdominal flap, 186-187
  axillary, 164
  lateral, 184-185, 188
  transposterior, 193
Acini
  in embryo, 36
  microanatomy of, under estrogen influence, 39
Ackerman classification of histologic types, 134
Active nonspecific immunotherapy, 128, 129
Active specific immunotherapy, 128, 129
Adenocarcinoma, infiltrating ductal, 178-179
Adenofibroma, 71
Adenomammectomy, 86
Adenosis, sclerosing, 73-76
Adjuvant therapy in primary breast cancer control, 126-129
Alveolar epithelium, carcinoma of, fibroadenoma and, 72
Alveoli, myoepithelial cell arrangement around small ducts and, 40
Anastomosis, end-to-side arterial, 228-230
Anatomy of breast
  general, 35-40
  sagittal, 37
  surgical, 35-53
Anger, 11
Anterior ramus, 47-48
Antigen, tumor-associated, 128
Anxiety, 10, 17-18
  as explanation of increased lagtime, 5
  about husband's reaction, 26
Apocrine metaplasia, cystic duct dilation with, 70
Architectural distortion, 56
  focal stellate, 59, 62
Areola
  bisection of, into equal parts, 196
  graft of, split-thickness, 242
  ischemia of nipple and, 120
  reconstruction of, 177
    depigmentation of, 170
  sharing of, from opposite breast, 242-243
  steel wire loop for marking, 100, 101, 102

Areola—cont'd
  tattooing of, 186-187, 244, 249, 250, 251
Arm, ipsilateral, edema of, 221
Arterial anastomosis, end-to-side, 228-230
Arterial blood supply to breast, 40-45
Arterial plexuses, principal, to nipple-areolar complex, 43
Arterioles, 44
Artery
  axillary, 228
  intercostal, 41, 42
  internal mammary, 41, 42
  lateral thoracic, 41, 42
  principal pathways of, to breast, 41
  thoracodorsal, 199
Asymptomatic women, 55
Attitudinal framework of mastectomy, 2-6
Augmentation mammaplasty, 110, 111, 112
  and reconstruction, 32
Auricular graft, 252
Avoidance as explanation of increased lagtime, 5
Axilla, distortion of, 225
Axillary abdominal flap, 164
Axillary artery, 228
Axillary lymphatics, 50
Axillary node
  metastases of, 144-145
  positive, 155-156
Axillary tail prosthesis, 174
Axillary vena comitans, 228

B

B cells, basal, 38
Bacillus Calmette-Guerin, 128
Bacitracin, 92
Banked nipple-areolar graft, 240
Basal B cells, 38
Behavior, sexual; see Sexual behavior
Beliefs about cancer and mastectomy, 2-3
Benign calcifications, 56, 58
Benign lesions of breast, classification of, 68
Bilateral capsulotomy, 170, 176-177, 178-179, 180-181, 182-183, 184-185
Bilateral hematomas, 118
Bilateral latissimus dorsi muculocutaneous flaps, 211

255

Bilateral reconstruction of breast with labial grafts, 245
Bilateral subcutaneous mastectomy, 96, 211
   and ptosis procedure, 114, 115
Bilumen prosthesis, Georgiade Surgitek, 171, 174
Biologic predeterminism, 140-142, 147-148
Biopsy, 9-11, 57-58
   one-stage, 9-11
   two-stage, 9
Bisection of breast into equal parts, 196
Blood, supply of
   to breast, 41
      arterial, 40-45
      musculocutaneous arterial, 44
      venous, 45-47
   to nipple, 42-43
Body image reactions in mastectomy, 12-13
Brachial plexus injury, upper motor neuron, 219
Brachiocutaneous nerve, 48
Brawny edema, 233
Breast
   bisection of, into equal parts, 196
   blood supply to; see Blood, supply of, to breast
   carcinoma of; see also Carcinoma, breast
      Ackerman classification of histologic types of, 134
      adjuvant therapy in primary control of, 126-129
      choice of operation in, 125-126
      classification of, 135
      Columbia Clinical Classification of, 144
      detection of, by patient and physician, 55
      development of, in opposite breast, 125-126
      histologic grading of, 142-143
      histologic types of, 134, 135-142
      histopathologic lesions in contralateral breast in, 152-163
      incidence of, 132, 148-149
      infiltrating, histologic types of, 136
      mammography in diagnosis of, 54-66
      nonpalpable, detection of, 55
      predetection behaviors in, 3-4
      predisposing characteristics of women with, 5-6
      risk of, based on mammographic appearance, 56-57
      variance in survival explained by prognosis for, 134
   classical stellate carcinoma of, 58, 59
   classification of benign lesions of, 68
   contralateral, 160-161
      areolar sharing from, 242-243
      carcinoma of, association of lesions with, 159
      development of breast cancer in, 125-126

Breast—cont'd
   contralateral—cont'd
      flap of, 164
      histopathologic lesions in, 152-163
      incidence of carcinoma in, 148-149
      reconstruction of, 235
   cystic change of, 70-71
   development of, 36
   embryology of, 35
   and femininity, 6-8
      cultural considerations of, 6-7
      internal sense of femininity and, 7-8
      subtractive sense of femininity and, 8
   fibrocystic disease of; see Fibrocystic disease of breast
   general anatomy and physiology of, 35-40
   hypertrophied; see Hypertrophied breast
   innervation of, 47-50
   loss of, 25-27
      anxiety about husbands and, 26
      concepts of femininity and, 25
      effect of, on sexual behavior, 26-27
      expressed concerns about, 25-26
      husband's reaction to mastectomy and, 26
      psychiatric or psychologic assistance in, 25-26
      quality of marriage and, 26
   lymphatics draining, 50-51
   and motherhood, 7
   mound of
      distortion of, with capsular contracture, 119
      reconstruction of, after mastectomy, 164-190
      symmetry of, in reconstruction, 232
   palpable carcinoma in one, and nonpalpable carcinoma in other breast, 59, 61
   parenchyma of, 37
      replacement of, with fat, 56
   phantom, sensations of, 15
   principal pathways to
      arterial, 41
      venous, 46
   reconstruction of; see Reconstruction, breast
   recurrent masses of, 89
   remaining, construction of tube from, 195
   sagittal anatomy of, 37
   skin of
      involvement with tumor, 126
      ischemia of, 117
   stellate carcinoma of; see Stellate carcinoma of breast
   surgical anatomy of, 35-53
   tissue of
      medial and lateral skin flaps dissected free from, 104
      necrosis of, 117-119

Breast—cont'd
  tissue of—cont'd
    remnants of, 117
    volumetric changes of, in nonpregnant, men-
      struating females, 39-40
Breast surgery, reconstructive; *see* Reconstruc-
  tion, breast
Breast Task Force, 127
Breast-sharing procedures, 193
Buccal mucosal grafts, 244-246

C

Calcifications
  benign, 56, 58
  malignant, 58
  subepithelial, 75
Camper, fascia of, 36
Cancer; *see* Carcinoma, breast
Capillary plexus, dermal, with precapillary
  sphincters, 45
Capsular contraction
  with firmness and possible breast mound dis-
    tortion, 119-122
  release of, 120-121
Capsulotomy, 166-167, 168, 169-172, 175, 186-
  187, 241
  bilateral, 170, 176-177, 178-179, 180-181,
    182-183, 184-185
Carcinoma, breast, 78-79; *see also* Breast, carcinoma of
  of alveolar epithelium, fibroadenoma and, 72
  of contralateral breast, association of lesions
    with, 159
  ductal, 135, 168
  of ductal epithelium, fibroadenoma and, 72
  fear of, 13, 23-24
  husband's reaction to, 24
  in situ lobular, 80
  infiltrating ductal; *see* Infiltrating ductal car-
    cinoma
  infiltrating lobular, 80
  intraductal, 79, 170, 182-183, 241
    comedocarcinoma variant of, 137, 138
    papillary variant of, 137
  invasive lobular, 216-217
  irregular, 147
  lobular, 135
    in situ, 82
    infiltrating, 135
    invasive, 140-142
    noninfiltrating, 135
  and mastectomy, beliefs about, 2-3
  nonpalpable, in one breast and palpable car-
    cinoma in other breast, 59, 61
  palpable, 59, 61
  scirrhous ductal, 59

Carcinoma, breast,—cont'd
  stellate; *see* Stellate carcinoma of breast
  tubular, 83
  well-delineated, 147
Cartilage
  conchal, 252
  implantation of, 250-252
CAT; *see* Computerized axial tomography
Cell
  basal B, 38
  chief, 38
  myoepithelial, 38
    arrangement of, around alveoli and small
      ducts, 40
  Paget, 124-125
  superficial (luminal) A, 38
Cellular immunotherapy, passive, 128-129
Cellular lesions in premenopausal and post-
  menopausal women, 160
Centripetal lymph flow, Rouvière's concept of, 51
Chemotherapeutic agents, 126-127
Chemotherapy, surgery followed by, 127
Chest, moulage of, for custom prosthesis, 173
Chief cells, 38
Circular plexus, 42, 43
Clothing problems and mastectomy, 17
Colloid variant of infiltrating ductal carcinoma,
  140, 141
Columbia Clinical Classification of breast carci-
  noma, 144
Comedocarcinoma
  intraductal, 81
  variant of, of infiltrating ductal carcinoma, 138
  variant of, of intraductal carcinoma, 137, 138
Communication
  in mastectomy, 9-10
  in reconstruction, 32
Composite graft, 252-253
Composite island flap, 209, 210
Composite tissue
  employed in reconstruction, 226
  transplantation of, microsurgical, 215-238
Computerized axial tomography (CAT), 55
Concerns
  about breast loss, 25-26
  about cancer, 23-24
  of women undergoing mastectomy, 13
Conchal cartilage, 252
Configuration of tumor border, 147
Contralateral breast; *see* Breast, contralateral
Convalescent period, 15
Cooper, ligaments of; *see* Ligaments of Cooper
Coping strategies, 24
Corynebacterium parvum, 128
Cribriform hyperplasia, 135
  intraductal epithelial, 77, 78, 158

Cultural considerations
  of breasts and femininity, 6-7
  of mastectomy experience, 1-8
Curvilinear submammary incision, 88-89
Custom prosthesis, moulage of chest for, 173
Custom stone model prosthesis, 173
Custom tricompartment prosthesis, 174
Cutaneous lymphatics, 50-51
Cyclic volumetric changes of breast in nonpreg-
    nant menstruating females, 39-40
Cyclical reactions to mastectomy, 11-12
Cyclophosphamide, 127
Cystic change in breast with extensive intraduc-
    tal epithelial hyperplasia, 70-71
Cystic disease, 67
Cystic duct dilation, 69-71
Cystic lesions, ultrasound in differentiation of
    solid lesions from, 55
Cystic masses in postmenopausal women, 71
Cystic mastitis, chronic, 67
Cytoxan; *see* Cyclophosphamide

D

Deep dermal plexus, 50
Defense mechanisms, 24
Delay in reporting symptoms to physician, 4-5
Delayed reconstruction, 150, 172
Denial, 5, 11, 24
Depigmentation of reconstructed areola, 170
Depression, 10, 11-12, 17
  during convalescence, 15
Dermal capillary plexus with precapillary sphinc-
    ters, 45
Dermal flap, 252
  approximation of, after insertion of prosthesis,
    105
  fat, 97
  in vascularity of nipple, 98
  width of, 103
Dermal graft, 182-188
Dermal pectoralis muscle flap, 99
Dermal pedicle, 97
Dermal pedicle nipple-areolar bearing flap, 104
Dermal plexus, deep, 50
Dermatitis, radiation, 219-221, 223
Dermis
  plexuses of, 50
  superficial dermus, 50
Dermis-fat-muscle flap, 193
d'Este, S., 197
Diagnosis of breast cancer, mammography in,
    54-66
Dilation, cystic duct, 69-71
Dimpling, 126
Disbelief, 11
Dissection of axilla, 225

Distant flaps transported on wrist carriers, 193
Distress reactions to mastectomy, 10, 12
Double-lumen prosthesis, subpectoral placement
    of, 94
Duct
  cystic, dilation of, 69-71
  lactiferous, in embryo, 36
  small, myoepithelial cell arrangement around
    alveoli and, 40
Ductal adenocarcinoma, infiltrating, 178-179
Ductal carcinoma, 135, 168
  infiltrating; *see* Infiltrating ductal carcinoma
  noninfiltrating, 135
  scirrhous, 59
Ductal epithelium, carcinoma of, fibroadenoma
    and, 72
Duke Breast Cancer Detection Demonstration
    Project, 55, 64
Duke University Medical Center, 22
DY (Wolfe) classification of risk to develop breast
    carcinoma based on mammographic ap-
    pearance, 56-57, 58, 59, 60
Dysplastic disease, dense, stellate carcinoma of
    breast obscured by, 59, 60

E

Ear(s), grafts from, 247-249
Earlobe, grafts from, 252-253
Early reconstruction, 149-150
Edema
  brawny, 233
  of ipsilateral arm, 221
Embryo, 6-week-old, mammary ridges in, 36
Embryology of breast, 35
End-to-end anastomosis, 228-230
End-to-side anastomosis, 228-230
Epidermis of nipple-areolar complex, 49
Epithelial hyperplasia, 137
  cribriform intraductal, 158
  extensive intraductal cystic change in breast
    with, 70-71
  intraductal, 77-78, 135
  papillary intraductal, 157
  solid intraductal, 158
Epitheliosis, "premalignant," 162
Epithelium, carcinoma of, fibroadenoma and, 72
Estradiol, 39
Estrogen, 38-39, 40, 76
  influence of, microanatomy of acini under, 39
  receptors of, 128
  sclerosing adenosis in postmenopausal women
    with deficiency of, 74-76

F

Faith, religious, as coping mechanism, 24
Family history, association of, with proliferative
    lesions, 156

Fascia of Camper, development of, 36
Fat, breast parenchyma replacement with, 56
Fat necrosis, 68-69
Fear
  of cancer, 13, 23-24
  experienced by husband, 14-15
  of mastectomy, 3, 13
Femininity
  and breasts; *see* Breast and femininity
  concepts of, and breast loss, 25
  definition of, in terms of sexual behavior, 7
Fibroadenoma, 71-72
Fibrocystic disease of breast, 67, 90, 110, 112, 120-121
  extensive, and ptosis, 116
  history of surgical management of, 86-87
  proliferative, 221-225
  severe, 106
    with associated mastodynia, 120
    macromastia with, 111
    and ptosis, 115
  with severe mastodynia, 107-108
  surgical management of, 86-123
Fibrocystic mastopathy, 67
Fibrosis, productive, infiltrating duct carcinoma with, 136
Fibrous septa delinated by ligaments of Cooper, 38
Firmness, capsular contraction with, 119-122
Flaps, 164, 188-189
  abdominal, 186-187
  abdominal transposterior, 193
  axillary abdominal, 164
  composite island, 209, 210
  contralateral breast, 164
  dermal; *see* Dermal flap
  dermal pectoralis muscle, 99
  dermal pedicle nipple-areolar bearing, 104
  dermis-fat-muscle, 193
  distant, transported on wrist carrier, 193
  "free," 189
  lateral, necrosis of, 118
  lateral abdominal, 188
    medially based, 184-185
  lateral pedicle, 164
  latissimus dorsi musculocutaneous; *see* Latissimus dorsi musculocutaneous flap
  local, 191-193
  marking of, 103
  microvascular, technique of, reconstruction with, 225-232
  midabdominal, superiorly based, 194
  medial and lateral, dissected free from breast tissue, 104

Flaps—cont'd
  musculocutaneous, definition of, 197-198
  myocutaneous, definition of, 197-198
  paddle-shaped, in latissimus dorsi musculocutaneous flap, 203
  rotation, 192
  skin-fat, 193
  Tansini, 197, 198
  thoracic, 164
  thoracoabdominal; *see* Thoracoabdominal flap
  vascularized groin, 225, 227, 236-237
  vertical, configuration of, 212
5-Fluorouracil, 127
Focal mastitis, 73
Focal stellate architectural distortion, 59, 62
Foramen, Langer's, development of, 36
Fracture, multiple rib, from radiation therapy, 219
"Free flap," 189
Frustration, 11
Full-thickness skin grafts
  labial, 244
  from lower abdomen, groin, and inner thigh area, 247

G
Gel-filled prosthesis, Silastic, 164
Georgiade Surgitek prosthesis, 93, 96, 105, 106, 108, 109, 112, 115, 116, 120-121, 168, 170, 174, 180-181, 182-183, 184-185
  bilumen, 171, 174
  double-lumen, 93, 96, 105, 106, 108, 109, 112, 115, 116, 120-121
  inflatable, 178-179
  "piggyback," 170, 172, 174, 176-177, 178-179, 180-181, 241
  Silastic, 92
Graft
  auricular, 252
  banked nipple-areolar, 240
  buccal mucosal, 244-246
  composite, 252-253
  dermal, 182-188
  from ear, 247-249
  from earlobe, 252-253
  full-thickness skin
    labial, 244
    from lower abdomen, groin, and inner thigh area, 247
  interpositional vein, 225-230, 237
  labia majora, 245, 246, 250, 252
  labia minora, 245
  labial, 186-187, 250
    bilateral reconstruction with, 245
  nipple-areolar, 169
    stored, 240-242

Graft—cont'd
  nipple-areolar—cont'd
    transfer of, to groin, modified mastectomy and, 166-167
  retroauricular skin, 247-249
  split-thickness; *see* Split-thickness graft
  vein, 228-230
Graft-vs-host reaction, 129
Grief, 11
Groin
  full-thickness skin grafts from, 247
  transfer of nipple-areolar graft to, modified mastectomy and, 166-167
Groin flap, vascularized, 225, 227, 236-237
Gross pathology, comparison of microscopic pathology to, 222

H

Healthy, well-vascularized skin, definition of, 220
Heller, superficial venous plexus of, 45
Hematoma, 117, 120
  bilateral, 118
Histologic grading of breast carcinoma, 142-143
Histologic type of breast cancer, 135-142
  Ackerman classification of, 134
  infiltrating, 136
Histopathologic lesions
  in contralateral breast, 152-163
  in subcutaneous mastectomy specimens, clinical significance of, 67-85
History, family, association of, with proliferative lesions, 156
Hospital experience, postsurgical, in mastectomy, 11-13
Hormone, receptors for, 128
Hormone-dependent tumors, 128
Host defense response, 147-148
Husband
  anxiety about effect of breast loss on, 26
  fears of, 14-15
  reaction of, to cancer, 24
  reaction of, to mastectomy, 14-15, 24, 26
Hyperplasia
  cribriform, 135
  cribriform intraductal epithelial, 158
  epithelial, 137
  intraductal epithelial, 70-71, 77-78, 135
  lobular, 76, 140
  papillary, 135
  papillary intraductal epithelial, 157
  solid intraductal epithelial, 158
Hypertrophied breast
  determination of new nipple site in recontouring of, 100
  subcutaneous mastectomy with, 95-109

Hypertrophy, moderate, with associated ptosis, 109

I

Immediate reconstruction, 149, 165
Immunology, tumor, 147-148
Immunotherapy
  active nonspecific, 128, 129
  active specific, 128, 129
  passive cellular, 128-129
Implant
  Silastic, 234-235
  subpectoral, 92-95
In situ lobular carcinoma, 80
Incidence of breast carcinoma, 148-149
  progressive increase in, 132
Incision
  curvilinear submammary, 88-89
  inframammary, 86
  lateral "S," 166
  submammary, 86
  surgical, for access to subpectoral plane, 93
  thoracomammary, 86
Infiltrating breast carcinoma, histologic types of, 136
Infiltrating ductal carcinoma, 59, 63, 64, 135, 138-140, 171, 178-179
  colloid variant of, 140, 141
  with comedocarcinoma variant, 138
  medullary variant of, 140, 141
  papillary variant of, 137-138
  with productive fibrosis, 136
  tubular variant of, 139
Infiltrating lobular carcinoma, 80, 135
Inflatable prosthesis, 178-179
Inframammary incision, 86
Injury, upper motor neuron brachial plexus, 219
Inner thigh area, full-thickness skin grafts from, 247
Innervation
  of breast, 47-50
  sympathetic, of nipple-areolar complex, 49
Intercostal arteries, 41, 42
Intercostal lymphatics, posterior, 50-51
Intercostal nerve, 47
  first, 48
  second, 48
  surgical anatomy of, 47
  third, 48
Intercostal vein, 45
Intercostobrachial nerve, 48
Internal mammary lymphatics, 50
Interpersonal problems of women undergoing mastectomy, 15-16
Interpositional vein grafts, 225-230, 237
Intraductal carcinoma, 79, 170, 182-183, 241

Intraductal carcinoma—cont'd
  comedocarcinoma variant of, 137, 138
  papillary variant of, 137
Intraductal comedocarcinoma, 81
Intraductal epithelial hyperplasia, 77-78, 135
  cribriform, 158
  extensive, cystic change in breast with, 70-71
  papillary, 157
  solid, 158
Invasive lobular carcinoma, 140-142, 216-217
Ipsilateral arm, edema of, 221
Irregular carcinoma, 147
Ischemia
  of breast skin, 117
  of nipple and areolar area, 120
Island flap
  composite, 209, 210
  latissimus dorsi musculocutaneous, 196-197

L

Labia majora graft, 245, 246, 250, 252
Labia minora graft, 245
Labial graft, 186-187, 250
  bilateral reconstruction with, 245
  full-thickness, 244
Lactiferous ducts in embryo, 36
Lagtime, 4-5
Langer's foramen, development of, 36
Lateral abdominal flap, 188
  medially based, 184-185
Lateral flap dissected free from breast tissue, 104
Lateral pedicle flap, 164
Lateral rami mammarii, 49
Lateral "S" incision, 166
Lateral skin flap, necrosis of, 118
Lateral thoracic artery, 41, 42
Lateral thoracic vein, 45
Latissimus dorsi muscle, 199
Latissimus dorsi musculocutaneous flap, 165, 184-185, 188-189, 191-214, 236-237
  anatomy of, 199
  bilateral, 211
  clinical experience with, 208-213
  evolution of, 197-199
  with lengthy vascular pedicle, 231
  outline of, 200
  paddle-shaped flap in, 203
  soft tissue replacement in, 191-197
  suturing in place, 206
  technique of, 207-208
  vascularized, 224, 230-232
Lesion
  association of, with carcinoma of contralateral breast, 159
  benign, of breast, classification of, 68

Lesion—cont'd
  cellular, in premenopausal and postmenopausal women, 160
  detection of, 55
  histopathologic
    in contralateral breast, 152-163
    in subcutaneous mastectomy specimens, clinical significance of, 67-85
  nonpalpable, mammography in detection of, 56, 57, 62-64
  proliferative, association of family history with, 156
  solid and cystic, ultrasound in differentiation of, 55
Ligaments of Cooper, 37
  development of, 36
  fibrous septa delineated by, 38
Linear microcalcifications, 58
Lobular carcinoma, 135
  in situ, 80, 82
  infiltrating, 80, 135
  invasive, 140-142, 216-217
  noninfiltrating, 135
Lobular hyperplasia, 76, 140
Lobules, persistent, and lobular hyperplasia, 76
Local flap, 191-193
Longitudinal veins, 45
Loop plexus, 42, 43
Looseness of skin, 94-95
Loss of breast; *see* Breast, loss of
Lower abdomen, full-thickness skin grafts from, 247
Luminal A cells, 38
Lumpectomy, 3
Luteal phase of menstrual cycle, breast volumetric changes in, 40
Lymph flow, centripetal, Rouvière's concept of, 51
Lymphatics, 50-51
  axillary, 50
  cutaneous, 50-51
  draining the breasts, 50-51
  internal mammary, 50
  posterior intercostal, 50-51

M

Macromastia, 106
  with severe fibrocystic disease of breast, 111
Malignancy, mammographic signs of, 56
Malignant calcifications, 58
Malignant microcalcifications, 56
Mammaplasty
  augmentation, 32, 110, 111, 112
  reduction, 106, 110, 111, 112, 171
Mammary lymphatics, internal, 50
Mammary ridges in 6-week-old embryo, 36

Mammography, 55-64
  of asymptomatic women, 55
  benefits and risks of, 64
  in detection of nonpalpable lesions, 56, 57, 62-64
  in diagnosis of breast cancer, 54-66
  and physical examination, 55
  risk to develop breast cancer based on, 56-57
  signs of malignancy in, 56
Marital problems of women undergoing mastectomy, 16-17
Marital relationship postsurgically, 14
Marriage, quality of, and breast loss, 26
Masses
  of breast, recurrent, 89
  cystic, in postmenopausal women, 71
Mastectomy
  attitudinal framework of, 2-6
  and cancer, beliefs about, 2-3
  and clothing problems, 17
  cultural context of, 1-8
  cyclical reactions of, 11-12
  distress reactions of, 12
  experience of, 8-18
  fears and concerns of, 3, 13
  husband's reaction to, 14-15, 24, 26
  long-term effects of, 17-18
  modified, with transfer of nipple-areolar graft to groin, 166-167
  postsurgical experiences of, 11-15
  presurgical experiences of, 11
  prosthetic and clothing problems of, 17
  psychologic effects of, 1-21
  radical; see Radical mastectomy
  reactions
    of others to, 16
    recalled, 23-27
    to viewing self in, 12
  reconstruction of breast mound after, 164-190
  reduction, 110, 111, 112
  scar of, 182-183
  segmental, 125
  self-concept and body image concerns of, 12-13
  sexual and marital problems of, 16-17
  short-term effects of, 15-17
  simple, 3
  social and interpersonal problems of, 15-16
  stress and communication in, 9-10
  subcutaneous; see Subcutaneous mastectomy
  subtractive process of, 8
  unilateral, 132
Mastitis, 67, 73
Mastodynia, 73, 90, 106
  severe, fibrocystic disease of breast with, 107-108, 120

Mastopathy
  fibrocystic, 67
  "precancerous," 162
Mechanic's waste, 95, 97
Medial flap dissected free from breast tissue, 104
Medial rami mammarii, 49
Medially based lateral abdominal flap, 184-185
Medullary variant of infiltrating ductal carcinoma, 140, 141
Menstrual cycle, breast volumetric changes in luteal phase of, 40
  proliferative phase of, 39-40
Menstruating, nonpregnant females, cyclic volumetric changes of breast in, 39-40
Menstruation, 40
Metaplasia, apocrine, 70
Metastasis, 142, 146
  axillary node, 144-145
Methotrexate, 127
Microcalcifications, 56
  linear, 58
  malignant, 56
  punctate, 58
Microscopic pathology, comparison of gross pathology with, 222
Microsurgical composite tissue transplantation for reconstruction, 215-238
Microvascular flap technique, reconstruction with, 225-232
Midabdominal flap, superiorly based, 194
Modified radical mastectomy; see Radical mastectomy, modified
Morbidity associated with radical mastectomy, 125
Motherhood and breasts, 7
Motor neuron brachial plexus injury, upper, 219
Moulage of chest for custom prosthesis, 173
Mucosal grafts, buccal, 244-246
Multicompartment prosthesis, 174
Multifocal fibroadenoma, 71
Multifocal mastitis, 73
Muscle, latissimus dorsi, 199
Muscle flap; see Flap
Musculocutaneous arterial blood supply to breast, 44
Musculocutaneous flap
  definition of, 197-198
  latissimus dorsi; see Latissimus dorsi musculocutaneous flap
Myoepithelial flap, definition of, 197-198
Myoepithelial cells, 38
  arrangement of, around alveoli and small ducts, 40

N

N1 (Wolfe) classification of risk to develop breast cancer based on mammographic appearance, 56-57, 59, 61
National Surgical Breast Project, 145
Necrosis
  of breast tissue, 117-119
  fat, 68-69
  of lateral skin flap, 118
Nerve
  brachiocutaneous, 48
  intercostal; *see* Intercostal nerve
  intercostobrachial, 48
  thoracodorsal, 199
Neuron brachial plexus injury, upper motor, 219
Nipple
  bisection of, into equal parts, 196
  blood supply to, 42-43
  involvement of, 126
  new site of, in recontouring of hypertrophied breast, 100
  projection of, 232-236, 253
  reconstruction of, 177, 249-253
  sharing of, 251
  vascularity of, dermal flap in, 98
Nipple-areolar bearing flaps, dermal pedicle, 104
Nipple-areolar complex, 35-36
  epidermis of, 49
  ischemia of, 120
  management of, in reconstruction, 239-253
  position of, in reconstruction, 239-249
  principal arterial plexuses to, 43
  reconstruction of, 188, 232-236
  sloughing of, 119
  sympathetic innervation of, 49
  as thick split-thickness graft, 166-167
Nipple-areolar graft, 169
  banked, 240
  stored, 240-242
  transfer of, to groin, modified mastectomy and, 166-167
Node
  axillary
    metastases to, 144-145
    positive, 155-156
    survival rates according to number examined, 146-147
Nodule, multiple, ptosis and, 114
  noninfiltrating ductal carcinoma, 135
Noninfiltrating lobular carcinoma, 135
Nonpalpable carcinoma
  detection of, 55
  in one breast and palpable carcinoma in other breast, 59, 61

Nonpalpable lesions, mammography in detection of, 56, 57, 62-64
Nonpregnant menstruating females, cyclic volumetric changes of breast in, 39-40

O

On the Removal of Benign Tumors of the Mamma without Mutilation of the Organ, 86
One-stage biopsy, 9-11
Operative procedure
  choice of, in breast cancer, 125-126
  for subcutaneous mastectomy, 88-109
Osteitis, radiation, 219, 223

P

P1 (Wolfe) classification of risk to develop breast cancer based on mammographic appearance, 56-57, 59, 62
P2 (Wolfe) classification of risk to develop breast cancer based on mammographic appearance, 56-57, 62-64
Paddle-shaped flap in latissimus dorsi musculocutaneous flap, 203
Paget cells, 124-125
Palpable carcinoma in one breast and nonpalpable carcinoma in other breast, 59, 61
Paper tape, skin-adherent, redraping of skin with, 95
Papillary hyperplasia, 135
  intraductal epithelial, 77, 78, 157
Papillary variant
  of infiltrating ductal carcinoma, 137-138
  of intraductal carcinoma, 137
Parenchyma, breast, 37
  replacement of, with fat, 56
Passive cellular immunotherapy, 128-129
Passive serotherapy, 129
Pathology, gross and microscopic, comparison of, 222
Patient; *see also* Women
  detection of breast cancer by, 55
  local tissues of, use of, in reconstruction, 174-183
Pectoralis muscle flap, dermal, 99
Pedicle, lengthy vascular, latissimus dorsi musculocutaneous flap with, 231
Pedicle flap, lateral, 164
Periareolar plexus, 42-43
Phantom breast sensations, 15
L-Phenylalanine mustard, 127
Physical examination and mammography, 55
Physician
  delay in reporting symptoms to, 4-5
  detection of breast cancer by, 55
Physiology of breast, 35-40

"Piggyback" prosthesis, Georgiade Surgitek, 170, 172, 174, 176-177, 178-179, 180-181, 241

Plastic Surgery of the Breasts and Abdominal Wall, 197

Plexus
  circular, 42, 43
  dermal, 50
    capillary, with precapillary sphincters, 45
    deep, 50
  injury to, upper motor neuron brachial, 219
  loop, 42, 43
  periareolar, 42-43
  principal arterial, to nipple-areolar complex, 43
  radial, 42-43
  superficial venous, of Heller, 45-47
  venous; *see* Venous plexus, superficial
Positive axillary nodes, 155-156
Posterior intercostal lymphatics, 50-51
Postmenopausal women
  cellular lesions in, 160
  cystic masses in, 71
  estrogen-deficient, sclerosing adenosis in, 74-76
  persistent lobular hyperplasia in, 76
Postoperative radiation, 233
Postsurgical experiences in mastectomy, 11-13, 14-15
Postsurgical marital relationship, 14
Postsurgical weakness, 15
Prayer as coping mechanism, 24
"Precancerous" mastopathy, 162
Precapillary sphincters, dermal capillary plexus with, 45
Predetection behaviors in breast cancer, 3-4
Predeterminism, biologic, 140-142, 147-148
Predisposing characteristics of women with breast cancer, 5-6
"Premalignant" epitheliosis, 162
Premenopausal women
  cellular lesions in, 160
  cystic change of breast in, 71
Preoperative evaluation for subcutaneous mastectomy, 87-88
Presurgical experiences of mastectomy, 9-11
Primary tumor, size of, 145-146
Progesterone, 38-39, 40
Prognosis
  of breast cancer, variance in survival explained by, 134
  for reconstruction, 131-151
    determination of, 133-148
Prolactin, 39
Proliferative fibrocystic disease, 221-225
Proliferative lesions, association of family history with, 156

Proliferative phase of menstrual cycle, breast volumetric changes in, 39-40
Prosthesis, 174
  approximation of dermal flaps after insertion of, 105
  axillary tail, 174
  custom, moulage of chest for, 173
  custom stone model, 173
  custom tricompartment, 174
  double-lumen, subpectoral placement of, 94
  Georgiade Surgitek; *see* Georgiade Surgitek prosthesis
  immediate insertion of, left subcutaneous mastectomy with, 166
  insertion of, 188
  multicompartment, 174
  "piggyback,"; *see* Georgiade Surgitek prosthesis, "piggyback"
  round, 172
  selection of, 172-174
  Silastic, 192
  Silastic gel-filled, 164
  triangular silicone gel, 174-177
Prosthetic problems of women undergoing mastectomy, 17
Psychiatric assistance in breast loss, 25-26
Psychologic assistance in breast loss, 25-26
Psychologic interviews of women undergoing reconstruction, 22-27
Psychologic reactions in mastectomy, 1-21
Ptosis
  correction of, 220, 234-235
  and extensive fibrocystic disease of breasts, 116
  moderate hypertrophy with associated, 109
  and multiple nodules, 114
  procedure of, 175, 184-185
    and bilateral subcutaneous mastectomy, 114, 115
  and severe fibrocystic disease of breasts, 115
  simple, correction of, in conjunction with subcutaneous mastectomy, 113
Punctate microcalcifications, 58

R

Radial plexus, 42-43
Radiation, postoperative, 233
Radiation dermatitis, 219-221, 223
Radiation osteitis, 219, 223
Radiation therapy, multiple rib fractures from, 219
Radical mastectomy, 3, 125, 182-183, 184-185, 186-187, 200, 207, 212, 216-217, 218-219, 224, 233, 234-235
  and axillary node metastasis, 145

Radical mastectomy—cont'd
  modified, 125, 166, 168, 170, 171, 175, 176-
    177, 178-179, 180-181, 216-217
  morbidity associated with, 125
  typical deformity resulting from, 209
Rami mammarii, 49
Ramus, anterior, 47-48
Rationale for reconstruction, 131-133
Reaction
  cyclical, to mastectomy, 11-12
  distress, to mastectomy, 12
  graft-vs-host, 129
  of husband; see Husband, reaction of
  of others to mastectomy, 16
  recalled, to mastectomy, 23-27
  to reconstruction, 31-32
  to viewing self in mastectomy, 12
Receptor
  estrogen, 128
  hormone, 128
Reconstruction, breast
  of areola, 177
    depigmentation of, 170
  and augmentation mammaplasty, 32
  bilateral, with labial grafts, 245
  of breast mound
    after mastectomy, 164-190
    symmetry in, 232
  composite tissue employed in, 226
  of contralateral breast, 235
  delayed, 150, 172
  determination of prognosis in, 133-148
  diagram of method of, 192
  early, 149-150
  expectations of, 28-30
  experience of, 22-23
  factors complicating, 221
  first-stage, 225-232
  immediate, 149, 165
  microsurgical composite tissue transplantation
    for, 215-238
  with microvascular flap technique, 225-232
  negative reactions to, 32
  nipple, 177, 249-253
  nipple-areolar, 188, 232-236
    management of, 239-253
    position in, 239-249
  process by which woman decides to seek, 28
  psychologic interviews of women undergoing,
    22-27
  rationale, prognosis, and timing of, 131-151
  reactions to, 31-32
  as search for restitution, 22-34
  second-stage, 232
  surgical method of, 165-169, 174-188
  third-stage, 232

Reconstruction, breast—cont'd
  timing of, 30, 148-150
  use of patient's local tissues in, 174-183
Reconstructive breast surgery; see Reconstruc-
    tion, breast
Redraping of skin with skin-adherent paper tape,
    95
Reduction mammaplasty, 106, 110, 111, 112,
    171
Religious faith as coping mechanism, 24
Restitution
  positive feelings associated with, 31-32
  reconstruction as search for, 22
Rete pegs, 44
Retroauricular skin graft, 247-249
Rib fractures, multiple, from radiation therapy,
    219
Risk-reward ratio, 29
Rotation flaps, 192
Round prosthesis, 172
Rouvière's concept of centripetal lymph flow, 51

S
"S" incision, lateral, 166
Sagittal anatomy of breast, 37
Scar
  mastectomy, 182-183
  surgical excision of, dermal graft and, 183-
    188
Scirrhous ductal carcinoma, 59
Sclerosing adenosis, 73-76
Screening
  of asymptomatic women, 55
  detection of breast cancer, mammography as,
    54
Segmental mastectomy, 125
Self-concept in mastectomy, 12-13
Self-esteem, 16
  loss of, 12
Self-respect, 16
Sensory discrimination of epidermis of nipple-
    areolar complex, 49
Septa, fibrous, delineated by ligaments of Coo-
    per, 38
Serotherapy, passive, 129
Sexual behavior
  definition of femininity in terms of, 7
  effect of breast loss on, 26-27
Sexual problems of women undergoing mastec-
    tomy, 16-17
Shock, 11, 12
Silastic gel-filled prosthesis, 164
Silastic implant, 234-235
Silastic prosthesis, 164, 192
Silicone gel prosthesis, triangular, 174-177
Size of primary tumor, 145-146

Skin
  breast
    involvement of, with tumor, 126
    ischemia of, 117
  healthy, well-vascularized, definition of, 220
  looseness of, 94-95
  redraping of, with skin-adherent paper tape, 95
Skin graft
  full-thickness, from lower abdomen, groin, and inner thigh area, 247
  retroauricular, 247-249
Skin-adherent paper tape, redraping of skin with, 95
Skin-fat flaps, 193
Sloughing of nipple-areola complex, 119
Social problems of women undergoing mastectomy, 15-16
Soft tissue, replacement of, in latissimus dorsi musculocutaneous flap, 191-197
Solid intraductal epithelial hyperplasia, 158
Solid lesions, ultrasound in differentiation of cystic lesions from, 55
Spence, tail of, 36, 37
Sphincter, precapillary, dermal capillary plexus with, 45
Split-thickness grafts
  areolar, 242
  thick, nipple-areola as, 166-167
Steel wire loop for marking areola, 100, 101, 102
Stellate architectural distortion, focal, 59, 62
Stellate carcinoma of breast
  classical, 58, 59
  obscured by dense dysplastic disease, 59, 60
Stone model prosthesis, custom, 173
Stress in mastectomy, 9-10
Subcutaneous mastectomy, 86, 110, 111, 112, 149, 166-167, 169, 170, 171, 175, 178-179, 182-183, 184-185, 218-219, 220, 234-235
  bilateral, 96, 211
    and ptosis procedure, 114, 115
  correction of simple ptosis in conjunction with, 113
  with hypertrophied breast, 95-109
  with immediate insertion of prosthesis, 166
  operative procedure of, 88-109
  preoperative evaluation for, 87-88
  selection of patients for, 87
  specimens of, clinical significance of histopathologic lesions observed in, 67-85
Subepithelial calcifications, 75
Submammary incision, 86
  curvilinear, 88-89
Subpectoral implantation, 92-95

Subpectoral placement of double-lumen prosthesis, 94
Subpectoral plane, surgical incision for access to, 93
Subtractive process of mastectomy, 8
Superficial A cells, 38
Superior-lateral base, thoracoabdominal transposition flap with, 194
Superiorly based midabdominal flap, 194
Superior-medial base, thoracoabdominal flap with, 193
Surgery
  followed by chemotherapy, 127
  reconstructive breast; see Reconstruction, breast
Surgical anatomy of breast, 35-53
Surgical excision of scar and dermal graft, 183-188
Surgical incision for access to subpectoral plane, 93
Surgical method of reconstruction, 165-169
Surgical techniques of reconstruction, 174-188
Sympathetic innervation of nipple-areolar complex, 49
Symptom, delay in reporting, to physician, 4-5

T
Tail of Spence, 36, 37
Tansini flap, 197, 198
Tape, skin-adherent paper, redraping of skin with, 95
Tattoo of areola, 186-187, 244, 249, 250, 251
Telangiectasis, 233
Therapy
  adjuvant, in primary breast cancer control, 126-129
  radiation, multiple rib fractures from, 219
Thermography in detection of lesions, 55
Thigh area, inner, full-thickness skin grafts from, 247
Thoracic artery, 41, 42
Thoracic flap, 164
Thoracic vein, lateral, 45
Thoracoabdominal flap, 164-165, 184-185, 193
  with superior-medial base, 193
  transposition, with superior-lateral base, 194
Thoracodorsal artery, 199
Thoracodorsal nerve, 199
Thoracodorsal vessels, 184-185
Thoracomammary incision, 86
Timing of reconstruction, 30, 131-151
Tissue
  composite, employed in reconstruction, 226
  transplantation of, microsurgical composite, for reconstruction, 215-238

Tomography, computerized axial, in detection of lesions, 55

Tranquilizers during convalescence, 15

Transplantation, microsurgical composite tissue, 215-238

Transposition flap, thoracoabdominal, with superior-lateral base, 194

Transposterior flap, abdominal, 193

Triangular silicone gel prosthesis, 174-177

Tricompartment prosthesis, custom, 174

Tube, construction of, from remaining breast, 195

Tubular carcinoma, 83

Tubular variant of infiltrating ductal carcinoma, 139

Tumor
border of, configuration of, 147
breast skin involvement with, 126
hormone-dependent, 128
immunology of, 147-148
primary, size of, 145-146

Tumor-associated antigens, 128

Two-stage biopsy, 9

U

Ultrasound in differentiation of solid from cystic lesions, 55

Unilateral mastectomy, 132

Upper motor neuron brachial plexus injury, 219

V

Vaccinia, 128

Vascular pedicle, lengthy, latissimus dorsi musculocutaneous flap with, 231

Vascularity of nipple, dermal flap in, 98

Vascularized groin flap, 225, 227, 236-237

Vascularized latissimus dorsi musculocutaneous flap, 224, 230-232

Vein
intercostal, 45
lateral thoracic, 45
longitudinal, 45
transverse superficial, 45

Vein graft, 228-230
interpositional, 225-230, 237

Vena comitans, axillary, 228

Venous blood supply, 45-47

Venous pathways of breast, principal, 46

Venous plexus, superficial
common patterns of, 46
of Heller, 45

Venules, 44

Vertical flap configuration, 212

Volumetric changes, cyclic, of breast in nonpregnant, menstruating females, 39-40

W

Weakness, postsurgical, 15

Well-delineated carcinoma, 147

Well-vascularized healthy skin, 220

Wire loop, steel, for marking areola, 100, 101, 102

Wolfe classification of risk to develop breast cancer based on mammographic appearance, 56-57

Women; *see also* Patient
asymptomatic, 55
local tissues of, use of, in reconstruction, 174-183
nonpregnant menstruating, cyclic volumetric changes of breast in, 39-40
postmenopausal; *see* Postmenopausal women
premenopausal; *see* Premenopausal women

Wrist carrier, distant flap transported on, 193